OXFORD MEDICAL PUBLICATIONS

AGING: A CHALLENGE TO SCIENCE AND SOCIETY

Volume 1

Biology

AGING: A CHALLENGE TO SCIENCE AND SOCIETY

Volume 1

Biology

Edited by

D. DANON

Head, Section of Biological Ultrastructure,
The Weizmann Institute of Science, Rehovot, Israel

N. W. SHOCK PhD

Chief, Gerontology Research Center, National Institute on Aging,
National Institutes of Health, Baltimore

and

M. MAROIS

Professor at the Faculty of Medicine of Paris
President of the Council of l'Institut de la Vie, Paris

Published on behalf of l'Institut de la Vie and the
World Health Organization Regional Office for Europe by

OXFORD UNIVERSITY PRESS

OXFORD   NEW YORK   TORONTO

1981

Oxford University Press, Walton Street, Oxford OX2 6DP

London Glasgow New York Toronto
Dehli Bombay Calcutta Madras Karachi
Kuala Lumpur Singapore Hong Kong Tokyo
Nairobi Dar es Salaam Cape Town
and associate companies in
Beirut Berlin Ibadan Mexico City

The authors alone are responsible for the views
expressed in this publication

British Library Cataloguing in Publication Data
Aging. – (Oxford medical publications),
Vol. 1: Biology
1. Aging
I. Danon, D   II. Shock, N W
III. Institut de la vie   IV. World Health
Organization. Regional Offiice for Europe
V. Series
612.6'7   QP86   79-41662
ISBN 0-19-261254-9

Printed in Great Britain at the University Press, Oxford
by Eric Buckley
Printer to the University

Foreword

by Leo A. Kaprio, M.D., WHO Regional Director for Europe

Compared to Methuselah's legendary 969 years, the span of life of ordinary mortals is rather modest; practically all the people who will be alive in the year 2000 will have been born in the present century, although there will be a significant number who were born during the first two decades. Indeed, in the developing countries of the world in the year 2000, there will be an estimated 26 million people aged 80 or more, a number which exceeds the 1970 world total in that age group.

The phenomenon of an aging world population is the consequence of scientific and social advances, which have resulted in a decrease in fertility together with an increase in the average duration of life. Over the remaining years of the century, the efforts of the World Health Organization will be concentrated on extending these achievements to all mankind with a view to attaining health for all by the year 2000.

If this goal is to be realized, the World Health Organization will require the cooperation not only of social policy makers, but also of the world scientific community. The strength of the Institut de la Vie is its success in drawing upon the resources of the latter. The present book is the outcome of a conference organized by the Institut in which distinguished scientists from many disciplines undertook a wide examination of the phenomenon of aging, ranging from the level of the cell to that of society. The Regional Office is glad to support the initiative of the Institut de la Vie in bringing this book to publication, especially since it provides those planning social interventions and research with a large body of expert knowledge in the field of aging.

The book is timely, since the community of nations has expressed a universal concern for the wellbeing of the world's older citizens, and the World Health Organization has been asked by its Member States to collaborate with the United Nations and voluntary organizations in preparing for a World Assembly on the Elderly which the United Nations will convene in 1982. The WHO Regional Office for Europe which has been responsible, since 1976, for WHO's worldwide programme on care of the aged and is coordinating the Organization's contribution to the 1982 World Assembly. A major objective of the programme is to cooperate with organizations and institutes to promote the exchange of scientific and other information. This book is certainly in line with that objective.

The challenge to science and society is to seek to advance humanity through a determined effort of will and intellect aimed at securing the physical, mental, and social well-being of our old people, our future selves. I hope that this book will help sustain enthusiasm for such an endeavour.

Preface

L'Institut de la Vie was founded in 1960. Its object is to safeguard and encourage the harmonious development of all human life. Its calling is universal, as life knows no frontiers. The institution analyses aspects of the human condition and deals with some of the major problems confronting mankind.

This century has seen a considerable increase in the number of older people all over the world. At the beginning of the century the average life span was less than fifty years. It is now more than seventy years in developed societies and will continue to increase in the next decades. A concomitant decrease in fecundity has also increased the proportion of older people in the population.

According to Alfred Sauvy: 'the twenty-first century will be the century of the aging of mankind'. The challenge to mankind presented by the increase in life expectancy must be considered from the triple viewpoints of science, medicine, and sociology as new obligations devolve on society to improve the quality of life for older people.

L'Institut de la Vie organized a world conference in Vichy (France), bringing together 230 scientists from 25 developed and developing countries. The aim of the conference was to consider from a dynamic and multidisciplinary perspective the state of knowledge within the sciences and professions concerned with aging and with old people, and the implication of these findings for policy- and decision-makers. The ultimate aim was to improve the quality of life

The organization of the conference was meticulous. An international meeting, two meetings of the executive committee, and many meetings of the French committee were held to select a programme and choose participants. Working sessions for each main topic alternated with plenary assemblies were conclusions from each session were reported and followed by discussions. This book is the first volume of three based on the updated proceedings of the conference. The scientific, medical, and social conclusions are undoubtedly of major importance. They are beneficient and will influence the policies of international organizations.

Maurice Marois

Acknowledgements

The Board of Governors of L'Institut de la Vie expresses its profound gratitude to (in alphabetical order):

L'Association des Régimes de Retraites Complémentaires, La Caisse des Dépôts et Consignations, La Caisse Générale de Retraite des Cadres par Répartition, La Caisse Interprofessionnelle de Prévoyance des Cadres, La Caisse de Retraite Interentreprises, Le Centre International de Gérontologie Sociale, La Fédération Nationale de la Mutualité Française, Les Laboratoires Dausse, La Mutuelle Générale de l'Education Nationale, L'Union des Caisess Centrales de la Mutualité Agricole, La Ville de Vichy, La Compagnie Fermière de L'Etablissement Thermal de Vichy

and to the *Comite de l'Allier*

President: Monsieur le Préfet Dablanc

G. Assemat, President de la Compagnie Fermière de Vichy
D. Brunel, Directeur Général de la Compagnie Fermière de Vichy
J. Cluzel, Sénateur
J. C. Dischamp, Recteur de l'Académie
G. Frelastre, Conseiller Général de l'Allier
J. Keller, Sous-Préfet de Vichy
J. Lacarin, Maire de Vichy
C. M. Loisy, Président des Sciences Médicales de Vichy
G. Mayniel, Doyen de l'Université
G. Peronnet, Député, ancien Ministre
A. Rabineau, Senateur
G. Rougeron, Président du Conseil Général
H. Theillou, Commissaire du Gouvernement

Comité Feminin d'Accueil

Présidente d'honneur: Madame Dablanc
Présidente: Madame Keller
Vice-Présidente: Madame de Garidel Thoron

Madame Assemat	Madame Frelastre
Madame de Bourbon Busset	Madame Peronnet
Madame Brunel	Madame Rougeron
Madame Cluzel	Madame Roux
Madame Combe	Madame Theillou

for their material and moral support which have made the conference on which this book is based possible.

The conference was prepared by:

an international meeting in September 1975, with the participation of (in alphabetical order)

E. Azouri	M. Marois
W. M. Beattie Jr.	P. Mauvais
C. Bergogne	J. M. A. Munnichs
J. E. Birren	G. C. Myers
H. B. Brotman	B. Neugarten
L. Crawford	H. L. Orbach
J. Deboise	E. Peysson
C. Eisdorfer	J. Piotrowski
J. Fessard	F. de Saint-Julien
J. Flesch	A. Sauvy
A. J. J. Gilmore	E. Shanas
G. Grenander	H. L. Sheppard
W. Z. Hirsch	C. Spielman
J. A. Huet	A. Svanborg
C. L. Johnston	H. Thomae
J. P. Junod	J. van de Putte
G. Kiesau	J. Vignalou
U. Lehr	M. Yoshikawa

and by:

two meetings of Comité Exécutif in January 1976 and in December 1976 and by many meetings of Comité Français.

Comité Exécutif	*Comité Français*
W. M. Beattie Jr.	P. de Baudus de Fransures
D. Danon	C. Bergogne
A. J. J. Gilmore	A. Borveau
J. A. Huet	P. Chevalier
J. M. A. Munichs	J. Deboise
P. Paillat	J. Flesch
J. Piotrowski	D. Forestier
N. W. Shock	A. Grandguillotte
A. Svanborg	J. de Haldat du Lys
H. Thomae	J. A. Huet
J. Vignalou	G. Maurice
	P. Mauvais
	P. Paillat
	F. de Saint-Julien
	C. Spielman
	J. P. Tisseyre
	J. Vignalou

Secrétaire Général: M. Marois
Secrétaire Général Adjoint: J. Fessard

*The conference on which this volume is based was
sponsored by L'Institut de la Vie*

Contents

List of contributors

Richard C. Adelman, PhD, Executive Director, Temple University Institute on Aging, Philadelphia, Pennsylvania, U.S.A.

Reuben Andres, MD, Chief, Clinical Physiology Branch, Gerontology Research Center, National Institute on Aging, National Institutes of Health, Public Health Service, U.S. Department of Health, Education, and Welfare, Bethesda and Baltimore City Hospitals, Baltimore, Maryland, U.S.A.

Arthur K. Balin, MD, PhD, The Wistar Institute of Anatomy and Biology and the University of Pennsylvania, Philadelphia, Pennsylvania 19104, U.S.A.

Arthur Bank, MD, Professor of Medicine and Human Genetics and Development, Cancer Research Center and Departments of Medicine and of Human Genetics and Development, Columbia University, New York, U.S.A.

Edwin L. Bierman, MD, Professor of Medicine, Head, Division of Metabolism, Endocrinology, and Gerontology, Department of Medicine, University of Washington, School of Medicine, Seattle, U.S.A.

François Bourlière, MD, DSc, Professor of Physiology, University of Paris V, Institut National de la Santé et de la Recherche Médicale, Unité de Recherches Gérontologiques, Paris, France.

Harold Brody, MD, PhD, Professor and Chairman, Department of Anatomical Sciences, State University of New York at Buffalo, School of Medicine, Buffalo New York, U.S.A.

Elsworth R. Buskirk, PhD, Professor of Applied Physiology and Director, Laboratory for Human Performance Research, The Pennsylvania State University, Pennsylvania, U.S.A.

Vincent J. Cristofalo, PhD, The Wistar Institute, Philadelphia, Pennsylvania 19104, U.S.A.

David Danon, MD, Head, Section of Biological Ultrastructure, The Weizmann Institute of Science, Rehovot, Israel.

Arthur V. Everitt, PhD, Associate Professor in Physiology, University of Sydney, Sydney, New South Wales, Australia.

Eitan Fibach, PhD, Cancer Research Center and Departments of Medicine and of Human Genetics and Development, Columbia University, New York, U.S.A.

Caleb E. Finch, PhD, Cancer Research Center and Departments of Medicine and of Human Genetics and Development, Columbia University, New York, U.S.A.

David Friedman, PhD, Department of Cell Biology, The Weizmann Institute of Sciences, Rehovot, Israel.

Yair Gazitt, PhD, Cancer Research Center and Departments of Medicine and of Human Genetics and Development, Columbia University, New York, U.S.A.

Amiela Globerson, PhD, Associate Professor, Department of Cell Biology, The Weizmann Institute of Sciences, Rehovot, Israel.

Joost J. Haaijman, PhD, The Institute for Experimental Gerontology, Organization for Health Research (T.N.O.), Rijswijk, The Netherlands.

Vladimir Hachinski, MD, FRCP (C), Research Co-ordinator, University of Toronto Clinic, Division of Neurology, MacLachlan Stroke Unit, Sunnybrook Medical Centre, Toronto, Ontario, Canada.

Leonard Hayflick, PhD, Senior Research Cell Biologist, Children's Hospital Medical Center, Bruce Lyon Memorial Research Laboratory, Oakland, California, U.S.A.

James L. Hodgson, PhD, Associate Professor of Applied Physiology, Laboratory for Human Performance Research, The Pennsylvania State University, Pennsylvania, U.S.A.

Herbert J. Kayden, MD, Professor of Medicine, New York University, School of Medicine, New York, U.S.A.

Alexander Leaf, MD, Jackson Professor of Clinical Medicine, Chief of Medical Services, Massachusetts General Hospital, Harvard Medical School, Boston, Massachusetts, U.S.A.

Robert D. Lindeman, MD, Chief of Staff, Veterans Administration Medical Center, Louisville, Kentucky, U.S.A.

Alvard Macieira-Coelho, MD, PhD, Director of Research at INSERM, Institut de Cancérologie et Immunogénétique, Groupe Hospitalier Paul-Brousse, Villejuif, France.

Takashi Makinodan, PhD, Director, GRECC, Veterans Administration, Wadsworth Hospital Center, Los Angeles, California, U.S.A.

Paul A. Marks, MD, Frode Jensen Professor of Medicine, College of Physicians and and Surgeons of Columbia University, Department of Human Genetics and Development, New York, U.S.A.

George M. Martin, MD, Professor of Pathology, Departments of Pathology and Genetics, University of Washington, Seattle, Washington, U.S.A.

Uri Nudel, PhD, Cancer Research Center and Departments of Medicine and of Human Genetics and Development, Columbia University, New York, U.S.A.

Walter D. Obrist, PhD, Division of Neurosurgery, University of Pennsylvania, Philadelphia, Pennsylvania, U.S.A.

Charles E. Ogburn, MS, Department of Pathology, University of Washington, Seattle, U.S.A.

J. M. Ordy, PhD, Head, Department of Neurobiology, Delta Regional Primate Research Center, Tulane University, Covington, Louisiana, U.S.A.

J. Radl, The Institute for Experimental Gerontology, Institute for Health Research, (T.N.O.), Rijswijk, The Netherlands.

Roberta Reuben, PhD, Assistant Professor of Human Genetics and Development, Cancer Research Center and Departments of Medicine and of Human Genetics and Development, Columbia University, New York, U.S.A.

Richard A. Rifkind, MD, Professor of Medicine and Human Genetics and Development, Cancer Research Center and Departments of Medicine and of Human Genetics and Development, Columbia University, New York, U.S.A.

Russell Ross, PLD, Associate Dean for Scientific Affairs, Professor of Pathology, University of Washington, School of Medicine, Office of the Dean, Seattle, Washington, U.S.A.

George A. Sacher, BS, Division of Biological and Medical Research, Argonne National Laboratory, Argonne, Illinois, U.S.A.

Jane Salmon, MD, Cancer Research Center and Departments of Medicine and of Human Genetics and Development, Columbia University, New York, U.S.A.

Arnold B. Scheibel, MD, Departments of Anatomy and Psychiatry and Brain Research Institute, University of California at Los Angeles, Center for the Health Sciences, Los Angeles, California, U.S.A.

Madge E. Scheibel (deceased), Departments of Anatomy and Psychiatry and Brain Research Institute, University of California at Los Angeles, Center for the Health Sciences, Los Angeles, California, U.S.A.

Edward L. Schneider, MD, Laboratory of Cellular and Comparative Physiclogy, Gerontology Research Center, National Institute on Aging, National Institutes of Health, Public Health Service, U.S. Department of Health, Education, and Welfare, Bethesda and Baltimore City Hospitals, Baltimore, Maryland, U.S.A.

Leonard M. Schuman, MSc, MD, Professor and Director, Division of Epidemiology, University of Minnesota—Twin Cities, School of Public Health, Minneapolis, Minnesota, U.S.A.

Nathan W. Shock, PhD, Scientist Emeritus NIA, Chief, Gerontology Research Center, National Institute on Aging, National Institutes of Health, Public Health Service, U.S. Department of Health, Education, and Welfare, Bethesda and Baltimore City Hospitals, Baltimore, Maryland, U.S.A.

Nicolae Simionescu, MD, Institute of Cellular Biology and Pathology, Bucharest, Romania.

F. Marott Sinex, PhD, Professor and Chairman, Department of Biochemistry, Boston University, School of Medicine, Boston, Massachusetts, U.S.A.

Maxine F. Singer, PhD, Head, Nucleic Acid Enzymology Section, Laboratory of Biochemistry, National Cancer Institute, National Institutes of Health, Bethesda, Maryland, U.S.A.

Theodore H. Spaet, MD, Head, Professor of Medicine, Division of Hematology, Medical Department, Montefiore Hospital and Medical Center and the Albert Einstein College of Medicine, Bronx, New York, U.S.A.

Curtis A. Sprague, MS, Department of Genetics, University of Washington, Seattle, U.S.A.

Bernard L. Strehler, PhD, Professor of Biology, Ahmanson Center for Biological Research, University of Southern California, Los Angeles, California, U.S.A.

Masaaki Terada, MD, Assistant Professor of Human Genetics and Development, Cancer Research Center and Departments of Medicine and of Human Genetics and Development, Columbia University, New York, U.S.A.

Robert D. Terry, MD, Professor and Chairman, Department of Pathology, Albert Einstein College of Medicine, Yeshiva University, The Bronx, New York U.S.A.

Jordan D. Tobin, MD, Medical Officer, Metabolism Section, Clinical Physiology Branch, Gerontology Research Center, National Institute on Aging, National Institutes of Health, Public Heath Service, U.S. Department of Health, Education, and Welfare, Bethesda and Baltimore City Hospitals, Baltimore, Maryland, U.S.A.

Roy L. Walford, MD, Professor of Pathology, School of Medicine, University of California at Los Angeles, Los Angeles, California, U.S.A.

Myron L. Weisfeldt, MD, Professor of Medicine, Director, Cardiology Division, The Johns Hopkins Medical Institutions, Baltimore, Maryland, U.S.A.

CHAPTER I

Session 1

Aging of the nervous system—structure

Introduction H. Brody

As chairman of this first session in biology, I would like first of all to thank Professor Marois and the Institut de la Vie for their kind hospitality but most importantly for having brought together a number of people who have in the past and present contributed much to what we know of the biological aspects of aging within a number of basic areas.

I particularly want to congratulate those who planned this programme. The most important system has been selected first—the nervous system. Then, this section will consider cellular aspects of atherogenesis and aging of the cardio-vascular system, a system which as we know was created specifically to nourish the brain.

The development of the neurosciences has been particularly impressive during the past decade. It was inevitable that the possibilities for fruitful investigation in the aging nervous system should have become obvious to neuroscientists. After all, if aging can be considered within the entire concept of development and maturation of the total organism, changes in the later stages of life ought to be as interesting and important as those in early development. And with the deepening concern regarding behavioural changes in aging, structuralists now find themselves being asked by physiologists, pharmacologists, pathologists, and psychiatrists to provide them with more information on structure around which they may build a more reasonable approach to problems involving the nervous system.

We are particularly fortunate in being able to include presentations about structural aspects of the aging nervous system which make use of both old and new techniques of investigation.

In 1906, the two fathers of neuroanatomy shared the Nobel Prize for their pioneering work in the histological structure of the nervous system. Ramón y Cajal and Camillo Golgi are names which are synonymous with excellence in histological preparations and interpretation of the nervous system and much of what we know at the present time of the anatomical network system and means of contact and communication within the nervous system is based on information obtained from their basic staining techniques. The physiologists (such as Lorente DeNo) recognized this early and have particularly depended upon the Golgi preparation to explain intra-nervous-system circuitry, and it is only reasonable to expect that in view of the communication problem which develops in the older individual, the nerve cell expressed by its processes and communication system may be undergoing changes which may be better understood when our concept of change over time is explained by firm experimental evidence regarding the neuron's processes.

The work of Golgi exemplified some of the best in neuroanatomy at the turn of the century, but, since the 1950s, the Scheibels have been considered by neuroanatomists as the reincarnation of Golgi and are looked upon as the finest interpreters of the Golgi technique in the present-day field of neuroanatomy.

It is therefore a pleasure for me to introduce to you Dr. Arnold Scheibel, Professor of Anatomy and Psychiatry at the University of California at Los Angeles who has written a paper on *Structural alteration in the aging brain*.

Our second author has been a pioneer in ultrastructural studies of the dementia brain and has contributed much to our understanding of the structure of the senile placque and especially the neurofibrillary tangle. Dr. Robert Terry is Professor and Chairman of the Department of Pathology at the Albert Einstein College of Medicine in New York. His paper is entitled *Neurofibres in aging*.

Structural alterations in the aging brain   Madge E. Scheibel and Arnold B. Scheibel

With regard to myself, I hold for certain that after that age (30 years) both my mind and my body have lost rather than gained and recoiled rather than advanced. It is possible that, in those who employ their time well, knowledge and experience grow with their years: but vivacity, quickness, firmness, and those other qualities which are much more our own, more important and essential, decay and languish. (Montaigne)

Throughout the ages, man has sung reluctantly of the waning of his vigour with the coming of old age. Changes in physical strength and endurance, sexual capacity, and intellectual ability all follow an inevitable path, if in a particular blend unique to each individual. Few would deny that deterioration of mental function with age presents the most difficult challenge to the individual and those around him. It also represents a realistic challenge to medicine, universal in application, and pressing in terms of the scope of human suffering it encompasses.

The complexity of the human nervous system, with its wealth of elements and almost infinitely complex connections, makes it an especially difficult organ system in which to identify those changes which are of causal, as opposed to secondary, significance in the aging process. Gross changes in the brain have been recognized for over 150 years (Esquirol 1838) and, for fully half of that time, a group of microscopic alterations which develop with advancing age (Scheibel and Scheibel 1975).

Previous papers have emphasized certain age-related changes which occur in the cell bodies themselves and in the extraneuronal surround. Such changes are pathognomonic of senescence, but with the exception of actual cell loss, their pathophysiological significance remains enigmatic. We wish to share with you a group of changes which our methods have revealed in the dendritic processes of nerve cells. We feel these are of special, possibly of aetiological, significance in the development of psychomotor deficits of the aged, for one overriding reason. Dendrites, in furnishing 75–90 per cent of the total surface of any neuron, function as the great receptors for all connections afferent to each parent neuron. Progressive loss of the dendritic apparatus results in impoverishment of communication between nerve cells, and, with this, progressive decrement in the capacity to process information. The central nervous system is, of course, above all else, a device which deals in information and any significant degeneration of this capability must result in decline of output performance whether at the perceptive–cognitive, motor, or emotional levels.

In our studies we have used modifications of the chrome–silver methods of Golgi (1886) because of their unique capability for making visible the connective elements of the brain, i.e., the dendrites and axons. The method impregnates fully and in great detail only a fraction of the elements present in any field— seldom more than 5–10 per cent. Although this restricts its usefulness as a truly quantitative technique, its advantages outweigh this one deficiency. As a matter of fact, if it were to stain successfully every neuron present, the result would be a dense opaque field useless for microscopic study. As it is, the characteristic, selective nature of the impregnation allows us to visualize individual elements in delicate silhouette against a translucent and almost colourless background. The Golgi methods thereby provide us with a rather elegant morphological assessment of the size, shape, and surface of nerve cells with all of their projections and processes and at least some idea of the fibres which terminate on their surfaces. In conjunction with the higher resolution, if more limited view, provided by the electron microscope, we are provided with a remarkably panoramic and detailed conception of structural organization and interrelations in a selected area of the neural feltwork or neuropil.

In the material which follows, we shall concentrate on those age-related changes which we have found in the nerve cells of selected portions of the new (neocortex) (Scheibel and Scheibel 1975) and old (archicortex) (Scheibel and Scheibel 1976) portions of the cerebral hemispheres, since these areas represent the initial foci of our studies. Follow-on studies of the thalamus and brain stem indicate that the general pattern at hierarchically lower centres is similar, although the senescing process at each level tends to have its own specific signature. The process of neural aging should be held apart from the more dramatic and catastrophic phenomena of the presenile and senile dementing syndromes. The former represents, so far as we know, one aspect of a general protoplasmic reaction; the latter are manifestations of disease processes which affect the nervous system either early (40–60 years) or later (beyond 65 or 70 years) in life, producing disabling effects on the psychomotor behaviour of the individual. None the less, the structural changes that develop in and around neurons are generally the same in both, differing only in speed of onset and intensity. We do not know what causes the dementing syndrome to develop either precociously or later in life, but whatever the nature of the process, it must bear some relationship to the more gradual changes that affect us all with age. The apparent generic similarity in pathohistology, and the fact that age-related structural changes vary more with the degree of psychomotor deterioration than with calendar age, persuade us that the dementing syndromes might be thought of as temporally-compressed and symptomatically-aggravated versions of a more general reaction of the individual neural apparatus to time's arrow.

If one studies tissue specimens from a series of brains of individuals who are of progressively greater age, one finds that the probability of morphological changes in the appearance of the nerve cells and their processes increases inexorably, even though, as already indicated, any one brain specimen may appear far more intact than another from a patient 15–20 years younger. The earliest changes which are visible in the neocortex using the methods of Golgi with the light microscope are patchy areas of loss of dendrite spines and localized swellings, usually at dendritic bifurcations and on the surface of the cell body. With progression, the general 'lumpiness' of the cell silhouette increases along with further spine loss. The horizontally oriented dendrites, i.e., the basilar shafts and the oblique branches of the apical dendrite, are now seen to be more intensively involved than the vertical components. Spine loss and irregular swelling of the cell body and dendrite shafts become more extensive, culminating in fragmentation of the dendrite stalks and progressive loss of the dendritic domain. Earlier loss of the horizontal components (Figs. 1(a)–(d), 2(b), and 3, stages 2 and 3) produces a rather familiar picture with isolated, unbranched apical stems and marked attenuation or disappearance of basilar branches. In some cases, all branches appear lost on one side, leading to an asymmetric 'amputated' appearance (Fig. 2(b); Fig. 3, stage 3). In other cases, the combination of total loss of the basilar dendrite system, together with swelling of the cell body, leads to a bell-shaped configuration of the neuron (Fig. 3, stage 4). Ultimately, the apical dendrite shaft becomes more tortuous and breaks up, followed by cell death.

When one compares the various cortical areas for vulnerability to age-linked pathology, it is clear that the cerebral neocortex does not react as a whole. In general, cortex of associative and elaborative areas (i.e., those presumably not involved in direct sensory and motor transactions with the long ascending and descending tract systems of the brain stem) appear maximally sensitive to these changes of senescence. Such areas include the anterior half of the frontal lobe, the superior and middle gyri of the temporal lobe, and portions of posterior parietal lobe. Primary sensory and motor areas appear somewhat more resistant to development of such pathology for reasons which are by no means clear.

From a comparative point of view, the archicortical structures, especially the hippocampal–dentate complex, also show a high degree of vulnerability to pathological change—a fact demonstrated not only by our Golgi methods, but in routine neuropathologically stained material as well. The general sequence of senescent change follows that already described for the neocortex, although the proportion of hippocampal pyramids showing advanced stages of cell injury and

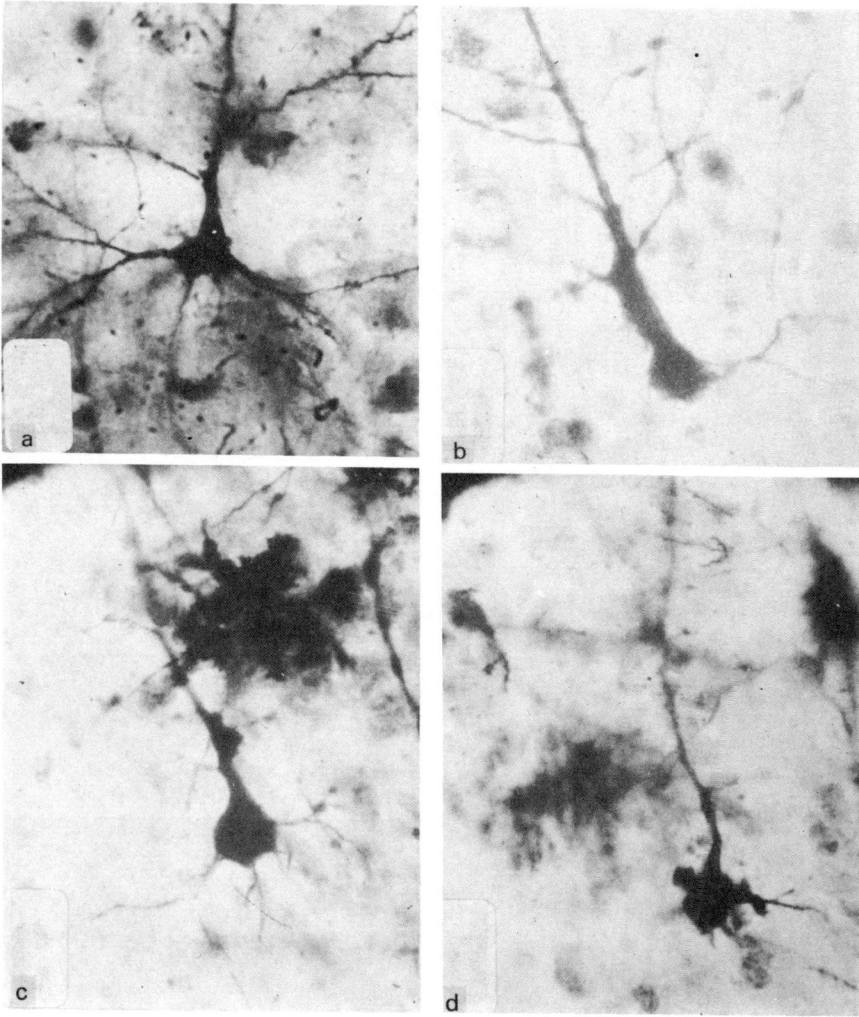

FIG. 1. Senescent changes in third- and fifth-layer pyramids of the inferior temporal gyrus in a 91-year-old man with early senile changes in behaviour. Note the apparent loss of dendrite spines and the sparsity of basilar dendrites, especially in b, c, and d. Irregular swelling and lumpiness are also obvious in b, c, and d. Stained by Golgi modification ($\times 150$).

complete cell loss appears even greater than that seen in associative neocortical zones (Fig. 5). The dentate granule cells of the dentate fascia are exceptional in that they have neither basilar dendrites nor a single apical shaft and accordingly do not show the familiar sequence of dendritic loss already described. Instead, the group of ascending dendrites which characteristically make up their domains show a patchy but progressive loss of spines combined with marked thinning of these shafts (Fig. 6) until they come to resemble clusters of asymmetric fibillary

FIG. 2. Contrast in structure of cortical neuropil between intellectually intact individuals (a and b) and those showing advanced senile behavioural changes (c and d). (a) Superior temporal cortex, fifth-layer pyramid from young adult accident victim. (b) Fifth-layer pyramid from same region in 60-year-old patient with marked senile behaviour. Note swelling of cell body and almost complete absence of horizontal dendrite systems. (c) Third and fourth layer from superior temporal cortex of intellectually intact 54-year-old man. (d) Third layer from superior temporal cortex of 72-year-old man with marked senile behaviour. Note paucity of cells and neuroglial overgrowth. Stained by Golgi modifications. (From Scheibel and Scheibel (1975). *Aging*, Vol. 1 (ed. H. Brady *et al.*) Raven Press, New York.)

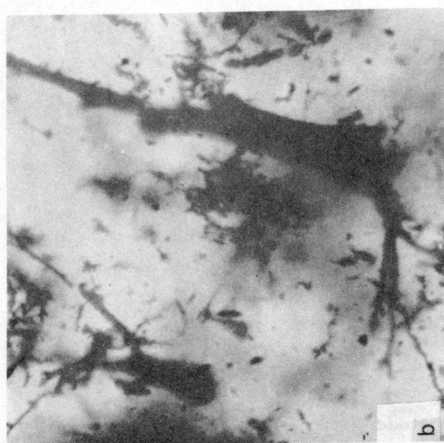

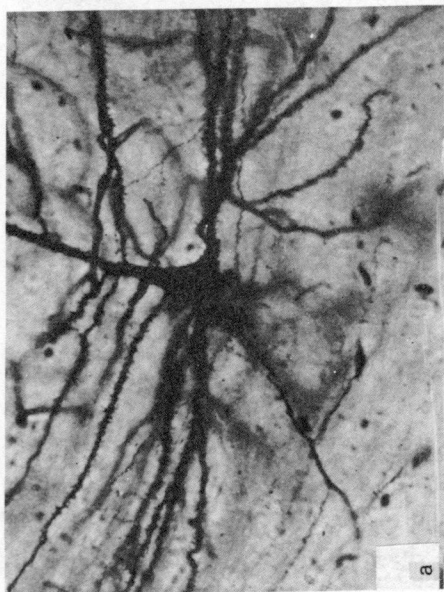

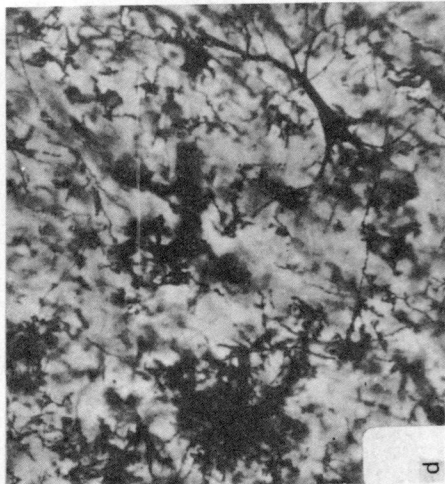

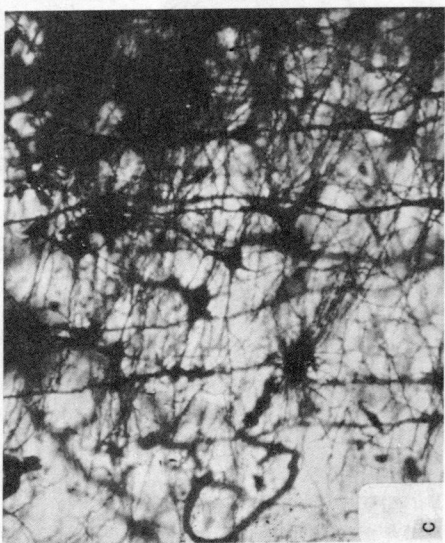

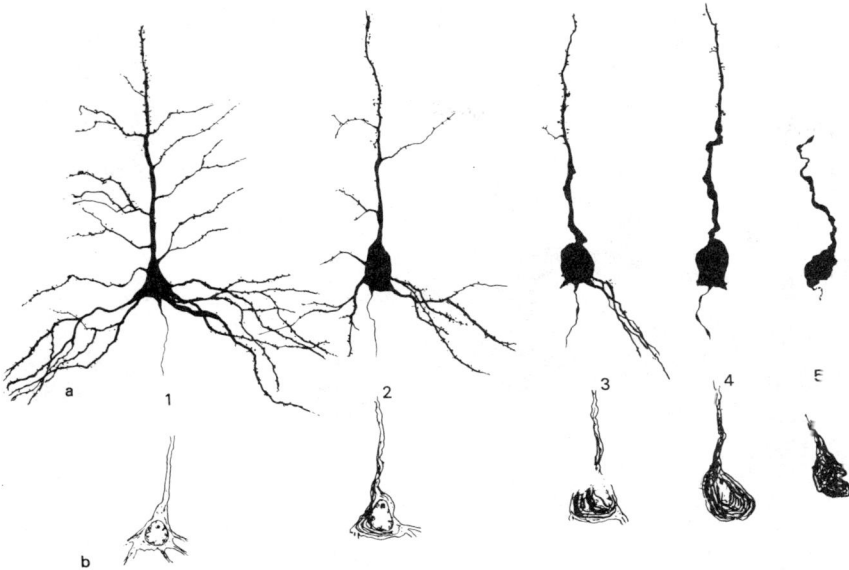

FIG. 3. Progression of senescent changes in cortical pyramids as seen in Golgi impregnations, A, and in reduced silver stain, B. The increasing development of neurofibrillary changes (abnormal microtubular material) in the cell body and dendrites in B is correlated with the changes of cell body silhouette and dendrites in B is correlated with the changes of cell body silhouette and dendritic domain in A. (From Scheibel and Scheibel (1975). *Aging*, Vol. 1 (ed. H. Brady *et al.*) Raven Press, New York.)

astroglia lined up with unaccustomed rigour. Eventually, the entire cell dendrite complex disappears and is replaced by glial overgrowth.

The adjacent entorhinal cortex, a zone of transition between old and new cortices, and one of the primary sources of afferents to dentate gyrus, has shown an idiosyncratic pathological feature in a few very old individuals in the appearance of spindle-like swellings along the apical shafts of deep pyramids (Figs. 7 and 8). They frequently appear at the same level in clusters of such shafts, thereby introducing the possibility of a local factor—possibly the microcirculation, being related to this positioning. While the cause for spindle formation remains obscure, dendrite shaft breakage invariably occurs at one end or the other of these structures. Further studies with techniques of higher resolution may reveal more critical data on the internal organization of these spindle-like structures.

On the possible significance of these studies

An abundant literature already exists documenting changes which are now known to characterize the aging or senile brain. These include structural changes of varying kinds in the cell body (lipofuscin pigment granules (Obersteiner 1903), granulovacuolar degeneration (Simchowitz 1911), and neurofibillary tangles (Alzheimer 1907)) and in the neuropil surrounding the nerve cells (the appearance

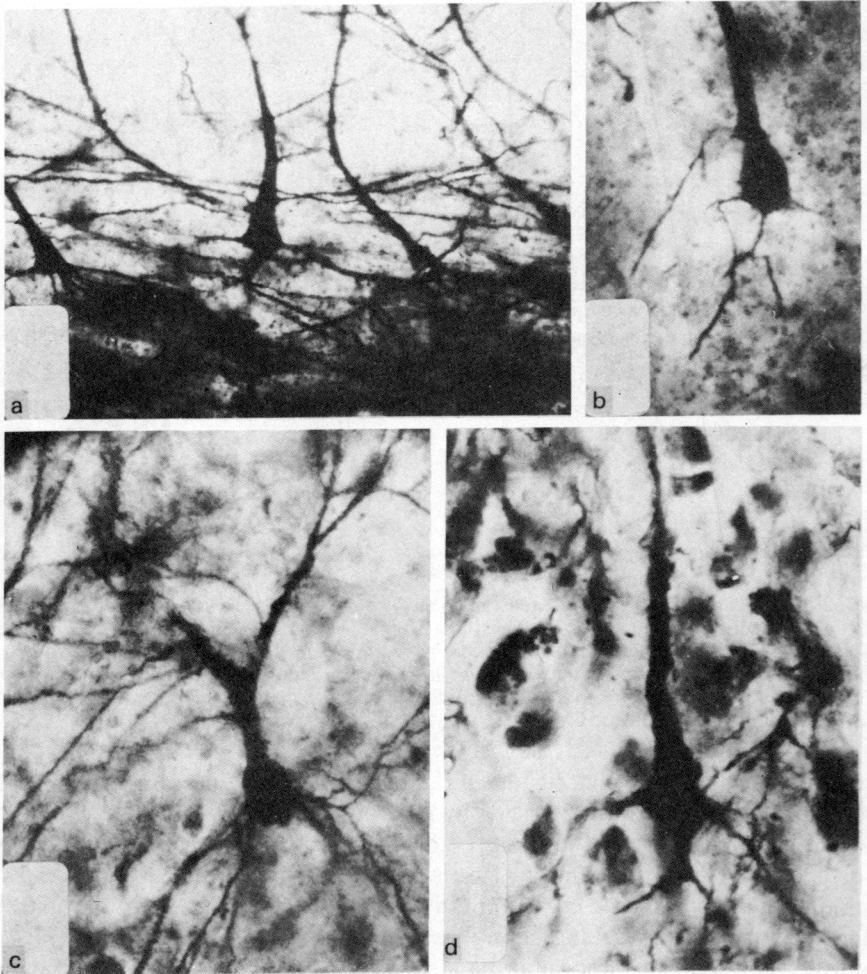

FIG. 4. Age-related changes in hippocampus. (a) Group of hippocampal pyramids in 102-year-old man showing dendritic distortions; (b) severe loss of basilar dendrites in 91-year-old man; (c) early changes in CA_2 pyramid of 91-year-old man; (d) pigment-filled cell bodies surround CA_3 pyramid losing its basilar dendrites and most of its spines. Stained by Golgi modification: a, ×150; b, c, and d, ×225.

of senile plaques (Blocq and Marinesco 1892; Simchowitz 1911)). The ultimate change appears when the nerve cell drops out and is replaced by a neuroglial overgrowth (gliosis). All of these changes bear a more or less linear relationship to the degree of psychomotor deficit, although their pathophysiological role is not yet clear. Cell loss, of course, represents a final irreversible state (since neurons do not reproduce themselves in the postnatal organism) and is clear evidence of an absolute decrement in functioning brain elements.

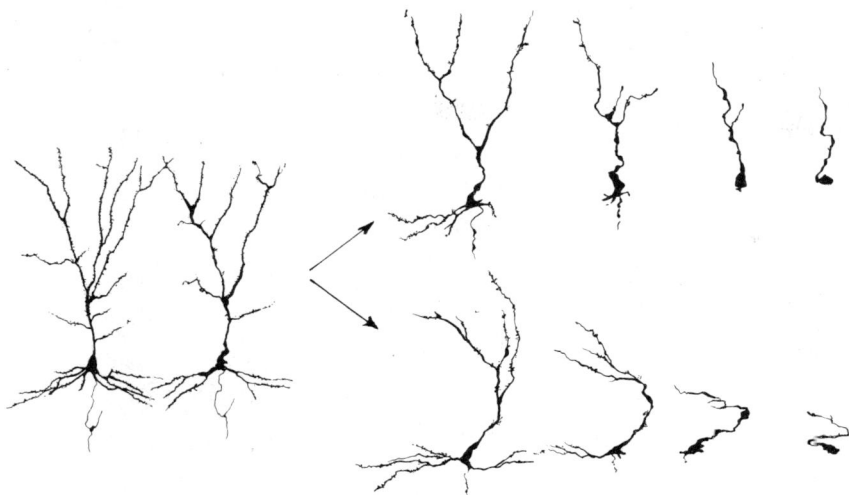

FIG. 5. Summary of progressive changes in hippocampal pyramid showing two possible sequences of senescent changes. (From Scheibel *et al*. 1974.)

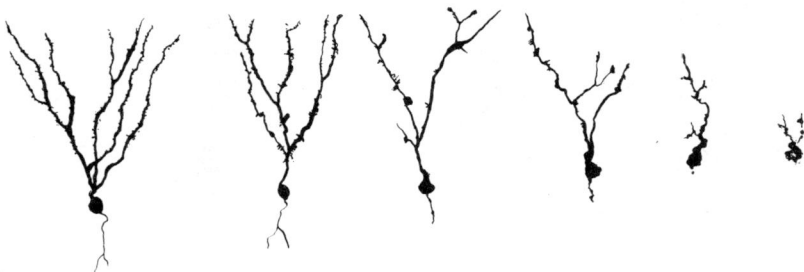

FIG. 6. Summary of progressive changes in dentate granule cells during senescence. (From Scheibel *et al*. 1974.)

Our findings provide evidence that the neuron may be functionally crippled long before the cell body itself shows visible evidence of dissolution. The inexorable loss of functional postsynaptic surface through decrement in the dendritic spine population, followed by progressive loss of the dendrite domain result in an increasing impoverishment of information input to the neurons with obvious impact on the information-processing capabilities of the brain as a total organ. A second and perhaps equally serious consequence of this increasing deprivation of afferent connections lies in the putative loss of biochemical substances—of more than informational value—carried transsynaptically from the presynaptic connections (Kreutzberg, Schubert, and Lux 1973). However, the ultimate significance of this type of interaction remains to be evaluated.

With regard to the progressive deprivation of dendritic surface, our data also suggest that a functionally significant fractionation may be discerned. The earlier

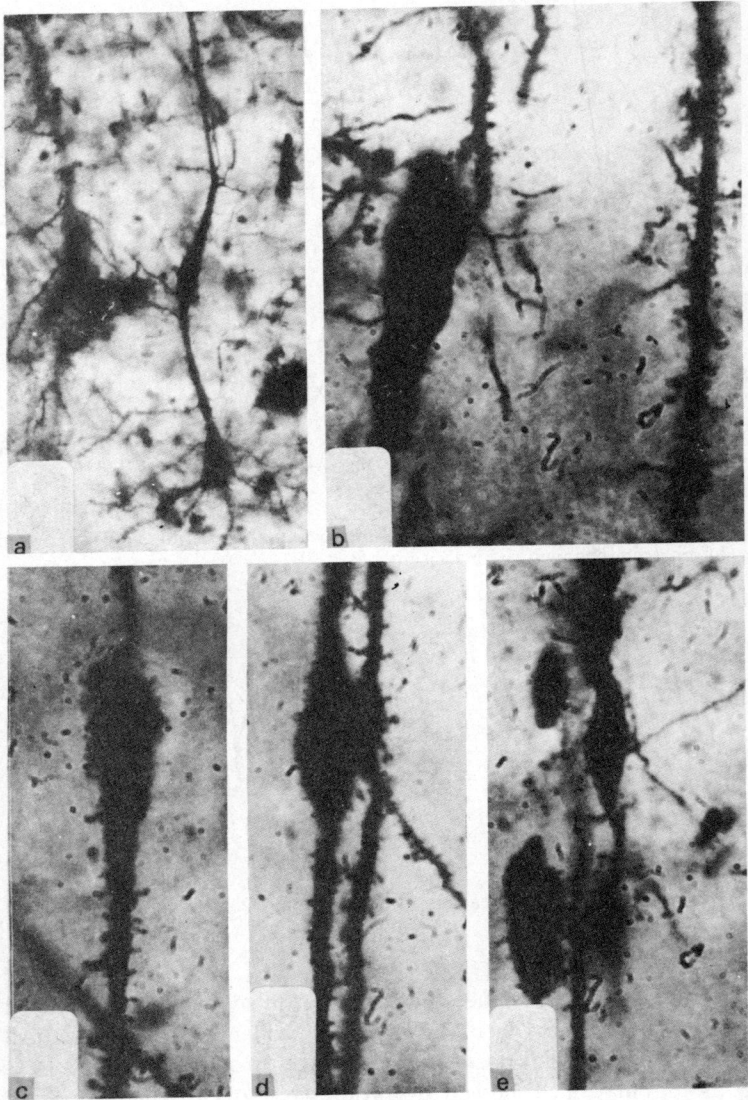

FIG. 7. Age-linked changes in pyramids of entorhinal cortex of 102-year-old man: (a) low-power view of entorhinal pyramidal cell with spindle body on apical shaft; (b) single spindle body with broken dendrite stalk and apparently normal adjacent spine-covered dendrite shaft; (c) detail of dendrite shaft with spindle body, both bearing spines; (d) details of two adjacent shafts, both spine-covered and both bearing spindle bodies at the same level; (e) fragmenting spindle bodies from several adjacent dendrite shafts. Stained by Golgi modifications: (a) ×60; (b), (c), and (d), ×360. (From Scheibel *et al.* 1974.)

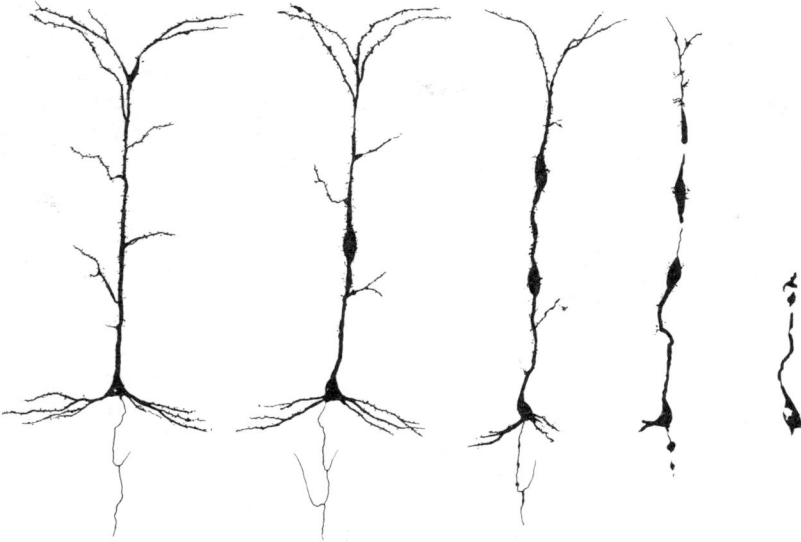

Fig. 8. Summary of progressive age-related changes in entorhinal pyramid during senescence. (From Scheibel *et al.* 1974.)

loss of horizontal dendritic components (basilar shafts and oblique branches of apical shafts), particularly in neurons of the cerebral neocortex, recals structural specificities earlier attributed to these dendrite systems. Previous experimental studies have singled out the horizontal elements as providing the principal receptive surfaces for presynaptic terminals of *intracortical origin* (Globus and Scheibel 1967). Attrition of horizontal components might therefore be expected to uncouple cortical elements from each other, resulting in progressive loss of those corticocortical links believed to be concerned with the more subtle and high-order processing functions of the hemispheres.

In addition, the basilar dendrite systems of neocortical pyramids, especially those of the fifth layer, have been found to generate extensive longitudinal associations of dendrites which we have called bundles (Scheibel, Davies, Lindsay, and Scheibel 1974). Based on correlated behavioural observations, we have suggested that dendrite bundles with their characteristic apposition of dendrite membrane to dendrite membrane may provide optimal loci for the laying down and storage of central programmes (Scheibel and Scheibel 1973). Since fifth-layer pyramids happen to be the source of most corticifugal axons, it follows that progressive loss of basilar dendrite systems might adversely affect both the range and complexity of 'higher-order' cerebral processing (due to their predominantly intracortically derived input) as well as the total scope of cortical output (due to progressive attenuation of the previously available armamentarium of output programmes).

Total nerve cell loss is becoming a useful measure of the degree of organic impairment of the cerebral cortical matrix since cell bodies are easily visualized by any one of a number of routine staining procedures, and because the cell counts themselves can be performed rather easily within certain limits of precision. However, for every nerve cell body which has disappeared, it seems likely that a number are undergoing various stages of senescent change from early spine loss to advanced degeneration of the dendritic domain. Most of these neurons are undoubtedly malfunctioning or non-functioning, so far as normal information-processing is concerned, yet the routine cell stains can give us little indication of this already existent pathology. The main exception here is the demonstration of intracellular inclusions of one sort or other, an enigmatic indicator at best, since some neurons such as those of inferior olive are already heavily charged with lipofuscin pigment granules by the tenth year of life.

As already noted, a more or less similar sequence of changes typical of senescence can be seen in the hippocampus and dentate gyrus of archicortex. In the hippocampus, particularly, cellular changes are widespread, the vast majority of pyramids swollen with pigment granules and showing nodulated and truncated dendrite domains. The fall-out of such cells may be particularly marked, and, whilst the pathogenic effects of this neuronal loss are not entirely clear owing to our inadequate knowledge of hippocampal function, hypotheses can at least be offered on the basis of some recent work in laboratory animals. This suggests a cognitive mapping function for the hippocampus, where cell clusters may encode data for a vast number of identifying characteristics of 'familiar' environments (O'Keefe and Dostrovsky 1971). While we are aware of the hazards involved in transferring data from one species to another, if the human hippocampus turns out to play a similar role, then the pathobiology of one of the most distressing symptoms of deepening senescence becomes understandable—i.e., the senile individual's progressive loss of orientation in time and space. It is possible that progressive loss of ensembles of hippocampal pyramids gradually erodes a major central representation of the individual's space–time envelope, leaving him lonely and confused, an anxious wanderer in an increasingly unfamiliar world.

Summary

Using a staining technique which enables visualization of all of the processes of nerve cells, dendritic and axonal, we have been able to follow the changes that human neurons undergo during the process of aging and senescence. There is progressive attrition of the dendritic receptive surface, starting with patchy loss of dendrite spines, followed by progressive loss of the elements of the dendritic domain, and culminating in total destruction of neural receptive apparatus and cell death. Much of the diminution in psychosocial capabilities which accompanies senescence is interpreted as resulting from progressive impoverishment of dendritic neuropil and the resulting loss of enormous numbers of synaptic connections. This results, in turn, in progressive decrement in the computational power of cerebral cortex and its program library. Equally characteristic deficits in geographical and temporal orientation are tentatively attributed to loss of ensembles of hippocampal pyramidal cells.

Addendum

Further information on patterns of aging and senescence in the human central nervous system has continued to become available, supporting and extending the above observations. Two examples will be presented briefly for their didactic value in illustrating possible correlations between structural changes in senescence and increasingly disordered motor function.

The giant pyramidal cells of Betz of the motor cortex appear particularly sensitive to the aging process. These huge neurons, seldom numbering more than 40 000 per hemisphere (Lassek 1954), generate large numbers of basilar dendrite shafts, some of which may spread laterally and obliquely through the cortex for 2–4 mm, equalling or exceeding the length of the apical shafts. Age-related changes in these neurons resemble those already described elsewhere and include patchy loss of dendrite spines, and irregular changes in the soma-dendrite silhouette indicating areas of swelling and/or constriction, followed by progressive loss of the dendritic domain. Basilar dendrite destruction precedes that of the apical system and the final stages of dissolution are marked by ensheathment of the pyknotic nerve cell bodies by proliferating astroglia.

By combining data from Golgi-impregnated material with that from Nissl and reduced silver-stained sections, it can be shown that 60–75 per cent of the total complement of Betz cells are damaged or destroyed by the seventh decade of life. In view of the remarkably limited number of such cells in each motor strip, a loss as marked as this might be expected to bear appreciable functional consequences.

Lassek (1954) has shown that the vast majority of Betz cells are located in those portions of motor cortex innervating the large extensor muscles of leg, thigh, and trunk, with very little representation in the geographically much more extensive zones concerned with hand, fingers, face, and mouth. Betz cell activity typically precedes any electromyographic evidence of muscle contraction and is characterized by a short burst of rapidly conducted spikes (Everts 1965, 1967). This phasic output pattern is unique to pyramidal cell activity since all other corticospinal output appears tonic in nature, with continuous variation in spike frequency and interspike intervals apparently carrying the relevant information. It appears increasingly likely that Betz cell activity is exclusively concerned with the brief initial lysis of anti-gravity tone in extensor muscles (Lundberg and Voorhoeve 1962), thereby allowing the desired motor sequence to be impressed upon the motor ensemble free of the constant constraint of maintained extensor tone. The latter is presumably reinstituted immediately following the motor sequence, or at each pause in the sequence of motor activities. It can therefore be postulated that with the failure of increasing numbers of Betz elements, motor activity must increasingly be superimposed upon a background of unrelieved extensor, antigravity tone. It is suggested that the increasing stiffness of the lower extremities and the slowing of motor activity with age may be due in part to this progressive failure of Betz cell activity (9).

Motor cell ensembles in the anterior horn of the spinal cord may show considerable change during the process of aging and senescence. Our data at this point suggest that such changes are not tightly linked to calender age but correlate more effectively with the degree of psychomotor and praxic change shown by the patient prior to death. As in other neural centres, the motor neurons show irregular swelling of somata and dendrites (the mature adult cells have no spines) with progressive fragmentation and loss of the dendrite shafts. As the dendrites undergo progressive degenerative changes, the sagittally-oriented dendrite bundles which form a prominent part of anterior horn neuropil (Matthews, Willis, and Williams 1971; Scheibel and Scheibel 1970) also show loss of substance. The functional role of these bundles is not clear. We have previously suggested that they are significantly, perhaps causally, related to the motor output programs generated by the neuropil zone, especially those of a stereotyped or repetitive nature (Scheibel and Scheibel 1973). Loss of such systems might be expected to interfere in increasing measure with effector patterns.

However, there is another aspect to the pattern of motor neuron loss which may be equally significant. Introductory analysis of Nissl stained material in conjunction with Golgi impregnations suggests that the smaller motor neurons show the most advanced senile changes and are the most likely to degenerate entirely. The larger neurons also show senile changes such as the accumulation of lipofuscin granules in the cytoplasm, swelling of the soma, fragmentation and loss of Nissl substance, increasingly eccentric position of the nucleus, etc. However, it appears as though they are able to tolerate greater degrees of structural change than the smaller neurons (Scheibel, unpublished). Assuming that these observations are borne out by further work, several interesting consequences can be deduced.

The population of small and medium-sized anterior horn cells are made up largely of gamma motor neurons and small alpha motor neurons. The function of the former is to bias muscle spindles to maintain spindle patterns during periods when the surrounding muscle belly is unloaded. As gamma elements are lost, spindle biassing fails with consequent restriction of information flow between receptor and central nervous system, a situation similar to that found in the postnatal organism. A likely result is decreasing precision of muscle activity due to defective sensory feedback.

A distinct set of functional consequences may also follow the selective loss of small alpha motor neurons. As indicated by that model of motor cell engagement known as the 'size principle' (Henneman, Somjen, and Carpenter 1965), motor neurons are activated by afferent volleys in a predictable sequence, the smallest cells responding earliest and with lowest threshold. These small motor neurons selectively innervate the richly vascularized, small muscle fibres capable of early, rapid, and sustained activity. Large motor neurons innervate large, pale, poorly vascularized fibres which contract later in the response sequence, and for brief periods only.

The combined result of this pattern of cell loss might well be to delay initiation of muscle contraction and to decrease the strength and precision of motor response. These changes characterize motor activity in the aging individual and it seems reasonable to assume that they represent a significant consequence of the alterations we have noted in the anterior horn. Secondary atrophic changes in muscle fibres originally supplied by the senescent and dying neurons result in decrease of total muscle mass and limitation of muscle strength and endurance, all commonly observed stigmata in the aged individual.

It should be stressed, in conclusion, that the sequences of structural alterations described above represent a general pattern only, and can be expected to vary with the general health of the individual, his genetic endowment, and perhaps the amount of neuromuscular challenge which he has faced over a significant portion of his life.

References

ALZHEIMER, A. (1907). *Cbl. Nervenheilk Psychiat.*, **18**, 177.

BLOCQ, P. and MARINESCO, G. (1892). *Semin. Med. Paris*, **12**, 445.

ESQUIROL, E. (1938). *Des maladies mentalis*, Vol. 2, p. 44. Paris.

EVARTS, E. (1965). *J. Neurophysiol.*, **28**, 216.

—— (1967). In *Neurophysiological basis of normal and abnormal motor activities* (eds. M. Yahr and D. Purpura), p. 215. Raven Press, New York.

GLOBUS, A. and SCHEIBEL, A. B. (1967). *J. comp. Neurol.*, **131**, 155.

GOLGI, C. (1886). *Sulla fina anatomia degli organi centrali del sistema nervosa.* Paris.

HENNEMAN, E., SOMJEN, G., and CARPENTER, D. (1965). *J. Neurophysiol.*, **28**, 560.

KREUTZBERG, G. W., SCHUBERT, S., and LUX, H. D. (1973). *Brain Res.*, **62**, 399.

LASSEK, A. (1954). *The pyramidal tract.* Thomas Springfield, Illinois.

LUNDBERG, A. and VOORHOEVE, P. (1962). *Acta Physiol. Scand.*, **56**, 201.

MATTHEWS, M., WILLIS, W., and WILLIAMS, V. (1971). *Anat. Rec.*, **171**, 313.

OBERSTEINER, H. (1903). *Arb. Neurol. Inst. Wien Univ.*, **10**, 245.

O'KEEFE, J. and DOSTROVSKY, J. (1971). *Brain Res.*, **34**, 171.

SCHEIBEL, M. E., DAVIES, T. L., LINDSAY, R. D., and SCHEIBEL, A. B. (1974). *Exp. Neurol.*, **42**, 307.

—— and SCHEIBEL, A. B. (1970). *Exp. Neurol.*, **28**, 106.

—— and —— (1973). *Int. J. Neurosci.*, **6**, 195.

—— and —— (1975). In *Aging* (eds. H. Brody *et al.*), Vol. 1, p. 11. Raven Press, New York.

—— and —— (1976). *Exp. Neurol.*, **53**, 420–30.

SIMCHOWITZ, T. (1911). *Nissl-Alzheimer Arbeiten*, **3**, 268.

Neurofibres and aging Robert D. Terry

Microscopic threadlike material has been noted within neurons for well over a century, perhaps beginning with Purkinje in 1837, but their reality, let alone their structure and function, was widely debated until quite recently. Optical bire-fringence of living cells has, however, proved their existence (Bear, Schmitt, and Young 1937), electron microscopy has revealed their structure, and chemical analysis has demonstrated their nature. The function of the neurofibres is still unproved, although earlier concepts relating the fibres to transmission of im-pulses (Bielschowsky 1905), or to cellular metabolic processes (Parker 1929), have been discarded, while axoplasmic transport is widely assumed to be their responsibility.

Abnormal neurofibrillary aggregates are prominent in the human brain of senile dementia of the very common Alzheimer type. It is this observation, now over 70 years old (Alzheimer 1907), that makes the subject appropriate in this volume on aging. My intention is to review briefly some of those aspects of the structure and chemistry of normal fibres which can be compared and contrasted with their abnormal analogues.

Normal fibres

Silver impregnation methods, such as those of Bielschowsky or Bodian for light microscopy, reveal a mesh of delicate fibres in normal mature neuronal perikarya and show longitudinally-oriented fibres in their neurites (Fig. 1). Glial fibres are demonstrable to the light microscopist with phosphotungstic acid—haematoxylin and certain aniline dyes. These glial elements are largely restricted

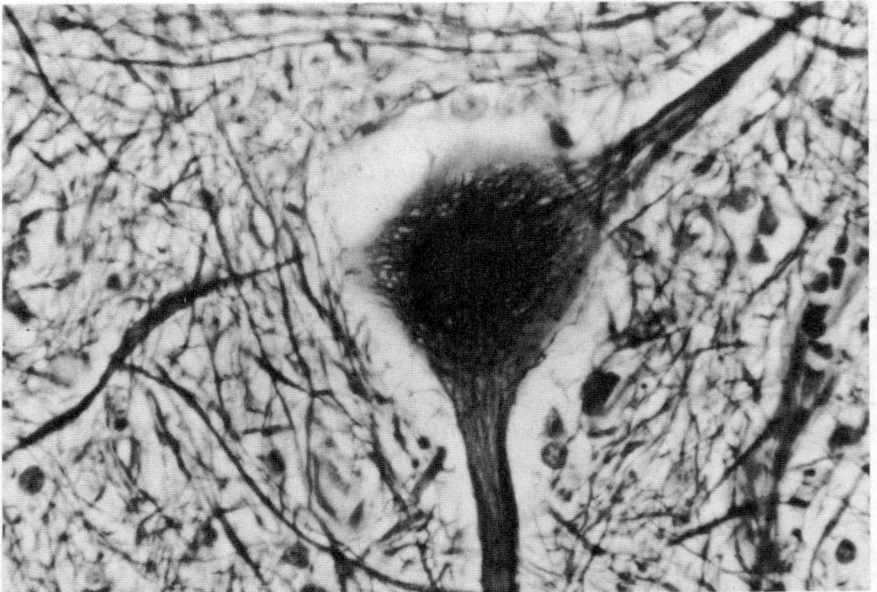

FIG. 1. This is a Bodian preparation of a normal human anterior horn cell. Neurofibres are clearly apparent, coursing through the perikaryon into the neurites. Each fibre here is very probably an aggregate of numerous neurofilaments, as described in the text.

to astrocytes and, to a lesser extent, the ependymal cells. Nothing can be learned of the size of these cellular organelles with these techniques, since the fibres tend to coalesce during the fixation and staining procedures.

Electron microscopy has demonstrated three types of intraneuronal fibre: tubules, filaments, and microfilaments. Best known are the neurotubules, which are essentially identical to microtubules in glial cells and, for that matter, in all eukaryotic cells. These are long, more or less straight structures, about 24 nm in outside diameter, with a wall 5 nm thick and a clear lumen 14 or 15 nm wide (Table 1, Fig. 2). High resolution images indicate that they have thirteen 5-nm granules in circular array to make up the cross-section (Ledbetter and Porter 1964). These granules are also aligned in longitudinal rows which form a right-handed helix around the lumen. The diameter is constant, and the tubule does not branch. Side arms, 20 to 50 nm long and about 3 nm thick, are arranged at frequent intervals along the length of the tubule. These are also called cross-bridges, although in most circumstances they do not link one tubule to another, but can often be seen to connect with other subcellular organelles.

While neurotubules are present in varying concentration throughout the neuron and its neurites, neurofilaments (Fig. 2) are more evident in axon and dendrite than in the cell body, where they are usually quite sparse. These neurofilaments are unbranched, are 9 to 11 nm in width, and are nearly solid with a small lumen which is usually not well visualized. Wuerker (1970) suggested that each filament is made up of four protofilaments, each in turn composed of a row of 3.5 nm granules. He proposed that the protofilaments are held together by short cross-bars about 2.5 nm wide. Side arms similar to those of the neurotubule are also to be found on the filaments. According to Peters and Vaughn (1967), tubules appear earlier than filaments in the developing axon. The mature axon, however, has more filaments than tubules.

Table 1 Major neurofilaments

	Neurotubules	Filaments	Paired helical filaments
Morphology			
Longitudinal section	linear	linear	linear
	even	even	narrowed every 80 nm
Cross-section	circular	circular	circular or arciform
Thickness	24 nm	10 nm	22 nm to 10 nm
Side arms	+	+	−
Stain			
Argentophilia	−	+	+
Congophilia	−	±	+
Stability			
Formalin (long)	−	+	+
Osmic acid	−	+	+
Glutaraldehyde	+	+	+
Cold	−	+	+
Ca++	−	+	+
Colchicine	−	+	?
Molecular weight	55 000 monomer	triplet	50 000 (?)
Net charge	acidic	acidic	acidic

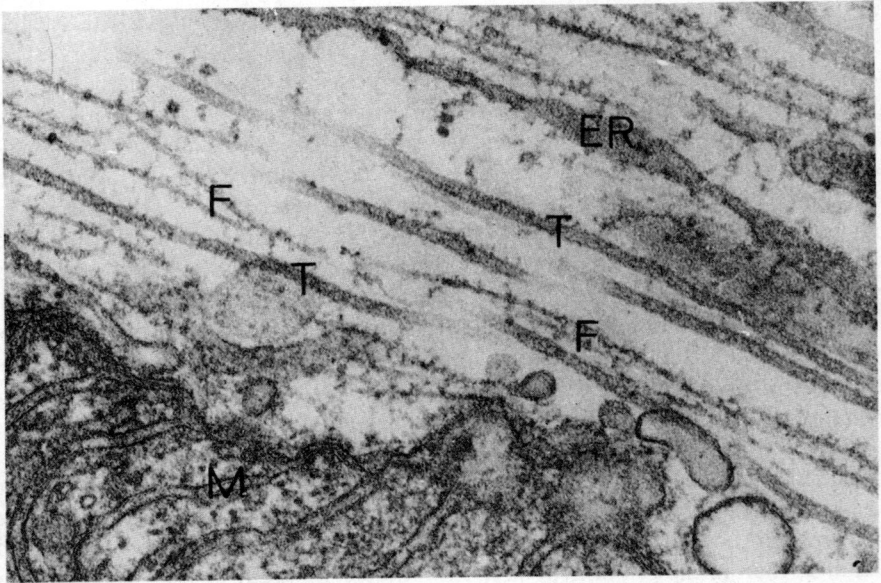

FIG. 2. An electron micrograph of axoplasm containing normal neurotubules and neurofilaments. Their side arms are apparent. E = endoplasmic reticulum; F = neurofilaments; M = myelin; and T = neurotubules. Magnification, × 70 000. [Photograph courtesy C. S. Raine, PhD.]

The third class of intraneuronal fibre is the microfilament, about which less is known in reference to its situation in the nervous system. These microfilaments are best seen in the growth cone of the developing neurite, but are also present, although not readily apparent, in the mature neuronal soma just inside the plasma membrane and just outside the nuclear envelope in relation to the nuclear pores (Metuzals and Mushynski 1974). The small, short fibres are only to 2 to 5 nm thick, and are apparently actin, or at least actin-like (Berl, Puszkin, and Nicklas 1973).

Glial fibres are most prominent in the fibrous astrocytes where their dimensions, as reported by electron microscopists, vary somewhat, perhaps depending on the sort of fixative that is used. Most commonly today, we prefix with an aldehyde, followed by osmic acid. This yields images indicating a filament thickness of 8 to 9 nm, which is slightly smaller than the neurofilament. Without the prefixation, the measurement is 6 to 7 nm (Terry and Weiss 1963). Wuerker (1970) reported that the glial filament is analogous to his model of the neurofilament, in that it is composed of four protofilaments held together by 1.5 nm cross-bars. The granules making up the protofilaments, he said, are each 2.5 nm in diameter. Each component is thus slightly smaller than in the neuronal filament. Some investigators (Gaskin and Shelanski 1976) believed that glial filaments may be identical to neurofilaments and also to 'intermediate filaments' in many other cell-types, suggesting that any minor size differences are due to coating of the fibre by cytoplasmic contributions. The lumen of the glial fibre is very subtle indeed, and is usually not apparent at all. Glial filaments, unlike neurofilaments and neurotubules, lack side arms. Perhaps for this reason the glial elements tend to become closely aggregated into packets which are not seen among neuronal fibres. Extensive chemical studies have been performed on the major fibre-types (Table 1), and detailed reviews can be found elsewhere (Bray 1974; Gaskin and Shelanski 1976; Roberts 1974; Shelanski, Liem, and Yen 1977).

The microtubule, perhaps because of its ubiquity, has been studied most intensively. The structures exist in the cytoplasm in equilibrium with their constituent protein, tubulin. This protein is usually purified from whole brain homogenate by a recycling operation in which tubules are repeatedly disassembled at 4 °C and reassembled at 37 °C (Borisy, Olmstead, Marcum, and Allen 1974; Shelanski, Gaskin, and Cantor 1973). Tubulin is an acidic, 6S dimer of 110 000 daltons, which binds two moles of guanine nucleotide (Weisenberg, Borisy, and Taylor 1968), one of which is very tightly bound. Spindle inhibitors such as colchicine shift the equilibrium from the tubule toward the dimeric form, binding stoichiometrically with the tubulin (Weisenberg *et al.* 1968). The α tubulin monomer is generally said to have a weight of 56 000 daltons, and the β monomer of 53 000 (Bryan and Wilson 1971; Feit, Slusarek, and Shelanski 1971), but some investigators contend that the monomers are of equal size and have slightly different net charges in SDS to account for their different rates of migration in an electrophoretic field (Wilson and Bryan 1974). Tubules depolymerize in the cold (Tilney and Porter 1967), or with increased pressure (Salmon 1975). The side arms which are reconstituted with neurotubules *in vitro* are probably made up of higher molecular weight proteins (Dentler, Granett, and Rosenbaum 1975; Murphy and Borisy 1975) in the range of 350 000 daltons.

Since there are decreased numbers of neurons and increased astrocytes in the aging human brain, there is probably a decreased concentration of tubulin here, but specific analyses in this regard apparently have not been done. McMartin and Schedlbauer (1975) have found that slices of aged mouse brain incorporate radioleucine normally into tubulin, and that this protein is at a normal level in these 25-month-old animals.

Neurofilaments (NF) are generally isolated from mammalian brain by flotation of myelinated axons from white matter, followed by an osmotic shock or triton to remove the myelin (Shelanski, Albert, DeVries, and Norton 1971). Several proteins are demonstrable in the subsequently purified fractions isolated in high ionic strength buffers (Liem, Yen, Salomon, and Shelanski 1978). Molecular weights of three relevant proteins are 68 000, 160 000, and 210 000. These comprise the neurofilament triplet. Unlike neurotubules, the neurofilaments do not depolymerize when treated with colchicine (Iqbal, Grundke-Iqbal, Wisniewski, and Terry 1977).

Glial fibrous acidic protein (GFAP) was originally isolated from brain tissue which had been altered by disease so that essentially the only remaining cells were fibrous astrocytes (Eng, Vanderhaegen, Bignami, and Gerste 1971). The molecular weight most commonly cited for this protein is about 50 000 daltons, although Bignami and Dahl (in press) believe it to be 54 000, and that the lower weight reflects proteolysis. One might predict a somewhat increased concentration of GFAP in the aged human brain, and an even higher concentration in the brain of senile dementia where astrocytic processes are particularly prominent. This astrocytic hypertrophy is a reaction to changes among neurons rather than a primary alteration of the glia.

Gaskin and Shelanski (1976) have emphasized several close similarities between GFAP and what until recently was thought to be neurofilament protein (NFP). In addition to the nearly identical size, Yen, Dahl, Schachner, and Shelanski (1976) point out numerous identical tryptic peptides as well as an *in vitro* reaction between an antibody raised against NFP and the antigen GFAP. Goldman, Farooq, and Norton (1977) have found that GFAP and NFP comigrate electrophoretically within a species, varying together from one species to another. These sorts of results, however, may well have come from contamination of the NFP fraction with large amounts of glial filament protein which resisted solubilization in the low ionic strength buffers then in use (Liem *et al.* 1978).

Immunological studies on these normal fibres and their component proteins are currently progressing rapidly in several laboratories, but the results are still confusing, and some are contradictory. GFAP is a potent antigen, and the antibody induced by it stains astrocytes specifically with both fluorescence (Bignami, Eng, Dahl, and Uyeda 1972) and peroxidase techniques (Ludwin, Kosek, and Eng 1976) on histological sections. Tubulin and neurofilament triplet proteins are less satisfactory as antigens, but several investigators have raised antibodies to them. It is becoming increasingly clear that, despite earlier reports to the contrary, the proteins of each type of fibre are probably separate and distinct, with little or no immunological crossover.

Abnormal fibres

Abnormal intraneuronal aggregates of argentophilic fibres (Fig. 3) are called Alzheimer's neurofibrillary tangles, having been first adequately described by Alois Alzheimer in 1907. In senile dementia of the Alzheimer form, that is about 50 per cent of senile patients (Tomlinson 1977), the tangles are present in great numbers in neurons of the neocortex and even more in the paleocortex. They are especially prominent in the pyramidal cells of the hippocampal subiculum and Sommer's sector. Tangles are very common in the amygdaloid nucleus and to a lesser extent in temporal and frontal cortex, cingulate gyrus, and other cortical areas. Smaller numbers are found in the hypothalamus and reticular substance (Hirano and Zimmerman 1962). The cerebellum and inferior olives are free of these lesions even in severe dementia, but a few tangles have been found in the anterior horn cells of the spinal cord in familial Alzheimer's disease (Feldman, Chandler, Levy, and Glaser 1963). It is very important that large numbers of cortical tangles correlate consistently with dementia (Farmer, Peck, and Terry 1976; Roth, Tomlinson, and Blessed 1966).

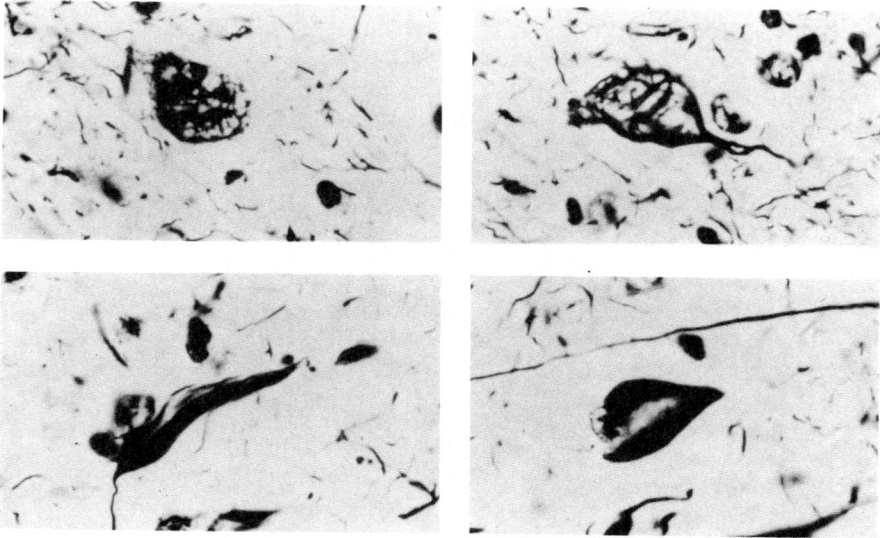

FIG. 3. These are Bodian preparations of neurofibrillary tangles from hippocampus and amygdaloid nucleus, and they display the variety of configurations to be found among these lesions. Each fibre in these images represents an aggregate of the paired helical filaments (PHF) described in the text.

Matsuyama, Namiki, and Watanabe (1966) found at least a few such lesions in very nearly all human brains beyond age 80, regardless of mental status. This indicates that the causal factor or factors, whether genetic, environmental, or infectious, are very widespread. It might also reduce to a semantic argument the question of whether this sort of tangle is pathologic or normal. Abnormality is related to the concentration of the lesions.

The tangles are made up of bundles of fibres each of which is now recognized as a pair of helically wound filaments (PHF), distinctly different from the configuration of any normal fibres. Each member of the pair is about 10 nm thick, and seems to be free of side arms. They twist about each other at regular intervals of about 80 nm, giving a period of 160 nm (Fig. 4). In cross-section they sometimes appear as a crescent with a concentric granule, but in other images they look circular. This latter form led some observers (Terry 1963) to believe that they were twisted tubules, although Kidd (1963) early proposed that they were indeed helically wound pairs. Convincing demonstration of their filamentous, helical nature was elicited with tilt stage electron microscopy and with scale models (Wisniewski, Narang, and Terry 1976). Normal neurotubules and neurofilaments are still present in parts of the neuronal soma not occupied by the tangle, which to a varying extent displaces these and other normal organelles.

These masses of PHF are found not only in neuronal perikarya but also in synaptic terminals, primarily axonal (Gonatas, Anderson, and Evangelista

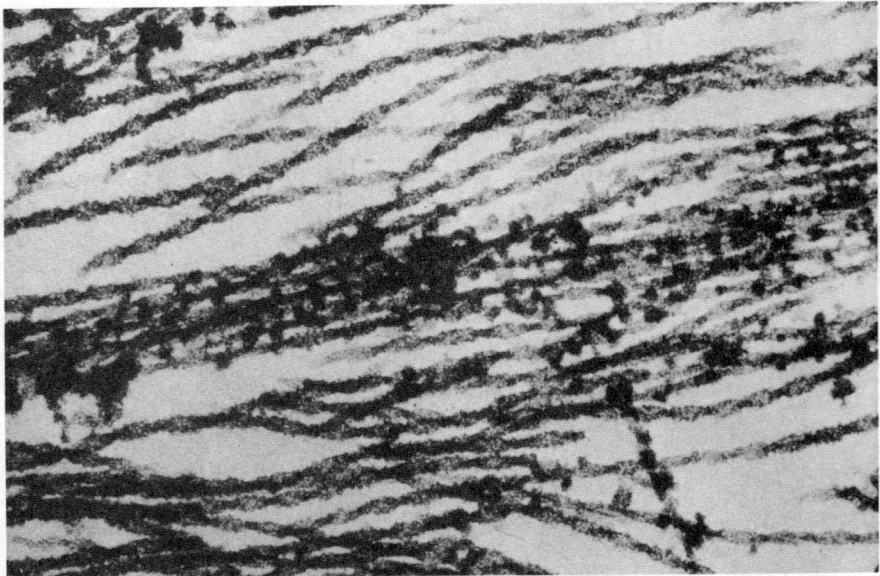

FIG. 4. An electron micrograph of PHF from a neurofibrillary tangle. The periodic crossings and the absence of side arms are characteristic of these abnormal organelles. Magnification, × 90 000.

1967) in neuritic or senile plaques (also characteristic of senility), and occasionally a few PHF are noted in myelinated axons. They have not, however, been described in the peripheral nervous system or in extraneuronal tissues. This point is of some interest since both microtubules, identical to neurotubules, and intermediate filaments similar to neurofilaments are present in a wide variety of extraneural cells. If one or another of these organelles were the direct precursor of the PHF, one might well have expected the latter to be more widespread in the affected patient.

Alzheimer's presenile and senile dementia are not, however, the only situations in which PHF are found in the brain. As seen in Table 2, they are present in extraordinary numbers in cases of Guam Parkinson–Dementia (Hirano, Malamud, and Kurland 1961). Adults over 35 or 40 years of age and surviving with Down's syndrome, which is a chromosomal disorder, often have many such lesions (Schochet, Lampert, and McCormick 1973). Many PHF tangles are present in neurons of the substantia nigra and locus caeruleus of patients with Parkinsonism of the sort which followed the viral encephalitis of von Economo (Wisniewski, Terry, and Hirano 1970). Similar lesions are common in the cerebral cortex of aging ex-prize fighters who display the 'punch drunk' syndrome (Corsellis, Bruton, and Freeman-Browne 1973). A few patients who have had subacute sclerosing panencephalitis, which is an infection due to a variant of measles virus, also develop tangles made up of PHF (Mandybur, Nagpaul,

Table 2 Neurofibrillary tangles

Material	Paired helical filaments	10-nm filament	Perikaryon	Neurites
Human				
Normal aging	+ (sparse)	−	+ (sparse)	+ (sparse)
Alzheimer's dementia	+	−	+	+
Guam Parkinsonism–dementia	+	−	+	−
Dementia pugilistica	+	−	+	−
Down's syndrome (late)	+	−	+	+
Postencephalitic Parkinsonism	+	−	+	−
Subacute sclerosing panencephalitis	+ (rare cases)	−	+	−
Lipofuscin storage	+ (rare cases)	−	+	−
Sporadic motor neuron disease	−	+	+	−
Vincristine neuropathy	−	+	+	+
Infantile neuroaxonal dystrophy	−	+	−	+
Steele–Richardson–Olszewski syndrome	−	15-nm tubule	+	−
Animal				
Aged monkey	+ (atypical, rare)	−	−	+
Zebra—congenital flexion	−	+	+	+
Aluminium encephalopathy	−	+	+	+
Spindle inhibitor encephalopathy	−	+	+	+
Lathyrogenic encephalopathy (IDPN)	−	+	−	+
Vitamin-E deficiency	−	+	−	+
Copper deficiency	−	+	+	−
Retrograde and Wallerian degeneration	−	+	+	+

Pappas, and Niklowitz 1977). Finally, as to the human (as far as we know to date), there have been a few cases of juvenile neuro-visceral lipid storage disease where occasional central neurons contain these particular lesions (Horoupian and Yang 1978). Thus viral infection, trauma, chromosomal disorder, and metabolic abnormality have all been implicated as possible causal agents.

The PHF have certain histological stain reactions similar to those of amyloid. That is, both PHF and amyloid fibres are congophilic, and become birefringent after staining with congo red. Furthermore, both react with thioflavin S (Schwartz, Kurucz, and Kurucz 1964), becoming fluorescent. There are, however, distinct ultrastructural and topographical differences, so that most observers do not believe that PHF are identical to amyloid, although this has been suggested many times since Divry's (1934) observation.

PHF identical to those of the human have not been reported in other species. We have found, however, very sparse clusters of abnormal fibres in pre-synaptic boutons of aged monkeys (Wisniewski, Ghetti, and Terry 1973). These paired filaments twist every 40 nm, and thus have a periodicity half that of the human. These lesions are so rare that this can not be regarded as a useful model, although these monkeys also have neuritic plaques otherwise very similar to those of the senile human.

De Boni and Crapper (1978) have reported that treatment of tissue cultures of human foetal cerebral cortex with an aqueous extract of Alzheimer brain tissue induces the formation of PHF in the cultured neurons. This is very important evidence pointing toward a transmissible agent involved in Alzheimer's disease.

Neurofibrillary tangles made up of simple filamentous aggregates are found in a wide variety of unusual circumstances (Table 2), but are not characteristic of the aging human brain. They can, however, be induced in certain experimental animals. Rabbits and cats are particularly susceptible to the intrathecal injection of aluminium salts, and this causes many large neurons, especially in the spinal cord and brain stem, to develop massive filamentous tangles (Terry and Peña 1965). This is of considerable interest in view of Crapper's finding (Crapper, Krishnan, and Dalton 1973) that the human brain in Alzheimer's disease has an abnormally high aluminium content associated with nuclear chromatin. There is no direct evidence, however, that aluminium causes aggregation of PHF in the human. There are only two published reports of human encephalopathy caused by aluminium, and in neither were there PHF, or even simple filamentous tangles (Lapresle, Duckett, Galle, and Cartier 1975; McLaughlin, Kazantzis, King, Teare, Porter, and Owen 1962). Spindle inhibitors such as colchicine or vinblastine also cause neurons to develop large bundles of 10 nm filaments as normal microtubules disappear (Wisniewski, Shelanski, and Terry 1968). This is an acute change often associated with cell death, while the lesion induced by aluminium salts is more durable and benign. In both the filaments have a structure identical to that of normal neurofilaments. Filament triplet proteins have been demonstrated in the aluminium-induced tangles (Selkoe, Liem, Yen, and Shelanski 1979).

Physiological studies on neurons with aluminium-induced filamentous tangles have been reported by Crapper and his colleagues (1976). They have found that post-synaptic excitatory and inhibitory mechanisms are abnormal, while there is no change in the axons' ability to propagate a potential or to release transmitter. Liwnicz, Kristensson, Wisniewski, Shelanski, and Terry (1974) found that these experimental tangles did not seem to affect axoplasmic flow. Data of this direct sort are not available on human neurons with PHF tangles, but analysis by Crapper, Dalton, Skopitz, Eng, Scott, and Hachinski (1975) of studies on evoked potentials in patients with Alzheimer's disease developing in Down's syndrome seem to confirm that cells with tangles tend to become electrically inactive because of post-synaptic failure. These workers suggest that this causes disfacilitation and disinhibition of residual neurons, and that this alters normal rhythms.

Isolation of human PHF is accomplished by first isolating neuronal perikarya (Iqbal and Tellez-Nagel 1972) from areas of autopsied human brain where microscopy indicated a high concentration of lesions. Subcellular fractionation of the neuronal pellet yields a fraction enriched in PHF (Davison and Winslow 1974; Iqbal, Wisniewski, Shelanski, Brostoff, Liwnicz, and Terry 1974). Electrophoresis of the PHF fraction on SDS-polyacrylamide gels indicates a molecular weight of 50 000 daltons for the major protein (PHFP). Two dimensional maps made with tryptic or chymotryptic digests of the PHFP show about 85 per cent coincidence with similarly treated human NFP (that is, the 50 000 dalton protein), and about 75 per cent coincidence with peptides from human β tubulin (Iqbal, Grundke-Iqbal, Wisniewski, and Terry 1978a). Fluorescamine micro-analysis of amino acids from PHFP shows that it is an acidic protein and has a composition lying between those of NFP and β tubulin, resembling the latter slightly more closely (Iqbal, Grundke-Iqbal, Wisniewski, and Terry 1978b). Antiserum prepared in the rabbit immunized with PHFP reacts *in vitro* with neurotubules and both tubulins, and on tissue sections with neurofibrillary tangles (Iqbal *et al.* 1978b). It is quite possible that this all represents severe contamination with glial filaments, and that PHF, themselves, have not yet been adequately examined chemically.

Quite recently, Iqbal *et al.* have reported that an antiserum has been prepared from a somewhat impure fraction of normal human brain microtubules, and that this antiserum reacts quite specifically with neurofibrillary tangles in light microscopic immunohistochemical preparations (Grundke-Iqbal, Johnson, Wisniewski, Terry, and Iqbal 1979). Despite the impurity of the antiserum, it is significant that there is an antigen in normal brain that is immunologically similar to one in the tangle.

The origin of the PHF in senile dementia is still unclear. The PHF seem to be closely related to a protein of normal brain tissue, but whether they are derived from one or another normal neurofibre, or whether they are made of a new protein, has not yet been fully ascertained. According to our working hypo-thesis, finding a modified or derived protein would lead to a search for the mechanism which produces an abnormal assembly. Should we find an entirely new or original protein, we would look for a slow virus or for activation of normally repressed inherited genetic information. It seems a little less probable to this observer that a new protein induced by a viral genome would be so similar to a normal family of proteins, but this possibility can not be excluded. It is more likely, however, that the PHF are the result of genetic derepression, or of post-transcriptional or post-translational modifications of one of the normal fibrous proteins. More complete analysis of the abnormal fibres will be necessary.

The functional effect of the abnormal fibres on cellular processes is entirely unknown. Neurotubules are widely thought to be involved in axoplasmic flow, and neurofilaments may be essential to the same process, either directly or through interaction with the tubules. Suzuki and Terry (1967) suggested that the neurofibrillary tangle may interfere with flow, but there is really no functional evidence in this regard except as stated for the aluminium-induced tangle (Liwnicz *et al.* 1974). The Scheibels (Scheibel and Scheibel 1975) have suggested that the tangles are responsible for atrophy of the dendritic arbor. Since, how-ever, these atrophic changes occur in the neocortex in the absence of tangles in normal human aging and in aged animals totally without tangles, this exclusive role must be discarded. The cellular lesion might block some other metabolic process, or synthesis of the PHF might deprive some other cellular process of essential substrate. It must be admitted, however, that the neurofibrillary tangle might simply be an epiphenomenon and not in itself harmful to the organism.

Since the PHF is such a distinctive, abnormal subcellular organelle, its appeal to the pathobiologist remains nearly irresistible. Its further investigation may shed real light on the nature and cause of one of mankind's most distressing disorders.

Acknowledgments

I am grateful to Drs Felicia Gaskin and Khalid Iqbal for their help and constructive criticism of the manuscript, and to Dr Henryk M. Wisniewski for several years of collaboration.

Our own work has been supported in part by grants NS-02255, NS-03356, and NS-08180 from the National Institutes of Health, plus funds generously provided by Mr Jerome Stone, the Nichamin Family Foundation, and others.

References

ALZHEIMER, A. (1907). *Zbl. Nervenheilk. Psychiat.*, **30**, 177.

BEAR, R. S., SCHMITT, F. O., and YOUNG, J. Z. (1937). *Proc. roy. Soc. (Lond.)*, **123**, 505.

BERL, S., PUSZKIN, S., and NICKLAS, W. J. (1973). *Science, N.Y.*, **179**, 441.

BIELSCHOWSKY, M. (1905). *J. Psychol. Neurol.*, **5**, 128.

BIGNAMI, A. and DAHL, D. (in press). In *Recent advances in spinal cord injury research*, (ed. N. F. Naftchi). Spectrum, Holliswood, New York.

——, ENG, L. F., DAHL, D., and UYEDA, C. T. (1972). *Brain Res.*, **43**, 429.

BORISY, G. G., OLMSTEAD, J. B., MARCUM, J. M., and ALLEN, C. (1974). *Fed. Proc.*, **33**, 167.

BRAY, D. (1974). *Endeavor*, **33**, 131.

BRYAN, J. and WILSON, L. (1971). *Proc. Nat. Acad. Sci. (USA)*, **68**, 172.

CORSELLIS, J. A. N., BRUTON, C. J., and FREEMAN-BROWNE, D. (1973). *Psychol. Med.*, **3**, 270.

CRAPPER, D. R. (1976). In *Aging*, Vol. 3 *Neurobiology of aging* (ed. R. D. Terry and S. Gershon), p. 405. Raven Press, New York.

——, KRISHNAN, S. S., and DALTON, A. J. (1973). *Science, N.Y.*, **180**, 511.

——, DALTON, A. J., SKOPITZ, M., ENG, P., SCOTT, J. W., and HACHINSKI, V. C. (1975). *Amer. med. Assoc. Arch. Neurol.*, **33**, 618.

DAVISON, P. F. and WINSLOW, B. (1974). *J. Neurobiol.*, **5**, 119.

DE BONI, U. and CRAPPER, D. R. (1978). *Nature (Lond.)*, **271**, 566.

DENTLER, W. L., GRANETT, S., and ROSENBAUM, J. L. (1975). *J. Cell Biol.*, **65**, 237.

DIVRY, P. (1934). *J. Belge Neurol. Psychiat.*, **34**, 197.

ENG, L. F., VANDERHAEGEN, J. J., BIGNAMI, A., and GERSTL, B. (1971). *Brain Res.*, **28**, 351.

FARMER, P., PECK, A., and TERRY, R. D. (1976). *J. Neuropathol. exp. Neurol.*, **35**, 367.

FEIT, H., SLUSAREK, L., and SHELANSKI, M. L. (1971). *Proc. Nat. Acad. Sci. (USA)*, **68**, 2028.

FELDMAN, R. G., CHANDLER, K. A., LEVY, L. L., and GLASER, G. H. (1963). *Neurol.*, **13**, 811.

GASKIN, F. and SHELANSKI, M. L. (1976). In *Essays in biochemistry* 1976 (ed. P. N. Campbell and W. N. Aldridge), Vol. 12, p. 115. Academic Press, New York.

GOLDMAN, J. E., FAROOQ, M., and NORTON, W. T. (1977). *Trans. Amer. Soc. Neurochem.*, **8**, 140.

GONATAS, N. K., ANDERSON, W., and EVANGELISTA, I. (1967). *J. Neuropathol. exp. Neurol.*, **26**, 25.

GRUNDKE-IQBAL, I., JOHNSON, A. B., WISNIEWSKI, H. M., TERRY, R. D., and IQBAL, K. (1979). *Lancet*, **i**, 578.

HIRANO, A., MALAMUD, N., and KURLAND, L. T. (1961). *Brain*, **84**, 662.

—— and ZIMMERMAN, H. M. (1962). *Amer. med. Assoc. Arch. Neurol.*, **7**, 227.

HOROUPIAN, D. S. and YANG, S. S. (1978). *Ann. Neurol.*, **4**, 404.

IQBAL, K. and TELLEZ-NAGEL, I. (1972). *Brain Res.*, **45**, 296.

——, WISNIEWSKI, H. M., SHELANSKI, M. L., BROSTOFF, S., LIWNICZ, B. H., and TERRY, R. D. (1974). *Brain Res.*, **77**, 337.

——, GRUNDKE-IQBAL, I., WISNIEWSKI, H. M., and TERRY, R. D. (1977). *J. Neurochem.*, **29**, 417.

——, ——, ——, and —— (1978a). *Brain Res.*, **142**, 321.

——, ——, ——, and —— (1978b). In *Aging*, Vol. 7 *Alzheimer's disease: senile dementia and related disorders* (ed. R. Katzman, R. D. Terry, and K. L. Bick), p. 409. Raven Press, New York.

KIDD, M. (1963). *Nature, (Lond.)*, **197**, 192.

LAPRESLE, J., DUCKETT, S., GALLE, P., and CARTIER, L. (1975). *C. R. Sc. Soc. Biol. (Paris)*, **169**, 282.

LEDBETTER, M. C. and PORTER, K. R. (1964). *Science, N.Y.*, **144**, 872.

LIEM, R. K. H., YEN, S.-H., SALOMON, G. D., and SHELANSKI, M. L. (1978). *J. Cell Biol.*, **79**, 637.

LIWNICZ, B. H., KRISTENSSON, K., WISNIEWSKI, H. M., SHELANSKI, M. L., and TERRY, R. D. (1974). *Brain Res.*, **80**, 413.

LUDWIN, S. K., KOSEK, J. C., and ENG, L. F. (1976). *J. comp. Neurol.*, **165**, 197.

MCLAUGHLIN, A. I. G., KAZANTZIS, G., KING, E., TEARE, D., PORTER, R. J., and OWEN, R. (1962). *Brit. J. indust. Med.*, **19**, 253.

MCMARTIN, D. N. and SCHEDLBAUER, L. M. (1975). *J. Gerontol.*, **30**, 132.

MANDYBUR, T. I., NAGPAUL, A. S., PAPPAS, Z., and NIKLOWITZ, W. J. (1977). *Ann. Neurol.*, **1**, 103.

MATSUYAMA, H., NAMIKI, H., and WATANABE, I. (1966). In *Proceedings of the Fifth International Congress of Neuropathology* (ed. F. Luthy and A. Bischoff), Series 100, p. 979. Excerpta Medica, Amsterdam.

METUZALS, J. and MUSHYNSKI, W. E. (1974). *J. Cell Biol.*, **61**, 701.

MURPHY, D. B. and BORISY, G. G. (1975). *Proc. Nat. Acad. Sci. (USA)*, **72**, 2696.

PARKER, G. H. (1929). *Amer. Naturalist*, **63**, 97.

PETERS, A. and VAUGHN, J. E. (1967). *J. Cell Biol.*, **32**, 113.

PURKINJE, J. E. (1837). In *Bericht über die Versammlung Deutscher Naturforscher und Ärzte in Prag*, September, 1837. Hasse, Prague.

ROBERTS, K. (1974). In *Progress in biophysics and molecular biology* (ed. A. J. F. Butler and D. Noble), p. 371. Pergamon Press, Elmsford, New York.

ROTH, M., TOMLINSON, B. E., and BLESSED, G. (1966). *Nature, (Lond.)*, **209**, 109.

SALMON, E. D. (1975). *Science, N.Y.*, **189**, 884.

SCHEIBEL, M. E. and SCHEIBEL, A. B. (1975). In *Aging*, Vol. 1 *Clinical, morphologic, and neurochemical aspects in the aging central nervous system* (ed. H. Brody, D. Harman, and J. M. Ordy), p. 11. Raven Press, New York.

SCHOCHET, S. S., LAMPERT, P. W., and MCCORMICK, W. F. (1973). *Acta Neuropathol.*, **23**, 342.

SCHWARTZ, P., KURUCZ, J., and KURUCZ, A. (1964). *J. Amer. Geriat. Soc.*, **12**, 908.

SELKOE, D. J., LIEM, R. K. H., YEN, S.-H., and SHELANSKI, M. L. (1979). *Brain Res.*, **163**, 235.

SHELANSKI, M. L., ALBERT, S., DEVRIES, G. H., and NORTON, W. T. (1971). *Science, N. Y.*, **174**, 1242.

SHELANSKI, M. L., GASKIN, F., and CANTOR, C. R. (1973). *Proc. Nat. Acad. Sci. (USA)*, **70**, 765.

——, LIEM, R. K. H., and YEN, S.-H. (1977). In *Mechanisms, regulation and special functions of protein synthesis in the brain* (ed. S. Roberts, A. Lajtha, and W. H. Gispen), p. 137. Elsevier–North-Holland Publishing Co., New York.

SUZUKI, K. and TERRY, R. D. (1967). *Acta Neuropathol.*, **8**, 276.

TERRY, R. D. (1963). *J. Neuropathol. exp, Neurol.*, **22**, 629.

—— and WEISS, M. (1963). *J. Neuropathol. exp. Neurol.*, **22**, 18.

—— and PEÑA, C. (1965). *J. Neuropathol. exp. Neurol.*, **24**, 200.

TILNEY, L. G. and PORTER, K. R. (1967). *J. Cell Biol.*, **34**, 327.

TOMLINSON, BERNARD E. (1977). Personal communication.

WEISENBERG, R. C., BORISY, G. G., and TAYLOR, E. W. (1968). *Biochem.*, **7**, 4466.

WILSON, L. and BRYAN, J. (1974). In *Advances in cell and molecular biology* (ed. E. J. DuPraw), Vol. 3, p. 22. Academic Press, New York.

WISNIEWSKI, H. M., SHELANSKI, M. L., and TERRY, R. D. (1968). *J. Cell Biol.*, **38**, 224.

——, TERRY, R. D., and HIRANO, A. (1970). *J. Neuropathol. exp. Neurol.*, **29**, 163.

——, GHETTI, B., and TERRY, R. D. (1973). *J. Neuropathol. exp. Neurol.*, **32**, 566.

——, NARANG, H. K., and TERRY, R. D. (1976). *J. Neurol. Sci.*, **27**, 173.

WUERKER, R. B. (1970). *Tissue Cell*, **2**, 1.

YEN, S. H., DAHL, D., SCHACHNER, M., and SHELANSKI, M. L. (1976). *Proc. Nat. Acad. Sci. (USA)*, **73**, 529.

Session 2

Aging of the nervous system—function

Introduction F. M. Sinex

The human species lives longer than any other vertebrate. As this long lifetime was evolved, the human organism may have had to cope more and more with limitations imposed by the inherent chemical instability of macromolecules, particularly those macromolecules which control gene expression, DNA and the proteins of chromatin. It is reasonable to ask if time-dependent change in such molecules plays a role in chronic diseases of old age such as senile dementia, degenerative joint disease, and diseases of the heart and blood vessels. Our laboratory at Boston University deals with the most costly and feared of these, the changes which occur in the brain with age and which may result in senility.

We have been evaluating five possible types of chemical change which might occur in the aging brain with the passage of time. These are changes in the structural or nonchromatin protein of the nucleus, change in covalent crosslinks between DNA and protein, and the possibility for glycosylation, racemization, and spontaneous loss of amide nitrogen. We have found that there is less freely melting DNA in the chromatin of older brains and we believe that this has resulted from alteration in the nature and placement of chromatin protein. However the largest differences observed seem to be in the interaction of chromatin with some of the non-chromatin protein of the nucleus and are found with relatively crude preparations, not highly purified chromatin.

We are attempting to apply what we have learned about the chromatin of aging rat brain to human brain. Our approach to senile dementia is not a conventional one. However, we believe that new findings in regard to the changes which occur in chromatin and other proteins with time warrant an exploration of dementia from this point of view.

Cerebral blood flow in normal aging and senility
Vladimir Hachinski and Walter D. Obrist

Methods of measuring cerebral blood flow

Cerebral blood flow (CBF) reflects brain function, thus CBF determinations offer a way of studying aging *in vivo*. Kety and Schmidt (1945, 1948a) introduced methods of determining global CBF in man in the 1940s. The method was based on the Fick principle, whereby the rate at which the cerebral venous content of an inert gas approaches the arterial blood content depends upon the volume of blood flowing through the brain. The subject inhaled small amounts of nitrous oxide and blood specimens for analysis were obtained from a peripheral artery and the internal jugular bulb. The CBF was expressed as millilitres of blood per 100 g of brain per minute and represented the total blood flow through the entire brain. It was only in the 1960s that reliable methods of measuring regional cerebral blood flow were developed. The most widely used method is by the introduction of a small amount of krypton 85 or xenon 133 dissolved in saline into the internal carotid artery (Lassen and Ingvar 1967, 1972). Xenon is chemically inert and diffuses very readily throughout the brain. Thus the clearance rate of the isotope is proportional to the CBF in any given area of the brain. The gamma ray decay curves of the isotope are monitored extracranially by a bank of probes varying in number from 8 to 254 (Paulson, Cronqvist, Risberg, and Jeppesen 1969; Sveinsdottir and Lassen 1975). Estimates of fast- and slow-flow components can also be made. Recently a method has been described for estimating the clearance rate and fractional blood flow of the fast compartment of the brain from the first ten minutes of xenon 133 clearance curves following a one-minute inhalation (Obrist, Thompson, Wang, and Wilkinson 1975). Up to 32 regional CBF values can be obtained by this method. Although less accurate than the carotid xenon method, it is repeatable, it measures CBF in both hemispheres simultaneously, and it monitors vertebral-basilar blood flow, which cannot be sampled with the intracarotid technique.

Changes in cerebral blood flow with normal aging

Dastur, Lane, Hansen, Kety, Butler, and Sokoloff (1963) in an extensive prospective study selected a number of healthy elderly subjects without any detectable medical, psychiatric, or neurological disease. In this group the CBF and $CMRO_2$ (cerebral metabolic rate of oxygen) were found to be the same as that of young healthy control subjects studied in the same way. A second group of elderly patients with minimal physical abnormalities but believed to be cerebrally intact, had significantly lowered CBF and $CMRO_2$ values.

Wang, Obrist, and Busse (1970) also studied two groups of healthy aged community volunteers. The mean CBF of the elderly subjects (52 ml/100 g/min) was significantly lower than that of healthy young adults (75 ml/100 g/min) studied by the same method. However, there was considerable overlap between the CBF values of the two groups: 33 to 72 ml/100 g/min in the elderly subjects and 57 to 92 ml/100 g/min for the young adults.

Although there may be a gradual slow decrease of CBF with age, the extent of this fall probably depends more on pathological changes than on age *per se*.

Cerebral blood flow in 'senility'

Esquirol's (1845) classification of mental diseases proposed a category of *'démence sénile'* which encompassed, but was not limited to, the intellectual deterioration of old age. A few years later, Griesinger (1867) attributed 'apathetic dementia' to diseases of the arteries, the so-called 'arteritis chronica' consisting of fatty degeneration, atheroma, and calcareous deposits:

This degeneration causes disorders of the circulation of the most various kinds—local anaemia with increasing diminution of the calibre of the arteries, encephalitic inflammation, and as it appears, various changes of nutrition of the cerebral substance, not yet known in detail.

The founder of the Vienna school of neuropathology, Carl Rokitansky (1850), in his four volume *Manual of pathological anatomy* lent further support to the idea that anaemia of the brain was a leading cause of mental deterioration. He stated that: 'A very remarkable instance of anaemia is that which arises from the contraction or obliteration of the vessels, which convey blood to the brain.' He thought that this resulted in the undernourishment and atrophy of the cerebrum. Despite the long history (Hachinski 1976) and persistent popularity of this view, atherosclerosis does not cause the insidious, slowly progressive dementia of old age ('senile' dementia). Most cases show Alzheimer-like degeneration of the brain at necropsy. There is no relationship between these parenchymal degenerative changes and arterial disease.

Arteriosclerotic narrowing of blood vessels, *per se*, is not sufficient to cause dementia. Arteriosclerosis is related to dementia, but in a more intricate fashion, namely in its role in the pathogenesis of brain infarcts. Hence the term 'multi-infarct dementia' (Hachinski, Lassen, and Marshall 1974) has been suggested when vascular disease is the cause of the mental decline. Recent pathological studies on the brains of elderly people provide a basis for classifying the aetiology of dementia, which has direct relevance for the interpretation of CBF findings. Corsellis has shown that the brains of demented old people can be distinguished from those with functional psychiatric disorders. Tomlinson, Blessed, and Roth (1970) distinguish two types of dementia in old age: (1) primary parenchymal degeneration, designated 'senile'; and (2) multiple cerebral infarction, designated 'arteriosclerotic'. Whereas the former is associated with typical Alzheimer changes (senile plaques and neurofibrillary tangles), the latter consists of multiple areas of cerebral softening secondary to ischaemic vascular disease. Fifty-eight per cent of the 50 elderly patients showed extensive senile plaque formation and/or neurofibrillary tangles. In contrast, only 32 per cent showed widespread cerebral softening with a volume exceeding 50 millilitres; a third of these patients also had severe Alzheimer changes. Less marked instances of one or both types of pathology were found in an additional 12 per cent of the cases.

Roth (1971) in a continuation of the same study, obtained significant correlations between the extent of pathological changes and a quantitative 'dementia score'. The severity of the dementia gave a product–moment correlation of 0.77

with the number of senile plaques per low-powered field, and 0.69 with the total amount (in ml) of cerebral softening. Differentiation of the two types of pathology was possible on purely clinical grounds, using the absence or presence of cerebrovascular disease as the main criterion. The distinction between the two types of dementia has been emphasized by Fisher (1968) and, more recently, by Hachinski, Lassen, and Marshall (1974). More sophisticated neuropsychological methods for differentiating the two types of dementia have been described by Perez, Rivera, Meyer, Gay, Taylor, and Mathew (1975).

O'Brien and Mallett (1970) were the first to suggest that CBF studies might distinguish the two types of dementia. Using the xenon 133 inhalation technique, they found a significantly greater reduction in CBF among demented patients with clinical evidence of cerebrovascular disease than in patients with dementia of non-vascular origin; in fact, the latter tended to have normal cerebral blood flows. They interpreted the decreased cerebral blood flow in vascular cases as a sign of global cerebral ischaemia. In view of the pathological evidence, however, it is more likely that the decreased CBF is due to a mosaic of underperfused and normally irrigated cerebral tissue rather than a global decrease in CBF.

The finding of the relatively greater decrease in CBF in early vascular dementia has been confirmed by using the xenon 133 intracaratoid injection technique and a compartmental analysis that distinguishes between grey and white matter (Hachinski, Iliff, Zilhka, Du Boulay, McAllister, Marshall, Russell, and Symon 1975). A group of patients with early mental impairment were studied. Dementia was classified clinically as multi-infarct or primary degenerative on the basis of the presence or absence of cerebral vascular disease as judged by an 'ischaemic score'. Both types of dementia showed a reduction in the relative size of the grey matter compartment. However, a significant blood flow reduction was obtained only in the multi-infarct group. This suggested that blood flow was adequate to meet the brain's lesser metabolic needs in the primary degenerative group, but inadequate for those with multi-infarct dementia. Of special interest is the correlation between the degree of dementia and CBF in the multi-infarct group, a relationship that was absent in patients of the primary degenerative type.

While confirming a generalized blood flow reduction in senile dementia and its correlation with the degree of mental impairment, Obrist, Chivian, Cronqvist, and Ingvar (1970) obtained significantly greater CBF decreases in the temporal and prefrontal areas where EEG abnormalities were maximal. This fronto-temporal focal decrease has also been observed by Ingvar and Gustafson (1970) and by Simard (Simard, Olesen, Paulson, Lassen, and Skinhøj 1971). It is consistent with the greater atrophy found in the temporal lobes of such patients (Tomlinson, Blessed, and Roth 1970).

Vascular reactivity to changes in arterial carbon dioxide tension ($PaCO_2$) is another potential means of distinguishing the two types of dementia. The normal response to elevation of $PaCO_2$ by the inhalation of 5–7 per cent CO_2 is a 30–50 per cent increase in CBF due to cerebral vasodilatation. Contrariwise, hyperventilation, which reduces $PaCO_2$, results in a corresponding decrease in

CBF due to cerebral vasoconstriction. In 1953, Schieve and Wilson reported differences in the CBF response to inhaled CO_2 between patients with clear-cut strokes and those with dementia who had no evidence of vascular disease. Whereas the latter group revealed a normal CBF increase, the patients with stroke had significantly smaller responses. Regretfully, the problem of CO_2 reactivity in dementia has received little further attention, particularly as it relates to differential diagnosis.

Although Simard and co-workers (1971) claim normal CO_2 reactivity in vascular dementia, their evidence is based on a single case subjected to hyperventilation. Dekoninck, Collard, and Jacquy (1975) obtained normal CBF responses to both hyperventilation and CO_2 inhalation among relatively healthy old people, and a reduction in reactivity among patients with cerebrovascular disease. A highly variable response was found in patients with dementia, but unfortunately the patients were not classified according to the presumed aetiology. Furthermore, they stated that 'during hypercarbia the PCO_2 was increased by 25 per cent; during hypocarbia the PCO_2 was decreased by 20 per cent.' It is not clear how or whether such precise changes in PCO_2 were achieved for individual patients.

Hachinski and colleagues (1975) carried out systematic observations on hyperventilation in dementia, and found a trend (not statistically significant) for smaller CBF decreases in patients of the multi-infarct type than in those with primary neuronal degeneration. CO_2 inhalation was not attempted. From this, it would appear that the vasoconstrictor response to hyperventilation does not clearly differentiate the two types of dementia. Whether there is a difference in the vasodilator response to CO_2 inhalation remains to be tested.

Still another potential means of studying dementia is the haemodynamic response to psychological stimuli. According to Ingvar, Risberg, and Schwartz (1975), CBF is normally augmented in the frontal and parietal areas during activation by mental tests. Comparable increases in blood flow were not obtained however, in demented patients with either Alzheimer's disease or normal pressure hydrocephalus. The functional response of regional CBF to psychological 'activation' could conceivably further our understanding of dementia.

Correlations with cerebral metabolism and electroencephalography

Measurements of cerebral metabolism and the cerebral electrical activity offer further *in vivo* information into the process of aging and dementia.

Differences in CBF between the two types of dementia are paralleled by variations in cerebral metabolic pattern. In a mixed series of 115 patients diagnosed as primary degenerative and multi-infarct dementia, Hoyer and Weinhardt (1976) observed a bimodal distribution of cerebral glucose uptake, comparable to the one obtained for blood flow. Because the cerebral metabolic rate for oxygen was more uniformly depressed, the glucose-to-oxygen ratio (G/O) paralleled differences in glucose uptake; i.e., a bimodal distribution was obtained.

When the patients were divided into two groups on the basis of their G/O ratio, it was found that those with a high G/O had relatively lower CBFs. The authors interpreted this as evidence for two distinct cerebral metabolic patterns in elderly demented patients. Since an elevated G/O ratio indicates a shift to anaerobic metabolism which is characteristic of cerebral ischaemia, it was speculated that the high G/O group represented cases of multi-infarct dementia. The possibility of differentiating the two pathological types of dementia on the basis of *in vivo* cerebral metabolic patterns clearly warrants further study.

The electroencephalogram (EEG) like cerebral blood flow, undergoes changes associated with age, the magnitude of change being primarily a function of health status. The EEG of healthy elderly subjects deviates minimally from that of young adults. On the other hand, elderly subjects with various physical and mental disorders, particularly those with diseases of the cardiovascular system and/or signs of organic dementia, undergo more pronounced alterations of their EEG. There is slowing of the dominate alpha rhythm from 10 to 9 or 8 Hz, and an increase in the prevalence of slower theta (4–7 Hz) and delta (1–3 Hz) waves. These findings correlate well with the severity of intellectual deterioration. Although the slowing is usually diffuse, the changes are usually maximal in the temporal lobe (Obrist 1972, 1975).

Summary

There is a minimal decline of CBF in entirely healthy elderly individuals. The decreases that can be observed in an unselected aging population are largely due to the systemic and cerebral disease.

Although Alzheimer-like degeneration of the brain, not arteriosclerosis, is the commonest cause of 'senility', a significant percentage of patients with intellectual impairment have treatable medical conditions (Marsden and Harrison 1972; Freeman 1976; Harrison and Marsden 1977). The treatment of hypertension and cardiac disorders (*Lancet* 1977), for example, could decrease the incidence of multi-infarct dementia.

Computerized tomography gives accurate anatomic details of the brain. The development of non-invasive methods of measuring CBF offers the potential of supplementing anatomic information with serial *in vivo* physiological measurements thus giving serial anatomo-functional maps of the brain in normal aging and in the various pathological processes producing 'senility'. As Cicero claimed: 'It is our duty to resist old age, to compensate for its defects by a watchful care, to fight against it as we would fight against disease', for 'senility' is not normal aging but often recognizable and sometimes treatable disease.

References

CORSELLIS, J. A. N. (1962). *Mental illness and the ageing brain*. Oxford University Press, London.

DASTUR, D. K., LANE, M. M., HANSEN, D. B., KETY, S. S., BUTLER, R. N., and SOKO-LOFF, L. (1963). In *Human aging: a biological and behavioural study*, p. 57. US. Government Printing Office.

DEKONINCK, W. J., COLLARD, M., and JACQUY, J. (1975). *Stroke*, **6**, 673.

ESQUIROL, J. E. D. (1845). In *Traite de maladies mentales*. (Engl. trans. by E. K. Hunt).

FISHER, C. M. (1968). In *Cerebral vascular diseases: sixth conference* (ed. J. F. Toole, R. G. Siekert, and J. P. Whisnant), p. 232. New York.

FREEMON, F. R. (1976). *Arch. Neurol.*, **33**, 658.

GRIESINGER, W. (1867). In *Mental pathology and therapeutics* (translated from the second German edition by L. C. Robertson and J. Rutherford), No. 33. New Sydenham Society Publication, London.

HACHINSKI, V. C. (1976). Cerebral arteriosclerosis and dementia. Evolution of a misconception. In *Actes, XXV Congres International, Histoire de la Medicine* (ed. de la Broquerie Fortier), Vol. 2, pp. 755–60.

——, LASSEN, N. A. and MARSHALL, J. (1974). *Lancet*, **2**, 207.

——, ILIFF, L. D., ZILHKA, E., DuBOULAY, G. H., McALLISTER, V. L., MARSHALL, J., RUSSELL, R. W. R., and SYMON, L. (1975). *Arch. Neurol.*, **20**, 315.

HARRISON, M. J. G. and MARSDEN, C. D. (1977). *Arch. Neurol.*, **34**, 199.

HOYER, S. and WEINHARDT, F. (1976). In *Cerebral vascular disease: Seventh International Conference* (ed. J. S. Meyer, J. Lechner, and M. Reivich), p. 84. Stuttgart.

INGVAR, D. H. and GUSTAFSON, L. (1970). *Acta Neurol. Scand.*, **43**, 42.

——, RISBERG, J., and SCHWARTZ, M. S. (1975). *Neurol.*, **25**, 964.

KETY, S. S. and SCHMIDT, C. F. (1945). *Amer. J. Physiol.*, **143**, 53.

—— and —— (1948a). *J. clin. Invest.*, **27**, 476.

The Lancet (1977). Editorial. *Lancet*, **1**, 27.

LASSEN, N. A. and INGVAR, D. H. (1961). *Experientia*, **17**, 42.

—— and —— (1972). In *Progress in nuclear medicine*, Vol. 1, p. 376. Karger, Basel, Switzerland.

LAVY, S., MELAMED, E., BENTIN, S., COOPER, G., and RINOT, Y. (1978). Bihemispheric decreases of regional cerebral blood flow in dementia: correlation with age matched normal controls. *Ann. Neurol.*, **4**, 445.

MARSDEN, C. D. and HARRISON, M. J. G. (1972). *Br. med. J.*, **2**, 249.

MELAMED, E., LAVY, S., SIEW, F., BENTIN, S., and COOPER, G. (1978). Correlation between regional cerebral blood flow and brain atrophy in dementia. *J. Neurol. Neurosurg. Psychiat.*, **41**, 894.

O'BRIEN, M. D. and MALLETT, B. L. (1970). *J. Neurol. Neurosurg. Psychiat.*, **33**, 497.

OBRIST, W. D. (1972). In *Aging and the brain* (ed. C. M. Gaitz), p. 117. Plenum Press, New York.

—— (1975). In *Behavior and brain electrical activity* (ed. N. Burch and H. L. Altshuler), p. 421. Plenum Press, New York.

—— (1978). Noninvasive studies of cerebral blood flow in aging and dementia. In *Alzheimer's disease: senile dementia and related disorders* (ed. R. Katzman, R. D. Terry, and K. L. Bick), p. 213. Longman, New York.

——, CHIVIAN, E., CRONQVIST, S., and INGVAR, D. H. (1970). *Neurology*, **20**, 315.

——, THOMPSON, H. D. Jr., WANG, H. S., and WILKINSON, W. E. (1975). *Stroke*, **6**, 245.

PAULSON, O. B., CRONQVIST, S., RISBERG, J., and JEPPESEN, F. I. (1969). *J. nucl. med.*, **10**, 164.

PEREZ, F. I., RIVERA, V. M., MEYER, J. S., GAY, J. R. A., TAYLOR, R. L., and MATHEW, N. T. (1975). *J. Neurol. Neurosurg. Psychiat.*, **38**, 533.

ROKITANSKY, C. (1850). *A manual of pathological anatomy*, Vol. III. The Sydenham Society, London.
ROTH, M. (1971). In *Recent developments in psychogeriatrics* (ed. D. W. K. Kay and A. Walk), p. 1. Ashford, U.K.
SCHIEVE, J. F. and WILSON, W. P. (1953). *Amer. J. Med.*, **15**, 171.
SIMARD, D., OLESEN, J., PAULSON, O. B., LASSEN, N.A., and SKINHØJ, E. (1971). *Brain*, **94**, 273.
SVEINSDOTTIR, E., LARSEN, B., ROMMER, P., and LASSEN, N. A. (1977). In *Cerebral blood flow and metabolism. J. Nucl. Med.*, **18**, 168–74.
TOMLINSON, B. E., BLESSED, G., and ROTH, M. J. (1970). *Neurol. Sci.*, **11**, 205.
WANG, H. S., OBRIST, W. D., and BUSSE, E. W. (1970). *Amer. J. Psychiat.*, **126**, 1205.

Neurotransmitters and aging in the human brain J. M. Ordy

Introduction

Role of the brain in aging

Aging is one of the most universal and inevitable social and scientific challenges confronting man. Although aging may be generalized throughout the body, increasing attention has been directed toward the role of the brain and endocrine organs as 'pacemakers' of aging. As major interrelated control systems of the body, the brain plays a unique role in adaptation to the environment through reflexes, conditioning, and higher forms of learning, based on electrical and chemical codes. Through the release of hormones, the endocrine organs play a key role in growth, reproduction, metabolism, homeostasis, and adaptation (Ordy and Kaack 1976). Significant correlations have been established among life span, brain size, and metabolism among species (Cutler 1976). It has been proposed that, by making organisms more independent of their environment (Ordy and Kaack 1976), the brain and endocrines have played a critical role in the evolution of life in phylogeny by maintaining and extending the life span (Sacher 1975).

Role of neurotransmitters as chemical regulators of physiology and behaviour

It is generally recognized that the sensory, learning, memory, drive, and motor capacities of man reach a peak in early adulthood, remain relatively constant throughout maturity, and then appear to decline during senescence (Botwinick 1973). Although tentative, age-dependent impairments in neural and endocrine control mechanisms have been proposed as the basic physiological sources of age-dependent changes not only in behaviour but in the total animal (Shock 1974; Ordy and Brizzee 1975; Ordy and Kaack 1976). Compelling evidence for this hypothesis includes: (1) age decrements in speed and accuracy of behaviour increase as performance complexity increases (Birren and Schaie 1976); and (2) age decrements in physiological functions which involve the co-ordinated activity of several organ systems are greater than functions that are relatable to a single organ (Schock 1974). Neurotransmitters and hormones have widespread effects as chemical regulators of co-ordinated physiological activity throughout the body. Although exact electrical and chemical codes remain to be clarified, particularly in the central nervous system (CNS), neurotransmitters and hormones have now been assigned an important role in sensory processes, learning, memory, motivation, and motor co-ordination during development, maturity, and aging (Ordy and Kaack 1975; Iversen and Iversen 1975). Age-dependent changes in the brain also include an increasing incidence of mental impairments and brain disorders during senescence. Specific changes in brain biogenic amines have been identified in some psychopathology and certain neurological disorders (Maas and Garver 1975; Moskowitz and Wurtman 1975; McGeer and McGeer 1976).

Basic elements of nervous circuits and neurotransmitters
Anatomically, the mammalian nervous system has been subdivided into the central nervous system (CNS), which includes the brain and the spinal cord, the peripheral nervous system (PNS) which includes 12 pairs of cranial nerves and 31 pairs of spinal nerves, and the autonomic nervous system (ANS) which comprises the sympathetic and parasympathetic divisions for the regulation of the internal environment. At the cellular level, the basic 'wiring diagram' of the mammalian nervous system is composed of receptor or afferent neurons (Golgi I) whose cell bodies are located outside the CNS, interneurons (Golgi Type II), whose cell bodies and short axons are located within the CNS, and motor neurons (Golgi I) with long axons, extending over 2 feet in man, whose cell bodies are located within the CNS. Since there is 'contiguity and not continuity' in sensory inter-motor-neuron networks, nerve impulses with information must be transferred across a *synapse*. This chemical information transfer by neurotransmitters across the synapse has great significance since it enormously increases the integrative capacity of the nervous system to respond to external and internal stimuli. The fundamental or basic 'wiring diagram' of the CNS, PNS, and ANS of the mammalian nervous system (including the role of the synapse) is illustrated in Fig. 1.

'Language' of neurons—excitation, conduction, transmission
According to current views in neurophysiology of 'higher neural activity', regardless of the reflex and behavioural complexity, all integrative responses are ultimately a result of the interactions of excitation and inhibition among spinal, subcortical, and cortical networks of the nervous system. This basic form of coding and communication extends from the receptor neurons to interneurons and to the effectors. Basically, it consists of neuronal excitation, conduction, and the liberation of synaptic neurotransmitters that have either excitatory or inhibitory influences on postsynaptic membranes of other neurons or effectors. Although the 'language' of neuronal excitation and conduction is primarily electrochemical, neurotransmission across synaptic junctions proceeds chemically in a dynamically polarized manner from axonal terminals across synaptic

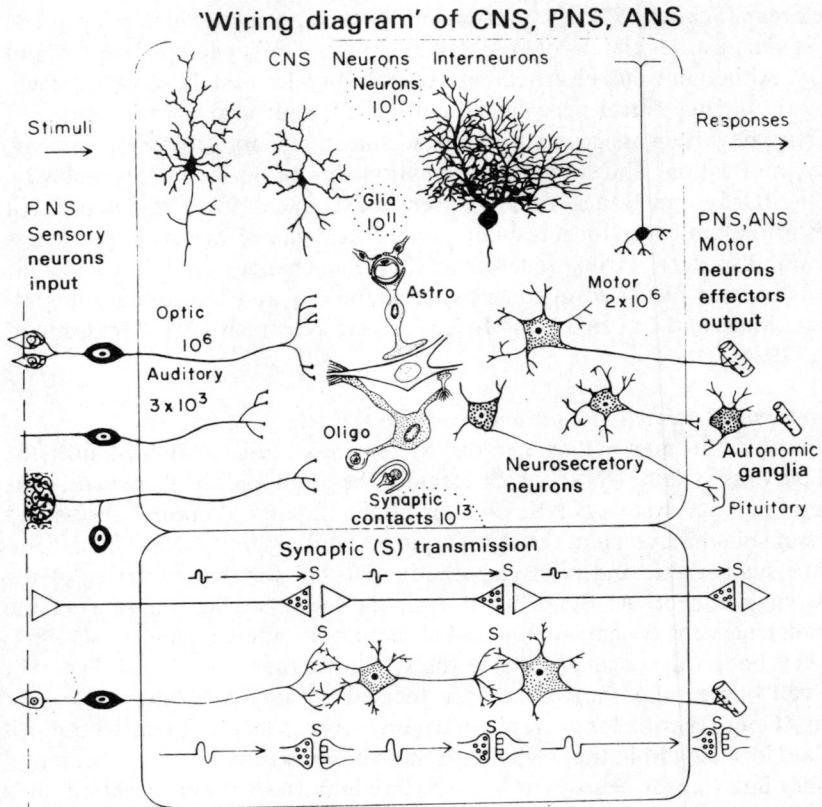

FIG. 1. Basic 'wiring diagram' of mammalian CNS, PNS, ANS nervous system, including role of synapse.

junctions to dendrites, cell bodies, axons, or effectors. Since transmission across the synapse is chemical, a great deal of recent research has included neurotransmitters and associated enzymes at the synapse as possible cellular sites of 'plasticity' in the nervous system. Through its structural and functional asymmetry, the synapse provides the postsynaptic excitation and inhibition for changing the firing rates and coding of other neurons. These changes in rate can serve as basic neural coding of information in the nervous system. The fundamental features of excitation, conduction, and neurotransmission in the neuron are illustrated schematically in Fig. 2.

Neurotransmitters and associated enzymes in CNS

A number of chemical substances, generally referred to as neurotransmitters or biogenic amines, have been proposed as physiological regulators among

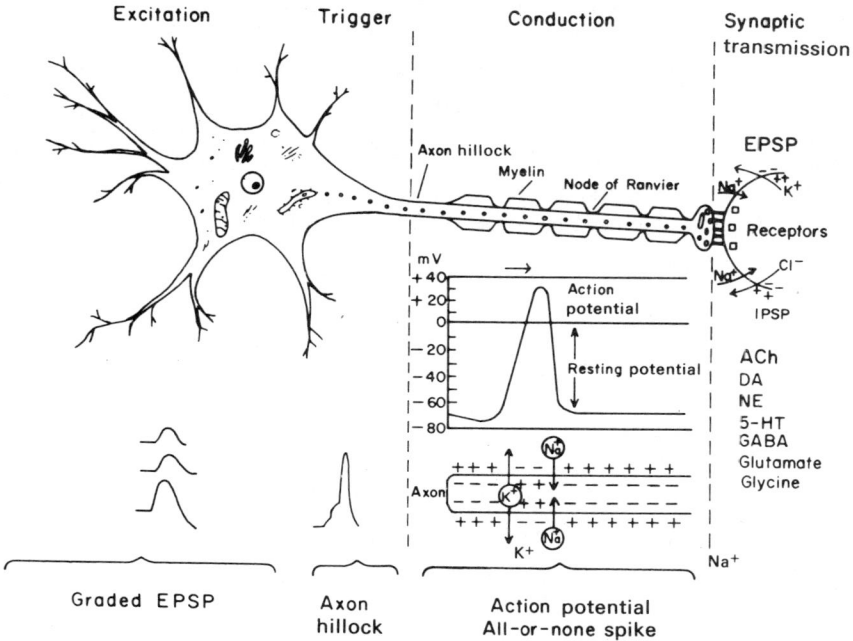

Fig. 2. Fundamental features or 'language' of excitation, conduction, and transmission of neuron.

neurons and between the nervous system and effectors. A major effort in neuro-chemistry has been devoted to the chemistry of synaptic transmission. The history and current knowledge of the biochemical events involved in synaptic transmission have been reviewed extensively in articles, books, and several volumes of the *Handbook of neurochemistry* (Lajtha 1969–72).

Essentially, arrival of an action potential at its presynaptic terminal results in release of a chemical transmitter, its diffusion across the synaptic cleft, and its interaction with receptors in the postsynaptic cell membrane. Transmitter release and receptor interactions involve ionic permeability changes in membranes. The ions, their changes and direction of movement, determine whether a transmitter is excitatory or inhibitory. Mechanisms of inactivation or re-uptake remove the transmitters from synaptic sites of action. Earlier criteria for identification of acetylcholine (ACh), and norepinephrine (NE) (as excitatory and inhibitory transmitters respectively) in isolated ganglia of the ANS, have been extended to the identification of 'putative' transmitters in the CNS. These criteria include: (1) enzymes in presynaptic terminals for synthesis; (2) storage granules; (3) release mechanisms in terminals; (4) synaptic mimicry or post-synaptic receptor response to presynaptic iontophoretic application; (5) enzymes for inactivation; or (6) mechanisms of presynaptic re-uptake. Based on studies with some mammalian species and invertebrates, the following substances and their associated enzymes of synthesis and degradation have been tentatively identified as putative transmitters in the mammalian CNS: (1) acetylcholine (ACh), cholinacetyltransferase (ChAc), and acetylcholin esterase (AChE); (2) the catecholamines norepinephrine (NE) and dopamine (DA) with the enzymes tyrosine hydroxylase (TH), DOPA decarboxylase (DDC), and monoamine oxidase (MAO); (3) serotonin (5-HT) with catechol-*o*-methyl-transferase (COMT); and (4) the amino acids—gamma amino butyric acid (GABA), glutamic acid, and glycine. Fig. 3 illustrates the putative neurotransmitters and

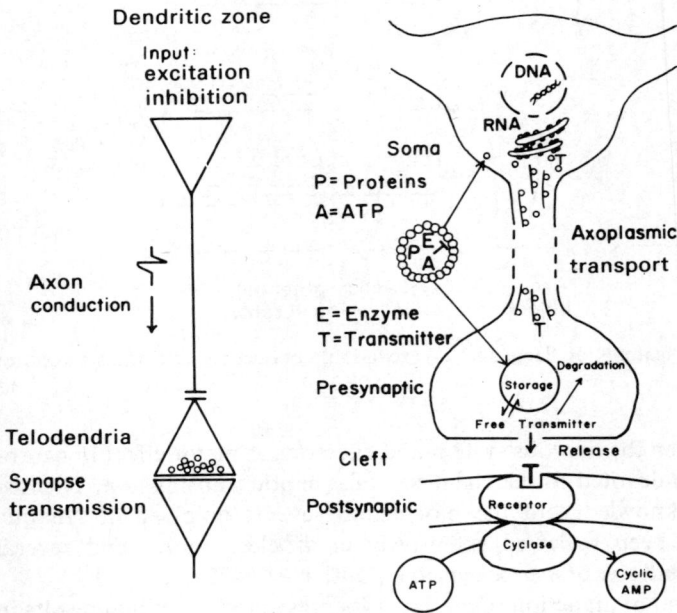

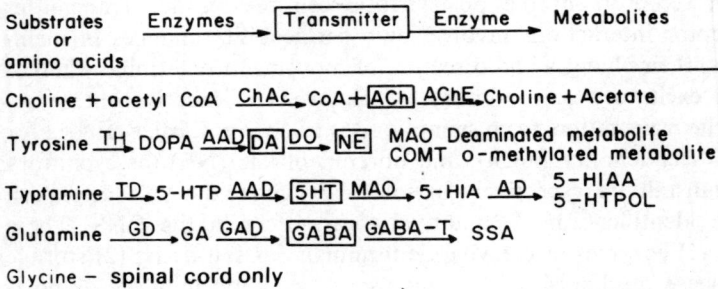

Fig. 3. Neurotransmitters and associated enzymes as physiological regulators in nervous system. Neurotransmitters (T) are synthesized in endoplasmic reticulum and transported via neurotubules to synaptosomes.

associated enzymes in their roles as physiological regulators in the mammalian nervous system.

Organization of chemical neurotransmitter pathways in the brain

Historically, concepts of chemical transmission were first developed in the ANS of the PNS. The identification, based on specific criteria for chemical neurotransmitters in the CNS, represents a relatively recent development. The identification and mapping of chemical neurotransmitter 'pathways' is based on the more recent developments of histochemical fluorescent techniques pioneered by Scandinavian workers (Dahlstrom and Fuxe 1964). With the histochemical fluorescent techniques, neurons and axonal fibres with their terminals containing specific chemical transmitters stored in vesicles, can be visualized and the neuroanatomical pathways of neurons with identified transmitters can be plotted throughout the brain. The histochemical fluorescent techniques have been used successfully for staining NE, DA, and 5-HT pathways in the brain. Since there is still no direct staining technique for ACh, mapping its distribution is based indirectly on staining the hydrolyzing enzyme AChE. The localization of GABA pathways is based on uptake of radioactively-labelled GABA and visualization of activity in autoradiograms. Thus far, chemical pathways for GABA and glycine remain to be established (Iversen and Iversen 1975).

With the development of histochemical fluorescent techniques, considerable progress has been made in mapping chemical pathways in the brain based on selective staining of neurons, axons, and their terminals containing particular neurotransmitters. Almost all studies of chemical neurotransmitter pathways in the brain have been based predominantly on the rat (Ungerstedt 1971; Livett 1973). However, some studies have been reported using cats (Jouvet 1972), and some non-human primates and man (Friede 1966; Olson, Boreus, and Seigen 1973). Although current identification of chemical neurotransmitter pathways in the brain is based primarily on rodents, the cat, and a few studies with non-human primates and man, Fig. 4 illustrates the presumptive distribution of DA-, NE-, 5-HT-, and AChE-containing neuron pathways in the primate brain.

Role of neurotransmitters and associated enzymes in physiology and behaviour

Remarkable progress has been made recently in neurochemical correlates involved in the regulation of physiology and behaviour. Although the historical antecedents of neurochemistry include: (a) the chemical composition; and (b) metabolism in the brain, a major effort has been devoted to (c) the chemistry of synaptic transmission, for reasons which include the following:

(1) Through its structural and functional asymmetry, neurotransmitters and their associated enzymes at the synapse provide the possible site of 'plasticity' or modifiability in the nervous system.

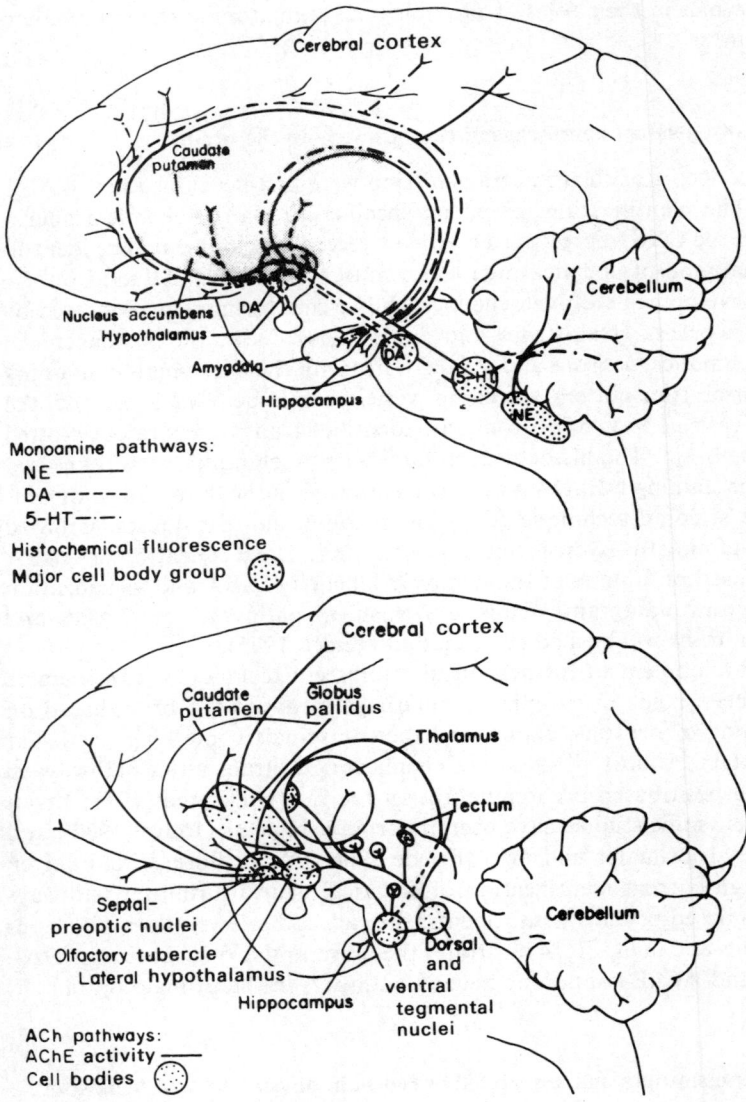

FIG. 4. Organization and distribution of chemical neurotransmitter pathways for norepinephrine (NE), dopamine (DA), and serotonin (5-HT) based on histochemical fluorescence, including location of cell body groups (top). Presumptive acetyl choline (ACh) distribution, based on AChE, with cell bodies.

(2) The reliance on chemical neurotransmitters by the brain is one important way in which the biochemistry and physiology of the brain differs from all other organs.

(3) In the field of neuropharmacology, dramatic progress has been made in the manipulation of neurotransmitters and their enzymes in relation to changes in physiology and behaviour.

On the basis of lesions or pathologies in specific neurochemical pathways, and the use of drugs, significant correlations have been made between behavioural changes and alterations in neurotransmitters. Considerable progress has been made in relating changes of DA in the basal ganglia to motor activity; changes in hypothalamic NE to arousal, feeding, drinking; changes in 5-HT in the tegmental nuclei and raphe to sleep–wake cycles; and changes in ACh in the limbic system, ascending reticular, thalamic centres, and cerebral cortex to excitation of EEG and behavioural arousal (Iversen and Iversen 1975). It seems relevant to note that almost all of these studies on the role of neurotransmitters in physiology and behaviour have been conducted on organisms during development and maturity rather than during aging. Although remarkable interdisciplinary progress has been made in neurobiology on brain development, interdisciplinary and neurochemical studies on the human brain during aging are still quite scarce and fragmentary.

Major chronological life span changes in the human brain as temporal points of reference for neurochemistry

Major emphasis in this review of recent neurochemical studies has been on life span changes in neurotransmitters. However, a more comprehensive interpretation can be made if these age-dependent changes in neurotransmitters are also related to changes in behaviour, electrical activity of the brain, morphology, neuropathology, and other neurochemical changes.

(a) *Behaviour.* According to behavioural studies, sensory, learning, memory, drive, and motor capacities of man reach a peak in early adulthood, remain relatively constant throughout maturity, and appear to decline in senescence (Botwinick 1973; Ordy and Brizzee 1975; Birren and Schaie 1976).

(b) *Electrophysiology.* In neurophysiological studies of the human brain during aging, significant life span changes have been reported in the electrical activity of the human brain as reflected in the cerebral evoked response. Visual, auditory, and somatosensory evoked potentials have been recorded from normal human subjects ranging in age from 1–81 years. Significant changes occur in latency, amplitude, and wave components during development, maturity, and aging (Beck, Dustman, and Schenkenberg 1975). These cerebral-evoked response changes particularly during development and aging, coincide with changes in sensory thresholds of information processing in the visual, auditory, and somatosensory systems. Also, it has been reported that conduction velocity of axons in the PNS decreases significantly in old age.

(c) *Morphology*. Morphologically, it is generally recognized that the human brain undergoes a period of rapid growth, remains relatively stable throughout maturity, and appears to decline during sensecence. At birth the human brain weighs approximately 350 g and represents 30 per cent of the 1400-g asymptotic adult weight. According to some studies, human brain weight of males decreases from 1400 g by 5 per cent at the age of 70 to 10 per cent by age 80 and by 20 per cent at age 90 and above. By age 90 the human brain weight has been reported to be reduced to 1100 g, the same weight as that of a 3-year-old child (Minckler and Boyd 1968). Life span changes in human brain weight in relation to reproduction are illustrated in Fig. 5. Other major morphological changes in the human brain during aging include: decrease in brain volume and increase in brain ventricles; widening and deepening of sulci with a decrease in width and mass of gyri; loss of neurons and increase in glia; decrease in dendrites and synapse or neuropil density; and progressive accumulation of intra- and extra-neuronal lipofuscin age pigment (Brizzee 1975a; Brizzee, Klara, and Johnson 1975; Brizzee, Kaack, and Klara 1975; Brody 1976; Feldman 1976; Sandoz and Meier-Ruge 1976).

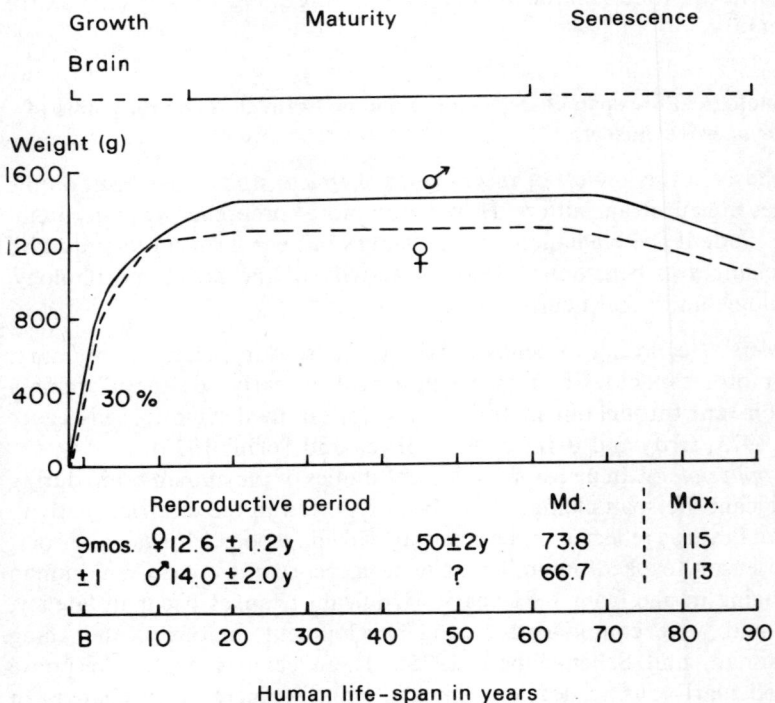

Fig. 5. Life span changes, including growth, maturity, and senescence in human male and female brain weight in relation to reproductive period.

(d) *Neuropathology.* Although the differentiation between normal aging and neuropathology remains to be clarified, increasing incidence of mental impairments and brain disorders have also been described in the human during senescence (Brizzee 1975b).

(e) *Other neurochemical changes in the human brain with age.* Although there is great recent interest in the neurochemistry of the human brain, the published neurochemical literature contains only a very limited number of studies and reviews dealing with life span changes in chemical composition, metabolism, and neurotransmitters in the brain during aging (Ordy and Kaack 1975; McGeer and McGeer 1975; Hermann 1975; Ordy, Kaack, and Brizzee 1975; Meier-Ruge, Reich Omeier, and Iwangoff 1976). Until very recently, the alleged rapid *postmortem* changes and the scarcity of normal human brain tissue specimens for chemical evaluations have been presumed to be major barriers rather than challenges for neurochemical studies.

Characteristic approaches to life span changes in neurotransmitters and associated enzymes

Although predominant efforts in the entire field of neurochemistry appear to be devoted to the chemistry of neurotransmitters in the mammalian brain, values for the human brain are scarce, fragmentary, and scattered throughout the literature (Ordy and Kaack 1975; Ordy, Kaack, and Brizzee 1975). Also it should be noted that values in the literature may not be based on chemical evaluations of carefully defined anatomical or chemical pathways in the brain. Regarding neurotransmitters and their enzymes during aging, five different types of approaches have been attempted to identify age-dependent changes of neurotransmitters in the brain.

(1) An initial approach has been to study some life span changes in neurotransmitters and associated enzymes in the adult human brain and to compare these values with those of early development (McGeer and McGeer 1975, 1976; Ordy, Kaack, and Brizzee 1975).

(2) A second approach has been to examine age-dependent changes in neurotransmitters from maturity to old age (Ordy and Kaack 1975; Ordy, Kaack, and Brizzee 1975).

(3) A third approach has been to examine age-dependent imbalances within a specific neurotransmitter–enzyme system during aging (Vernadakis 1973). Presumably, the asymptotic adult values represent an optimum balance between synthesizing enzyme activity, neurotransmitter concentration, and turnover, as well as catabolic enzyme activity within a particular neurotransmitter system.

(4) A fourth approach has been to examine imbalances among different neurotransmitter systems in the brain during aging. If interactions among different neurotransmitters are also optimal in the adult brain, adult interaction values can serve as points of reference that may be used for imbalances during aging and disease (McGeer and McGeer 1976).

(5) Since age-dependent changes in the brain include increasing mental impairments and brain disorders, a fifth approach has been to characterize neurotransmitter interactions in specific psychopathologies and neurological disorders.

Since they are scattered throughout the literature, Table 1 contains a summary of neurotransmitter concentrations as well as levels of synthesizing and catabolizing enzyme activity for some regions of the adult human brain. These values have been obtained from sources in the literature cited in this chapter.

Table 1 Neurotransmitters and associated enzymes in adult human brain†

Neurotransmitter	Associated enzymes	
	Synthesis	Degradation
Acetylcholine 0.5–0.6 μg/g (ACh) (human cerebral cortex)	Choline acetyltransferase 0.39 nmol/g/h (ChAc) (human cortex)	Acetylcholinesterase 0.29 nmol/g/h (AChE) (human cortex)
Dopamine 2.45–3.75 μg/g (DA) (human caudate)	DOPA decarboxylase 3.0 μmol/g/h (DOD) (human caudate)	Dopamine β hydroxylase 0.5 nmol/h/ml (D βH) (human CSF)
Norepinephrine 0.35–0.60 μg/g (NE) (human hypothalamus)	Dopamine β hydroxylase 0.5 nmol/h/ml (D βH) (human CSF)	Catechol-*o*-methyl transferase 0.5 μmol/g/h. (COMT) (human hypothalamus
Serotonin 0.2–0.23 μg/g (5-HT) (human hindbrain)	5-Hydroxytryptophan decarboxylase 3.0 nmol/g/h (AAD) (human hypothalamus)	Monoamine oxidase 8.4 μmol/g/h (MAO) (human hypothalamus)
γ-aminobutyric acid 3.1 μmol/h/g (GABA) (human caudate)	Glutamic acid decarboxylase 1640 nmol/g/h. (GAD) (human hypothalamus)	GABA-transaminase 9 nmol/kg/h (GABA-T) (monkey occipital cortex)
Glutamate 10 nmol/brain (mammalian brain)	Glutamate dehydrogenase 0.59 mg/ml (GD) (beef liver)	Glutamic acid decarboxylase 1640–56 nmol/g/h (GAD) (human hypothalamus)

† Neurotransmitter and associated enzyme values for the adult human brain were selected from regions with highest content or as the only values available. Values are based on published references.

Neurotransmitter, enzyme values in the adult human brain

(a) *ACh; ChAc—AChE.* A value of 0.5–0.6 μg/g tissue for ACh has been reported in the adult brain cerebral cortex. The synthesizing enzyme ChAc and the hydrolyzing enzyme AChE have a level of activity of 0.38 nmol/g/h and 0.29 nmol/g/h respectively in the adult human cortex.

(b) *DA; TH—DOD—DO.* DA has been measured in the adult human caudate at 2.45–3.75 g/g tissue. In that same region, DOD activity is 3.0 μmol/g/h. The degrading enzyme of DA which is also the synthesizing enzyme of NE is dopamine-β-oxidase (DO) and has an adult activity measured in the dog brain of 2.5–3.5 nmol/g/h.

(c) *NE; TH–DO--MAO–COMT.* The NE concentration is 0.35–0. μg/g tissue measured in the human hypothalamus. Its immediate synthesizing enzyme is

DO, as mentioned above, and has been measured in adult dog brain as 2.5–3.5 nM/g/h. However, the rate-limiting enzyme of the catecholamines DA and NE synthesis is TH, and it has a value of 33.6 nmol/h/100 g protein measured in the human caudate. The degrading enzymes of NE are MAO and COMT. Measured in the adult human hypothalamus, they have an activity of 8.4 μmol/g/h for MAO and 0.5 μmol/g/h for COMT.

(d) *5-HT; AAD–MAO*. The asymptotic adult value for 5-HT in the human hind-brain is 0.2–0.23 μg/g. Its synthesizing enzyme, 5-hydroxytryptophan decar-boxylase (amino-acid decarboxylase AAD), in the human hypothalamus has an activity level of 3.0 μmol/g/h. The catabolic enzyme, MAO, in the adult human hypothalamus has an activity level of 8.4 μmol/g/h.

(e) *GABA; GAD–GABA-T*. GABA has a value of 2–4 nM/g tissue as measured in the mammalian cortex. The synthesizing enzyme, GAD, measured in the human hypothalamus has a value of 1640 nmol/g/h and the degrading enzyme, GABA-transaminase (GABA-T) has a value of 9 nmol/kg/h as measured in the monkey occipital cortex.

(f) *Glutamate; GD–GAD*. Glutamate in the mammalian brain has a value of 10 nmol/brain. The synthesizing enzyme, GD, in beef liver has a value of 0.59 mg/ml and the degrading enzyme GAD has a value of 1640–56 nmol/g/h as measured in the human hypothalamus.

(g) *Glycine*. As in the case of GABA, glycine has been reported to be an im-portant inhibitory transmitter in the mammalian central nervous system. How-ever, glycine has been localized only in inhibitory interneurons in the spinal cord which are located in the medial gray matter and project to motor neurons in the ventral horn.

(h) *Histamine and aspartic acid*. According to recent studies, both of these amino acids have been implicated as neurotransmitters in the mammalian nervous system. However, at present, their status is doubtful and remains to be clarified. As a note of caution concerning neurotransmitter and enzyme values cited for the adult human brain in this review, it should be recognized that these values: (a) are tentative; (b) are not necessarily based on carefully-defined anatomical regions; and finally (c) include values from lower species which may not coincide with those in man.

Major life span trends in neurotransmitters and associated enzyme values
The life span changes in cholinergetic and monoaminergic transmitters and their enzymes that have been reported, are based on brain tissue samples obtained from accident victims ranging in age from 1–80 years, with no apparent history of neuropathology or other diseases. Thus far, life span changes in ACh for man have not been reported. Only two studies have reported on ACh values in the adult human brain. Post-maturity declines in ChAc and AChE activity have been reported for the human cerebral cortex. Small but statistically significant post-maturity declines in DA, NE, and 5-HT concentrations have also been reported for the caudate nucleus and for the hindbrain. Age-dependent declines in the activities of DOD, TH, and GAD in the substantia nigra, caudate nucleus,

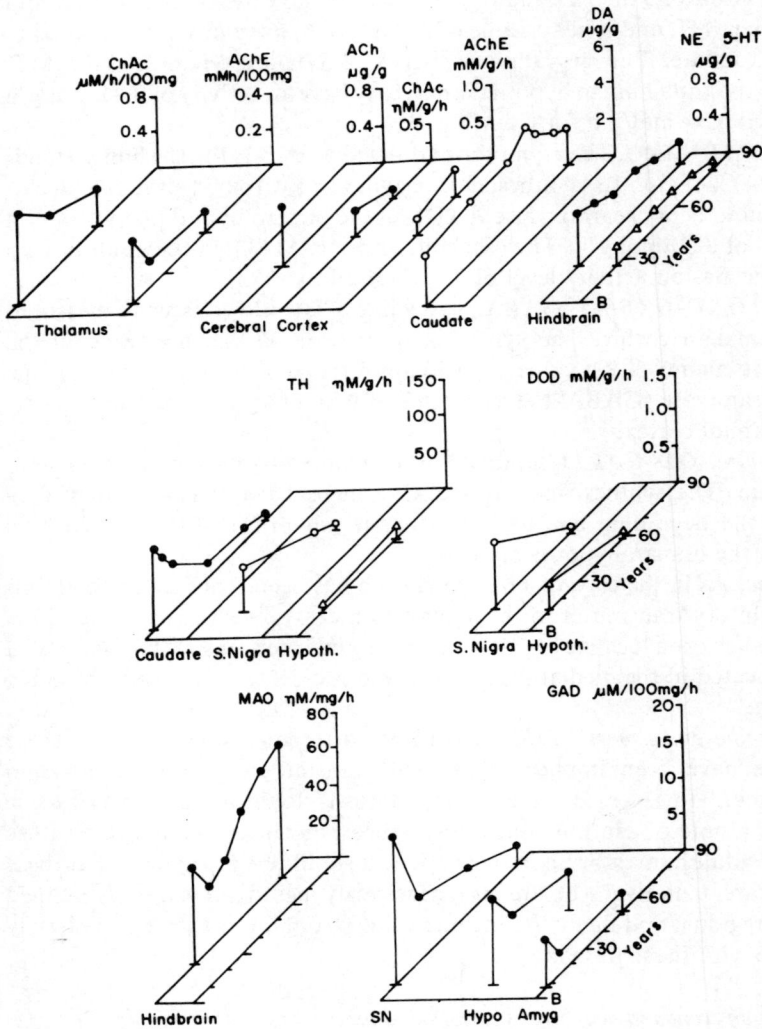

FIG. 6. Life span differences in neurotransmitters and enzymes in some regions of human brain, based on published references.

putamen, and hypothalamus have also been reported. Although requiring clarification in terms of regional differences, MAO has been reported to increase in activity with old age in many regions. Age-dependent decreases in enzyme activity associated with catecholamines, GABA, and ACh in the old human brain have also been reported recently (McGeer and McGeer 1976). In general, the published findings indicate that neurotransmitters and their enzymes appear to decline in many regions of the human brain during aging. Fig. 6 illustrates the reported life span changes in neurotransmitters and their enzymes in some regions of the human brain.

Imbalances within a neurotransmitter–enzyme system during aging

Depending upon the region of the brain, imbalances in neurotransmitters and their enzymes during aging appear as possible major sources of age-dependent chemical decline in the brain. Although such imbalances have not been explored in detail in the normal human brain, they have been established in the brain of the chicken during development and aging. The synthesizing enzyme ChAc and the hydrolyzing enzyme AChE of ACh were determined during development, maturity, and aging in the cerebral cortex, optic lobes, cerebellum, and midbrain. In the cerebral hemispheres, ChAc and AChE reached asymptotic levels by 3 months post-hatching; but after 3 months, ChAc decreased up to 3 years; whereas AChE decreased up to 20 months and then reached high levels of activity at 3 years. It appears that in old age of 3 years, activities of the two cholinergic enzymes were opposite from what they were during development, since the

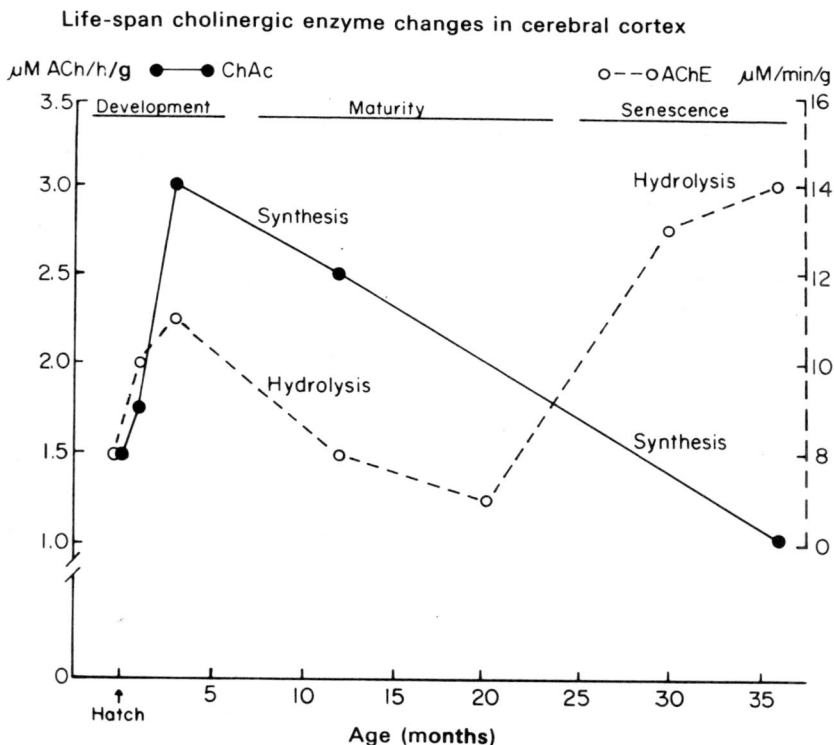

FIG. 7. ChAc and AChE enzyme activity during development, maturity, and aging in the cerebral hemisphers of chicken.

synthesizing enzyme ChAc had a very low level of activity whereas the hydrolyzing enzyme AChE appeared to be at a very high level of activity in the cortex. Since ChAc appears to be a more reliable index of ACh, the age-dependent declines in ChAc may reflect decreases in this synthesizing enzyme activity, loss of cholinergic neurons, or both. However, to establish more fully whether imbalances within the cholinergic system during aging represent a possible major source of age-dependent chemical decline in the brain, ACh levels, turnover, and ACh receptor alterations would also have to be established. Fig. 7 illustrates ChAc and AChE enzyme activity during development, maturity, and aging in the cerebral hemisphere of the chicken.

Imbalances among different types of neutrotransmitter systems during aging
As in the case of imbalances within a specific cholinergic neurotransmitter-enzyme system, imbalances among different types of neurotransmitter systems in the same region, or among different regions may also constitute possible major sources of age-dependent chemical changes in the brain. It has been proposed that regulation of extrapyramidal motor functions in the normal adult human brain depends on the balance between dopaminergic, cholinergic, and GABA-minergic activity. During aging, there appears to be a progressive imbalance among dopaminergic, cholinergic, and GABAminergic neurotransmitters in the basal ganglia of man resulting in motor impairments. According to some recent studies, such imbalances among different neurotransmitter systems are also prominent manifestations of such age-dependent brain and motor disorders as Parkinsonism and Huntington's chorea and possibly also of some mental impairments (McGeer and McGeer 1976).

Age-dependent changes in neurotransmitters in psychopathology and neurological diseases
In recent years, there has been some remarkable progress in studies of brain aminergic system interactions and psychopathology. These studies have focused on the role of such specific amines as NE, DA, 5-HT, and their metabolites in manic states, depression, and schizophrenia. Earlier theories of neurochemical correlates of psychopathology tended to emphasize alterations in one amine system alone without reference to interactions with other amine systems. More recently, it has become apparent that clarification of amine system interactions in the brain are essential for an understanding of normal behaviour (Iversen and Iversen 1975) as well as amine-mediated manic states, depression, schizophrenia, and abnormal behaviour (Mandell 1975).

Greater progress has been reported in clarification of the role of catecholamines in some specific neurological diseases. According to histochemical fluorescent studies, dopaminergic axons from the substantia nigra project to the caudate, putamen, and globus pallidus. Using immunohistochemical techniques for ChAc, it has been demonstrated that these structures, in turn, are found to contain cholinergic ACh interneuron cell bodies. From these basal ganglia nuclei GABAminergic neurons project back to the substantia nigra and other regions of the brain. In the normal adult circuits of the basal ganglia, a proper balance of these excitatory and inhibitory neuron interactions is essential for optimum motor performance. It has been established that even mild symptoms of Parkinson's disease are associated with significant striatal dopamine decreases. In Huntington's chorea, the caudate appears more affected pathologically than the putamen. In this disorder, there is greater decrease in ChAc, and consequently ACh, in the caudate nuclei. Symptoms of Parkinson's disease and Huntington's chorea appear related not only to significant decreases in dopamine, ChAc, or GAD but each of these diseases appears related to specific patterns of imbalance between dopaminergic and cholinergic neurotransmitter interactions, or between dopaminergic and GABAminergic interactions respectively in the basal ganglia (McGeer and McGeer 1976). In addition to the examination of imbalances in

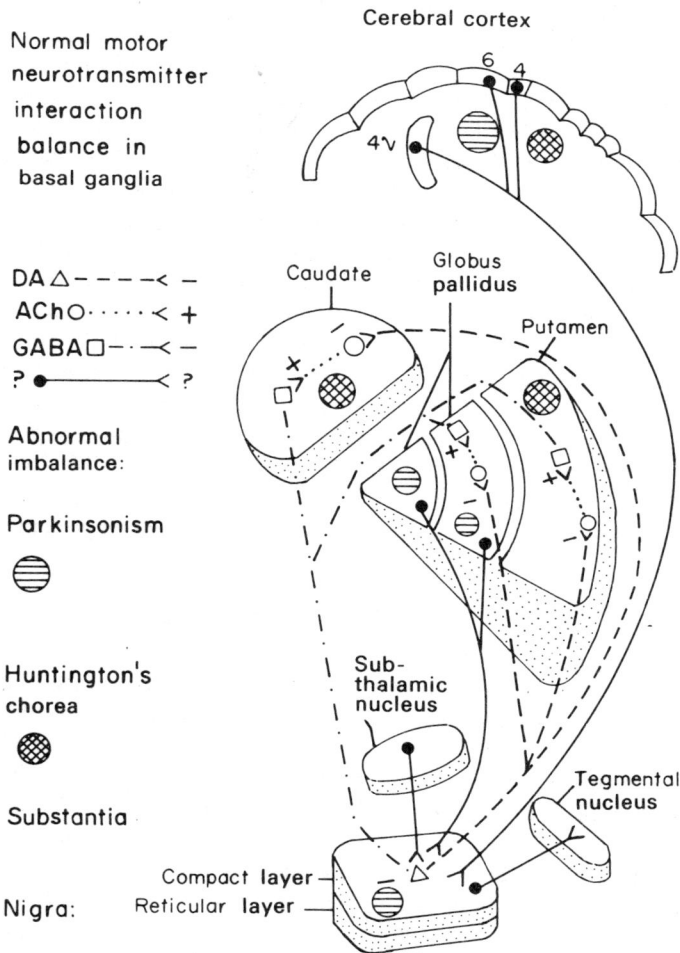

Fig. 8. Imbalances among dopaminergic, cholinergic, and GABAminergic transmitters in basal ganglia in Parkinsonism and Huntington's Chorea.

neurotransmitters in Parkinsonism and Huntington's chorea, characteristic alterations in catecholamines, enzymes, and metabolites have also been reported in other neurological disorders (Moskowitz and Wurtman 1975). Fig. 8 illustrates possible relationships and imbalances among dopaminergic, cholinergic, and GABAminergic interactions in the basal ganglia in Parkinsonism and Huntington's chorea.

Possible age-dependent changes in excitation, conduction, and neurotransmission in single neurons

Although elegant 'single-unit' neuron iontophoretic studies of neuronal excitation, conduction and transmission have been carried out in recent years in different regions of the mammalian brain, thus far these single-unit electrochemical studies have not been applied to possible age-dependent changes in excitation, conduction, and transmission in relation to chemical and morphological changes in single neurons. However, loss of dendritic spines with aging has been reported (Feldman 1976). Decreases in axonal transport mechanisms and conduction velocity in the PNS have also been reported (Birren and Schaie 1976). Decreases in enzyme activity and neurotransmitters, as reported in this review, also appear as prominent manifestations of neuronal aging. It seems likely that age-dependent changes in transmitter receptors and re-uptake mechanisms may also occur. Consequently, at the single unit neuron level, it seems likely that (a) the age-dependent decreases in dendritic spines, synapses, or neuropil density may result in age-dependent decreases in 'input' balance of excitation or inhibition; (b) alterations in axon transport mechanisms, myelin lamellae, and/or diameter may result in decreasing conduction velocity; and (c) changes in neurotransmitters, enzymes, or their imbalances at the synapses may result in changes in neurotransmission. Fig. 9 illustrates possible age-dependent changes in excitation, conduction, and transmission in single neurons associated with loss of dendrites, axon characteristics, and synaptic components.

Neurotransmitters and aging in non-human primate 'models'

Although of the same taxonomic order as man, it seems surprising that non-human primates have been used so infrequently in neurobiological research on aging. Many of man's most distinctive sensory, learning, and motor capacities are shared only by higher diurnal primates. There is an increasing encephalization or localization of distinctive sensory–cognitive–motor functions in the cortex of primates and man. Life span changes in these specific sensory, associative, and motor functions of the brain may be identified more readily in regions where neuronal contact specificity has been demonstrated to be uniquely precise.

An extensive literature has accumulated on the functional localization of sensory, associative, and motor functions in the primate brain. As far as age declines in complex sensory, learning, and motor skills are concerned in man, it is important to note for animal 'models' used in the neurobiology of aging, that

Neuron development, maturity, aging

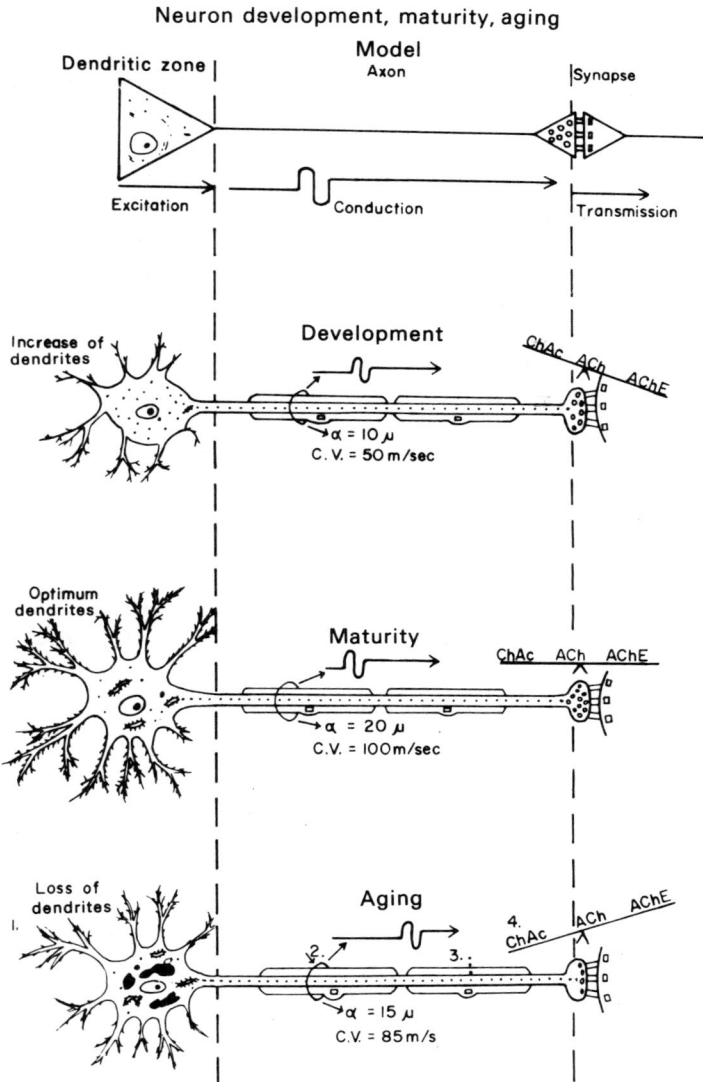

FIG. 9. Age changes in neuron include: loss of dendritic spines; lipofuscine pigment accumulation; loss of myelin lamellae; conduction velocity (C.V.); decreased transport of transmitter via neurotubules; imbalance in enzymes.

regulation of complex behaviour coincides with advanced neocortical development of the brain of higher diurnal primates and that this integration is not organized similarly at cortical and subcortical levels in lower species. Consequently, the specific decreases in sensory processes, learning, memory, and speed and accuracy of complex manipulatory behaviour with aging, which are prominent manifestations in old human subjects, may be demonstrable only in higher primates.

One of the most likely non-human candidates for increasing future use in neurobiological studies of aging is the rhesus monkey. Its maximum life span extends to 32 years. In one interdisciplinary study, observations were made in cross-sectional age samples on life span changes in visual acuity, discrimination learning, short-term memory, and motor performance in relation to cholinergic and adrenergic neurotransmitters and their enzymes: (a) in the visual, motor, and somatosensory areas of the cerebral cortex, (b) in the hypothalamus of the limbic system; and (c) the caudate nucleus of the basal ganglia. An examination of life span changes in NE, 5-HT, and H_2O indicated small but significant declines of NE in the somatosensory region of the cerebral cortex, the caudate, and more highly significant declines in the hypothalamus after 20 years of age. H_2O also declined in the motor cortex and caudate. 5-HT declined significantly in the hypothalamus after 20 years of age. Life span changes in AChE, MAO, and COMT were also examined in the visual, motor, and somatosensory regions of the cerebral cortex and the caudate nucleus. AChE remained relatively constant in the visual, motor, and somatosensory regions but declined significantly in the area of highest activity of the caudate after 20 years of age. In the case of MAO, there were significant age-dependent increases as well as decreases, depending upon region and age. COMT declined significantly in visual, motor, and somato-sensory regions after 18 years of age, whereas in the caudate, COMT declined more gradually after 20 years of age (Ordy 1975). Life span changes in NE, 5-HT, AChE, MAO, and COMT in the brain of the rhesus monkey are illus-trated in Fig. 10.

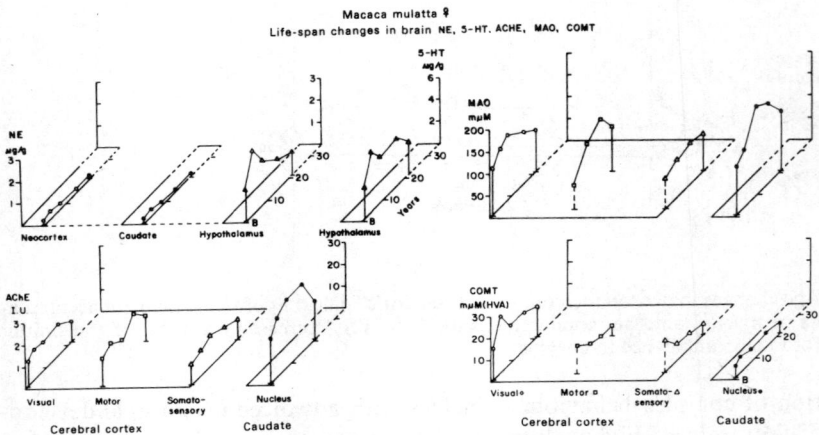

FIG. 10. Life span differences in norepinephrine (NE), serotonin (5-HT), acetyl choline esterase (AChE), monoamine oxidase (MAO), and catechol-*o*-methyl-transferase (COMT) in some regions of the brain of the rhesus monkey.

Age–stress interaction effects on brain neurotransmitters, behaviour, life span in rodent 'models'

In order to study the effects of environmental stress on post-maturity environmental modifiability or 'plasticity' of brain neurotransmitters, behaviour, and life span, subjects from an inbred strain of C57B1/10 male and female mice were exposed in an environmental chamber to intermittent electric foot shock across the entire life span. Maximum life span extends to 32 months in this strain. Brain AChE increased from 4–6 months and then decreased significantly from 16–24 months. Brain NE also increased from 4–16 months and then decreased by 24 months. There was a significant age–stress interaction effect on brain NE. Brain NE decreased in response to stress throughout the life span. Regarding the chemical and morphological 'plasticity' of the brain with age, in addition to the age-dependent changes in DNA, RNA, protein, AChE, and NE, there occurred, at each age level, shorter-lasting and possibly reversible fluctuations in neurotransmitters and other chemical constituents in response to environmental stress. The environmental modifiability or 'plasticity' of these brain chemical constituents remained into senescence but it was not constant across the life span. Depending upon type, duration, and intensity of a continuum from stimulation to stress, significant changes have been reported in age-specific mortality, mean life span, or the rate of aging (Ordy and Schjeide 1973).

General summary and conclusions

As stated earlier, the sensory, learning, memory, drive, and motor capacities of man reach a peak in early adulthood, remain relatively constant throughout maturity and then appear to decline during old age. More specifically, impairment of speed and accuracy of behaviour with age increases as performance complexity increases. Also, age decrements in physiological functions which involve the co-ordinated activity of several organ systems are greater than functions that involve a single organ. Neurotransmitters and hormones have widespread effects as chemical regulators of co-ordinated physiological activity throughout the body and on behaviour. Specific neurotransmitters and hormones have now been identified in sensory processes, learning, memory, motivation, and motor co-ordination during development, maturity, and aging (Ordy and Kaack 1975; Iversen and Iversen 1975).

The 'language' of neuronal excitation and conduction is primarily electrochemical. Neurotransmission across synaptic junctions proceeds chemically in a dynamically polarized manner from axon terminals across synaptic junctions to dendrites, cell bodies, axons, or effectors. Since transmission across the synapse is chemical, a great deal of recent neurochemical research has included studies of neurotransmitters and associated enzymes at the synapse as possible cellular sites of plasticity in the nervous system. Remarkable progress has been made recently in identifying neurochemical correlates, particularly neurotransmitters involved in the regulation of physiology and behaviour. However, this vast progress has been primarily in research on brain development from birth to maturity rather than from maturity to old age. Since post-mitotic neurons do not divide after birth and remain throughout life, senescence in the brain represents only a different aspect of the total life span ontogenetic programme. Regarding major life span changes in neurotransmitters and associated enzymes, values reported for the human brain are scarce, fragmentary, and scattered throughout the literature. Five different types of approach have emerged to identify age-dependent changes in neurotransmitters of the human brain.

(1) An initial approach has been to study life span changes in neurotransmitters and associated enzymes in the adult human brain and to compare these values with those of early development.

(2) A second approach has been to examine age-dependent changes in neurotransmitters from maturity to old age.

(3) A third approach has been to examine age-dependent imbalances within a specific neurotransmitter–enzyme system during development and aging.

(4) A fourth approach has been to examine imbalances among different types of neurotransmitter systems in the brain during aging.

(5) A fifth approach has been to characterize imbalances of neurotransmitter interactions in specific psychopathologies and neurological disorders during aging.

As yet, single-unit neuron iontophertic methods have not been applied to study possible age-dependent changes in excitation, conduction, and transmission in relation to chemical and morphological changes in single neurons. However, loss of dendritic spines, decreases in number of synapses, alterations in axonal transport mechanisms, number of myelin lamellae, and/or axon diameter have all been reported. Consequently, it seems likely that, at the single-unit neuron level, age-dependent decreases in excitation, conduction, and transmission may occur during aging. Age-dependent changes may include loss of neurons, changes in remaining neurons, or combinations of both.

Although findings on life span changes in neurotransmitters in the human brain are scarce and fragmentary, more comprehensive interpretations of the reported chemical changes can be made if these age-dependent changes in neurotransmitters of the CNS are also related to changes in behaviour, electrical activity of the brain, morphology, neuropathology, and other relevant neurochemical changes. According to behavioural studies, sensory, learning, memory, drive, and motor capacities of man decline in senescence. Significant age-dependent changes have been reported in the electrical activity of the human brain as reflected in visual, auditory, and somatosensory evoked cerebral potentials. Age-dependent decreases in axon conduction velocity of the PNS have also been reported. Morphologically, age-dependent declines occur in brain volume, loss of neurons, and decreases in neuropil density. Increases in lipofuscin also appear as prominent manifestations of aging. Whereas age-dependent changes in neurotransmitters may represent basic chemical changes in the human brain, ultimately these changes have to be related to the loss of neurons, possible increase of glia, as well as the decrease in neuropil density. These age-dependent changes in neurotransmitters also remain to be clarified in terms of age-dependent changes in neuronal network capacity for processing information and neural activity in different regions of the brain. For example, age-dependent changes in sensory processes, learning, and motor performance have been related to changes in electrical activity, neurotransmitters, other chemical changes, and to cell loss in specific regions of the cerebral cortex (Ordy and Brizzee 1975). However, although learning and memory may be localized in the cortex, learning or performance also imply dependence on drives and their reinforcement. Learning and drives have been 'linked' as an integrative, adaptive process through the limbic system, hypothalamus, pituitary, and endocrine organs. Consequently, age-dependent impairments in behaviour can be associated not only with changes in electrical activity, neurotransmitters and cell loss from the cerebral cortex, but also with changes in other regions of the brain and endocrine organs (Ordy and Kaack 1976). Recent studies suggest that age-dependent impairments in learning and short-term memory may be associated not only with cell loss in the cortex (Ordy, Brizzee, Kaack and Hansche 1978), but also with changes in modulation of memory consolidation in the remaining cells of the cortex by decreases in catecholamines of cells in the hypothalamus, or changes in other limbic regions that project to the cortex and influence remaining cells in the cerebral cortex. Age declines in short-term memory, electrical activity, neurotransmitters, and loss of neurons may also be affected even more indirectly by 'feedback' declines in circulating pituitary and other endocrine hormones that may influence hormone receptors of neurons in the brain. Target organ hormone receptors are known to decrease with age. Hormones are also known to influence catecholamine metabolism in the brain by altering the rate-limiting tyrosine hydroxylase activity and the re-uptake of catecholamines at membranes (Villee 1975). In future studies of aging, it seems likely that neurotransmitters and hormones will play an increasingly important role not only at the cellular level but in multidisciplinary attempts to bridge the gaps from behavioural to electrical, neurochemical, and morphological levels of observation in the new field of neurobiology and aging.

References

BECK, E. C., DUSTMAN, R. E., and SCHENKENBERG, T. (1935). In *Neurobiology of aging* (eds. J. M. Ordy and K. R. Brizzee), p. 175. Plenum Press, New York.

BIRREN, J. and SCHAIE, K. W. (eds.) (1976). *Handbook of the psychology of aging*, Vol. 2. Van Nostrand, Reinhold, New York.

BOTWINICK, J. (1973). *Aging and behavior*. Springer, New York.

BRIZZEE, K. R. (1975a). In *Neurobiology of aging* (eds. J. M. Ordy and K. R. Brizzee), p. 401. Plenum Press, New York.

—— (1975b). In *Neurobiology of aging* (eds. J. M. Ordy and K. R. Brizzee), p. 287. Plenum Press, New York.

——, KLARA, P., and JOHNSON, J. E. (1975). In *Neurobiology of aging* (eds. J. M. Ordy and K. R. Brizzee), p. 425. Plenum Press, New York.

——, KAACK, B., and KLARA, P. (1975). In *Neurobiology of aging* (eds. J. M. Ordy and K. R. Brizzee), p. 463. Plenum Press, New York.

BRODY, H. (1976). In *Neurobiology of aging* (eds. R. Terry and S. Gershon), p. 211. Raven Press, New York.

CUTLER, R. G. (1976). *J. Human Evol.*, **5**, 169.

DAHLSTROM, A. and FUXE, K. (1964). *Acta Physiol. Scand. Suppl. 62*, **232**, 1.

FELDMAN, M. L. (1976). In *Neurobiology of aging* (eds. R. Terry and S. Gershon), p. 211. Raven Press, New York.

FRIEDE, R. L. (1966). *Topographic brain chemistry.* Academic Press, New York.

HERMANN, R. L. (1975). In *Neurobiology of aging* (eds. J. M. Ordy and K. R. Brizzee), p. 307. Plenum Press, New York.

IVERSEN, S. D. and IVERSEN, L. L. (1975). In *Handbook of psychobiology* (eds. M. S. Gazzaniga and C. Blakemore), p. 153. Academic Press, New York.

JOUVET, M. (1972). *Ergeb. Physiol.*, **64**, 166.

LAJTHA, A. (ed.) (1969–72). *Handbook of neurochemistry*, Vols. 1–7. Plenum Press, New York.

LIVETT, B. G. (1973). *Brit. med. Bull.*, **29**, 93.

MAAS, J. W. and GARVER, D. (1975). In Advances in Biochemical Psychopharmacology, Vol. 13, *Neurobiological mechanisms of adaptation and behavior*, (eds. A. J. Mandell), p. 61. Raven Press, New York.

MANDELL, A. J. (ed.) (1975). Advances in Biochemical Psychopharmacology, Vol. 13, *Neurobiological mechanisms of adaptation and behavior.* Raven Press, New York.

McGREER, E. G. and McGEER, P. L. (1975). In *Neurobiology of aging* (eds. J. M. Ordy and K. R. Brizzee), p. 307. Plenum Press, New York.

—— and —— (1976). In *Neurobiology of aging* (eds. R. Terry and S. Gershon), p. 389. Raven Press, New York.

MEIER-RUGE, W., REICHLMEIER, K., and IWANGOFF, P. (1976). In *Neurobiology of aging* (eds. R. Terry and S. Gershon), p. 379. Raven Press, New York.

MINCKLER, T. M. and BOYD, E. (1968). In *Pathology of the nervous system*, Vol. I (ed. J. Minckler). McGraw-Hill, New York.

MOSKOWITZ, M. A. and WURTMAN, R. (1975). *New Engl. J. Med.*, **293**, 274.

OLSON, L., BOREUS, L. O., and SEIGER, A. (1973). *Z. Anat. Entwicklungsgesch*, **139**, 259.

ORDY, J. M. (1975). In *Neurobiology of aging* (eds. J. M. Ordy and K. R. Brizzee), p. 575. Plenum Press, New York.

—— and KAACK, B. (1975). In *Neurobiology of aging* (eds. J. M. Ordy and K. R. Brizzee), p. 253. Plenum Press, New York.

—— and —— (1976). *Special review of experimental aging research* (ed. M. F. Elias, B. E. Eleftheriou, and P. K. Elias), p. 255. EAR, Inc., Bar Harbor Maine.

——, ——, and BRIZZEE, K. R. (1975). In *Clinical, morphologic and neurochemical aspects in the aging central nervous system* (ed. H. Brody, D. Harman, and J. M. Ordy), p. 133. Raven Press, New York.

—— and BRIZZEE, K. R. (eds.) (1975). *Neurobiology of aging: an interdisciplinary life-span approach.* Plenum Press, New York.

—— —— KAACK, B., and HANSCHE, J. (1978). *Gerontology*, **24**, 276–85.

—— and SCHJEIDE, O. A. (1973). In Progress in Brain Research, Vol. 40, *Neurobiological aspects of maturation and aging* (ed. D. Ford), p. 25. Elsevier, Amsterdam.

SACHER, G. (1975). In *Primate functional morphology and evolution* (ed. R. Tuttle), p. 111. Mouton, The Hague.

SANDOZ, P. and MEIER-RUGE, W. (1976). *Abstracts from 29th Meeting of Gerontological Society*, p. 41.

SHOCK, N. W. (1974). In *Theoretical aspects of aging* (ed. M. Rockestein), p. 119. Academic Press, New York.

UNGERSTEDT, U. (1971). *Acta. Physiol. Scand., Suppl. 367.*

VERNADAKIS, A. (1973). In Progress in Brain Research, Vol. 40, *Neurobiological aspects of maturation and aging* (ed. D. Ford), p. 231. Elsevier, Amsterdam.

VILLEE, D. B. (1975). *Human endocrinology.* Saunders, Philadelphia.

Session 3

Aging of the cardiovascular system

Aging of the cardiac muscle Myron L. Weisfeldt

Introduction

This chapter presents data from isolated systems in which we have made an effort to characterize (1) changes with age in the intrinsic contractile properties of cardiac muscle, (2) age-associated changes in myocardial stiffness, and (3) changes with age in the inotropic responsiveness of cardiac muscle concluding with a comment on studies dealing with the issue of energy availability to the aged myocardium.

It is extremely difficult to separate the effects of aging from those of cardiac disease states. We have attempted to study a population of animals without evidence of cardiac disease, but this has proved difficult. One approach to this problem is to study a number of species throughout the life span in an effort to identify those aspects of myocardial function which show similar age-associated changes. The assumption is that cardiac diseases differ between species.

The overall conclusions which we have derived from the studies are as follows:

(1) Certain aspects of cardiac muscle function show significant age changes whereas other aspects of cardiac muscle function appear to show no physiologically significant change. Thus, it is possible to characterize the myocardium of the aged individual in terms of maintained or retained function and in terms of physiologically significant age changes.

(2) Not all age-associated changes are clearly deterimental or lead to a decline in cardiac function. This, I believe, will mean in the future the treatment of cardiac disease in the aged individual will be tailored to the limitations and attributes of the aged heart.

What are some of the major characteristics of aged cardiac muscle? I will present evidence that there are age changes in stiffness of cardiac muscle. These age-associated increases in stiffness are at least theoretically advantageous in terms of allowing cardiac muscle with diminished shortening ability to develop tension at a rate which is unchanged. The increase in stiffness combined with prolongation of the duration of contraction appears to allow cardiac muscle from the aged individual to develop the same amount of total force during contraction as is developed by cardiac muscle from a younger animal despite decreased intrinsic contractile ability in the former. Thus, in terms of contraction, the age-associated increase in cardiac muscle stiffness appears to be beneficial. Since an age-associated increase in stiffness characterizes resting cardiac muscle as well, the heart of the aged individual will be less able to adapt to an acute increase in workload because of decreased diastolic compliance or increased stiffness. Pulmonary oedema, or acute heart failure will appear more rapidly if the pumping ability of the left ventricle is exceeded. Another major finding is that myocardium from the senescent rat appears to have diminished inotropic response to those agents which require a cell membrane receptor.

In contrast, there appears to be no age-associated decrease in the inotropic response to agents which are at the present time felt not to require a cell membrane receptor to exert an inotropic effect. Clearly, extension of the present studies to the human will be necessary before application of such principles to man can actually be undertaken, but these studies suggest that aging may be an important factor in selection of inotropic agents. Thus, the overall picture which we develop for cardiac muscle in the aged rat highlights selectivity of age-related changes, the mechanism of these age-associated changes, and the implication of these changes for overall cardiovascular function and regulation.

In the majority of the studies, Wistar rats taken from the Gerontology Research Center colony maintained by the National Institute on Aging in Baltimore were employed. 24–27-month-old animals were compared to 6–12-month-old animals. All of these animals were maintained with constant dietary and environmental conditions as to temperature, humidity, and lighting. The animals were housed in small cages with five other rats of the same sex. The animals tended to be obese and they did have identifiable diseases which appeared throughout their life span; chronic renal disease, respiratory infections, and tumours were common. Though one selects apparently healthy animals for study, it is clear that other factors aside from aging *per se*, such as disease and lack of exercise, may be influencing the results of these studies. Again, I would note the importance of studying many species and in studying the relationship between disease states and apparent aging changes. Pathological studies of the hearts of rats taken from this colony show relatively little coronary vessel narrowing or intimal lesions in the large- to middle-size coronary arteries from non-breeder senescent rats (Weisfeldt, Wright, Shreiner, Lakatta, and Shock 1971). Direct measurement of intra-arterial pressure in animals from this colony in the unanaesthetized state has demonstrated no apparent hypertension within the senescent group (Rothbaum, Shaw, Angell, and Shock 1973). Some degree of myocardial hypertrophy is suggested by comparison of heart weights from young and old animals (Shreiner, Weisfeldt, and Shock 1969). In this colony there has been an 8–15 per cent increase in heart weight noted between 12 and 24 months of age. In recent studies performed by Dr. Frank Yin in our laboratory, tibial bone length has been utilized as a normalizing factor to compare the heart weights of adult and senescent rats. These studies suggest that the extent of increase in heart weight is no more than 10 per cent within this colony. Heart weight/body weight ratios as used by others in assessing the extent of myocardial hypertrophy with aging (Berg and Harmison 1955) have clearly been shown by these recent studies to be inappropriate and to lead to an overestimate of the actual extent of hypertrophy in the aged rat. In early classic studies by Wilens and Sproul (1938), age-associated myocardial fibrosis was noted. These observations have been confirmed by measurement of hydroxy-proline content. Although this appearance of increased fibrous tissue is significant, it does not amount to more than a doubling of the fibrous tissue even in the subendocardium where this fibrosis is most evident. Travis and Travis (1972) have examined hearts of senescent rats from the Gerontology Research Colony using the electron microscope. Similar studies have been performed in Sprague–Dawley rats by Tomanek and Karlsson (1973). In general, there is no prominent change in the myofibres themselves, although increased lipofucin was noted by both groups of investigations. In rats greater than 18 months of age there is an increased number of residual bodies near the mitochondria in the nuclear pole zone and the mitochondrial rows separating the myofibrillar masses. There are also signs of increased lysosomal activity particularly in the mitochondrial regions. There does not appear to be a marked age-associated decrease in the number of mitochondria as noted in other types of muscle with age (Herbener 1971).

Intrinsic contractile properties

Early studies by Shreiner and associates (1969) and Lee, Karpeles, and Downing (1972) using rats from this colony demonstrated an overall decrease in cardiac function with age in male rats. Neither study characterized the mechanism for this age-associated decrease in function. Studies of isolated cardiac muscle by Alpert, Gale, and Taylor (1967) provide essential information concerning intrinsic cardiac muscle function from the aged rat. These investigators demonstrated an age-associated decrease in the apparent maximal velocity of contractile element shortening assessed in afterloaded isotonic contractions and a parallel decrease in the myofibrillar ATPase activity. These investigators also made the observation that there was no age-associated difference in the ability of cardiac muscle to develop tension under isometric conditions (i.e. when the muscle is held fixed at the optimal muscle length and does not shorten with contraction). It is this apparent disparity between the index of contractility (velocity of shortening) and the ability to develop tension under isometric conditions which will be a major point. Lakatta, Gerstenblith, Angell, Shock, and Weisfeldt (1975b) studied the time course of isometric contraction of trabeculae carneae from 6-, 12-, and 24-month-old rats paced at 24 beats per minute at 29 °C in Krebs–Ringer bicarbonate solution modified by decreasing the calcium concentration to 1 mM and the magnesium concentration to 0.6 mM. Glucose (16 mM) was added. The muscles were studied at the length at which the contractile tension was maximal. There was no significant age-dependent difference in the length of muscles nor the cross-sectional area of these muscles. These studies again demonstrated that there was no age-associated change in the maximal tension developed under isometric conditions and, in addition, that there was no significant age-associated change in the rate of tension development (dT/dt) under these conditions. Of greater interest was the observation that there was a prolongation of the time to peak tension and the half relaxation time (that is the time for tension to fall from its peak value to one-half its peak value) during relaxation.

Our initial hypothesis was that the ability of the aged cardiac muscle to maintain peak active tension development, despite apparent decrease in intrinsic contractile ability, was a result of a prolonged period of activation due to delayed relaxation of cardiac muscle. This prolonged contraction duration is reflected in the time to peak tension and relaxation time. There is more time for the contractile elements to develop tension during a contraction–relaxation cycle. Other studies were performed and helped to support this hypothesis. Since catecholamines are known to shorten the duration of active state of cardiac muscle, and since aged myocardium appears to be somewhat depleted of catecholamines (Gey, Burkhard, and Pletscher 1965; Frolkis, Bezrukov, Bogatskaya, Verkhratsky, Zamostian, Shevtchuk, and Shtchegoleva 1970), the prolonged contraction duration could reflect only catecholamine depletion. To eliminate this possibility, muscles from other adult and senescent rats were studied under conditions of addition of 1×10^{-6} M dl-propranolol to the bathing fluid and after depletion of tissue catecholamines with 6-hydroxy-dopamine using the technique of Roberts (Lakatta, Gerstenblith, *et al.* 1975b). Under both conditions of effective sympathetic blockade and depletion of catecholamines, again we found at optimal length there was no age-associated decrease in active tension development or dT/dt, but there was a persistent prolongation of contraction duration. Thus, prolonged contraction duration appears to be an intrinsic property of cardiac muscle from the aged animal and not related to catecholamine depletion.

Secondly, electromechanical coupling of muscles from adult and senescent rats was studied in an effort to examine the time course of recovery of contractile ability of cardiac muscle. It was our hypothesis that a decreased mechanical response to an early electrical stimulus after a contraction (in the absence of evidence of decreased electrical responsiveness of the membrane) would provide indirect evidence of a decreased rate of recovery or prolongation of the phase of cardiac relaxation and recovery in the muscles from the senescent rats. Lee *et al.* (1970) have reported evidence that mechanical refractoriness at short interstimulus intervals results from an inadequate period of time for calcium accumulation at the releasing sites between depolarizations. We studied the electrical and mechanical responses to paired electrical pacing of isolated rat trabeculae carneae at increasingly short coupling intervals. These studies demonstrated a greater mechanical refractoriness in aged cardiac muscle at short coupling intervals whereas there was no age-associated change in electrical refractoriness as assessed by intracellular microelectrode recordings. Cardiac muscle from senescent rats demonstrated electrical responsiveness at coupling intervals in which there was no apparent mechanical response. This greater electrical–mechanical dissociation, again, suggested that there was an alteration in the time course of calcium movement and recovery during cardiac muscle relaxation. A third piece of evidence, which points to prolonged contraction duration as a result of delayed relaxation in senescent myocardium, was obtained through study of another state in which there is prolonged contraction duration: recovery from hypoxia (Weisfeldt, Armstrong, Scully, Sanders, and Dagget 1974). It has been suggested that this prolongation of contraction duration is due to decreased activity of the cardiac relaxing system during this period of time in which there is rapid influx of calcium into the myocardial cell. This conclusion is supported by measurements of passive viscoelastic properties, which show no change which could account for prolonged contraction duration during this period of recovery following hypoxia (Templeton, Adcock, and Willerton 1973). When adult and senescent cardiac muscle was exposed to hypoxia and reoxygenation, the prolongation of contraction duration during recovery was significantly greater in the aged muscles than in the adult muscles. This suggests that there is a significant age-associated change in the active relaxation system since even greater impairment of this system is seen under the stress of recovery from hypoxia. During hypoxia itself, no age associated changes in contraction duration or contractile function were noted. Thus, these pieces of indirect evidence suggest that there is an intrinsic age-associated change in cardiac muscle function such that there is a prolongation and delay in cardiac muscle relaxation. Recently Dr. Jeffrey Froehlich and Dr. Gary Gerstenblith and associates have completed detailed studies of the kinetics of calcium uptake by isolated microsomal preparations from cardiac muscle from adult and senile rats from this colony. These studies have not been reported in formal fashion, but I can say that these studies are consistent with the hypothesis we have entertained to this point. Like all other studies in which isolated subcellular fractions from tissue from adult and senile animals are compared, these studies can rightfully be criticized from the point of view of sampling problems. Clearly, the microsomal preparation from adult and senile rats may differ in any number of properties based on the composition or character of amount of the subcellular fractions which are isolated in the particular preparation in each age group. It is my personal feeling that it is only where there are detailed comparisons of subcellular fractions and physiological evidence to support the biochemical data that such studies are useful. Thus, the lack of age-associated change in active tension development by cardiac muscle from the aged rat appears to be related to a prolonged period of activation as a result of delayed cardiac muscle relaxation.

The studies discussed so far do not explain the maintenance of the rate of tension rise under isometric conditions. You will recall that throughout the studies both with and without sympathetic blockade and catecholamine depletion, there was no age-associated decrease in the maximal rate of isometric tension development, despite the previous studies suggesting an age-associated decrease in shortening velocity. Evidence has clearly suggested that there is significant shortening in so-called isometric preparations, and therefore, the rate of shortening should be an important determinant of the maximal rate of tension rise (Krueger and Pollack 1975). We thus hypothesized that there may be important age-associated changes in stiffness of cardiac muscle particularly during the contraction cycle. If the cardiac muscle of the senescent rat is in fact stiffer and if the stiffer element is functionally in series with contractile elements, then the maintenance of the rate of tension rise could be a reflection of a balancing between the tendency for decreasing shortening velocity to result in a lower maximum rate of tension rise and the increased stiffness of cardiac muscle from the senescent animal tending to increase the rate of tension rise. The results of these two effects in opposite direction could be a net lack of change in the maximal rate of tension rise under isometric conditions.

This hypothesis was suggested by early studies of resting compliance or muscle stiffness in trabeculae carneae from adult and senile rats (Weisfeldt, Loeven, and Shock 1971). Resting tension was measured in trabeculae carneae during step-wise increases in muscle length. Resting tension was normalized to the cross-sectional area of the muscle. Initially, the length of the muscle at zero resting tension (L_0) was determined. Then the length of the muscle was increased by 5 per cent at 4-minute intervals and the resting tension determined after a 4-minute period for stress relaxation. These studies showed that muscles from the senile rats had significantly greater resting tension at muscle length greater than 115 per cent of L_0. Muscle lengths at L_{max} expressed as a per cent of L_0 did not differ significantly between old and young rats, but there was a significantly higher resting tension in the muscles from the senile rats. Subsequent studies utilizing this preparation demonstrated an age-associated decrease in the magnitude of stress relaxation. The time-related fall in resting tension, stress relaxation, was greater in muscles from adult rats than in muscles from senile rats. Thus cardiac muscle from the senescent animal was characterized by an increase in resting stiffness which was at least in part attributable to an age-associated increase in viscous stiffness. Early studies of Templeton, Wildenthal, Willerson, and Reardon (1974) suggested that there was a direct relation between stiffness of resting cardiac muscle and stiffness of cardiac muscle during contraction. If such was the case for the age change in cardiac muscle (that the increase in resting stiffness which we observed in the trabeculae carneae predicts an increase in stiffness during contraction), then this increase in stiffness might well explain the maintenance of the rate of tension development. Following the methods developed by Templeton and associates, Spurgeon, Thorne, Yin, Weisfeldt, and Shock (1976) have measured the dynamic stiffness of isometric rat trabeculae carneae at L_{max} using a sinusoidal length forcing function.

To permit the measurement of stiffness during an isometric twitch a servo-motor system capable of producing fine gradations in length superimposed on the basic isometric preparation was designed. Such a system allowed no length changes in the preparation due to increasing force generated by the twitch itself. By means of a servo system, a length perturbation with any forcing function desired up to a peak amplitude of 0.25 mm at frequencies from dc to 100 Hz could be superimposed on the study length.

Tension and length were digitized and stored temporarily on digital tape. Two successive cycles of contraction (only one of which contained forcing function perturbations) were displayed on an oscilloscope. The unperturbed signal was subtracted from the perturbed leaving a pseudo high frequency component. By

subtracting unperturbed from perturbed twitches, an approximation of force development due only to the lengthy perturbation change throughout the time course of the muscle contraction was derived.

Combining the force and length data, a resulting dynamic stiffness, defined at dT/dL and denoted by (R), was obtained. The dT term is the perturbation force (g) divided by the cross-sectional area (mm^2) at the unperturbed study length, while dL is the perturbation length (mm) divided by the unperturbed study length. The value for R was calculated for each 20-ms interval beginning in the late diastolic period preceding stimulus, and proceeding for 16 perturbing cycles at the probing frequency during the isometric contraction.

The slope of the relationship between stiffness and tension during the entire phase of tension rise and fall, during single contractions, was greater in muscles from senescent male and female rats than their adult counterparts. The age dependence of this slope was independent of resting muscle length and was greater at higher frequencies of perturbations. This latter observation of greater age differences in stiffness at higher perturbation frequency, again suggests an age-associated increase in viscous stiffness. Since these studies demonstrate an age-associated increase in stiffness at any given level of tension throughout contraction, they support the hypothesis that the maintenance of the rate of tension development and perhaps also in part the maintenance of tension development ability is related to the age-associated increase in dynamic stiffness of cardiac muscle.

Similar measurements of dynamic stiffness of intact left ventricles of beagles have recently been made by Templeton, Ecker, and Mitchell (1972).

Eight young (27 ± 2.5 month) and seven old (128 ± 20.5 month) beagles were placed on complete cardiopulmonary bypass; the arterial pressure was constant at 80 mmHg and the heart contracted isovolumically at a rate of 120 beats per minute. Diastolic pressure–volume curves were established for each unpaced left ventricle, and the volume at the apex of the curve was used during the data collection. Stiffness was measured with a sinusoidal volume-forcing function, similar to the length-forcing function used in the rat. This system imposed a sinusoidal volume displacement of 1 cc at 20 Hz into the left ventricle of these animals. In each ventricle stiffness was linearly related to pressure during the cardiac cycle and was greater for any given pressure in the older beagles.

Thus, in two species, the rat and the dog, there is an age-associated increase in the dynamic stiffness of cardiac muscle. The mechanism for this increase is unclear, but could relate to properties of the connective tissue or contractile elements of the myocardium.

I have thus detailed, to this point, the evidence supporting the notion that with senescence there is a decrease in contractile ability which is at least in part compensated on a functional level by delayed relaxation and increased dynamic muscle stiffness.

Inotropic responsiveness

We turn now to the inotropic response of cardiac muscle from the senescent animal. The most important physiological inotropic factor is that mediated by the sympathetic nervous system through catecholamines, and we will therefore examine that response first.

The inotropic response of isolated rat trabeculae carneae from 6-, 12-, and 25-month-old rats at L_{max} was studied by Lakatta, Gerstenblith, Angell, Shock, and Weisteldt (1975a). Baseline dT/dt and active tension were again not age-related. However, the increase in dT/dt under isometric conditions was significantly less in the 25-month-old group than it was in the 6-month-old group at the same concentration of norepinephrine or isoproterenol. Although the baseline contraction duration was again longer in the muscles from the older group, the extent of shortening of contraction duration with catecholamines was similar in muscles from senile and adult animals. The combination of the decreased inotropic response (as indexed by dT/dt) and the similar extent of relative shortening of contraction duration resulted in striking differences in the extent of increase in active tension with catecholamine stimulation. Under conditions of 1.0 mM calcium and a pacing rate of 24 beats/minute there was, in fact, no increase in active tension in muscles from the 25-month-old group at norepinephrine concentrations up to 1×10^{-5} M; whereas, the muscles from 6- and 12-month-old rats showed an increase in active tension of 21 ± 4 and 22 ± 4.1 per cent, respectively. Catecholamines are thought to alter active state properties. First, they shorten the duration of active state by stimulating the cardiac relaxing system (Rolett 1974). Since contraction duration is shortened proportionately in the young and aged muscles, it appears that the sequence of biochemical events responsible for this effect is intact in aged cardiac muscle. Catecholamines are also believed to increase the intensity of active state (Rolett 1974) by increasing the amount of calcium delivered to the contractile element. As judged by the response of dT/dt, it appears that this effect is less in aged muscles. This could be due to either less calcium being delivered to the contractile element in the aged muscle, or to an impaired contractile element response to the calcium despite an equal amount of calcium being delivered. To explore these possibilities, the effect of age on the inotropic response to increasing concentrations of calcium from 0.5 to 2.5 mM was also determined. There was no age difference in the increase in developed tension or maximal rate of tension development to the level of calcium which gave a maximal response. These findings then suggest that the ability of the contractile elements to respond to increased calcium is intact and that the diminished inotropic response to catecholamines in aged myocardium probably results from an impairment in the ability of the catecholamines to increase the amount of calcium delivered to the contractile element.

Yin, Spurgeon, Raizes, Green, Weisfeldt, and Shock (1976) have recently demonstrated a similar age-associated decrease in the chronotropic response of aged beagles to catecholamines. The maximal heart rate achieved during isoproterenol stimulation was significantly lower in senescent than young adult dogs in the intact unanaesthetized state, after anaesthesia, and after atropine blockade. In the inotropic studies, we were unable to achieve or study maximal inotropy because of the appearance of arrhythmias. With the chronotropic effects, we can say that the dose-response curve shows that there is no age change in threshold or receptor sensitivity. The age difference appeared to relate to receptor number or factors distal to the receptor. Two other inotropic agents have also been examined in the trabeculae preparation from adult and senescent rats. Like the inotropic response to calcium, the inotropic response of the rat trabeculae carneae to paired pacing at 0.25 mM calcium demonstrated no age-associated decrease (Gerstenblith, Lakatta, Spurgeon, Shock, and Weistfeldt 1975). Thus, two inotropic agents not requiring a receptor were not associated with aging changes. In contrast, the inotropic response to ouabain, a digitalis glycoside, showed an age-associated decrease. Thus, two agents which exhibit an inotropic effect thought to be mediated via a cell membrane receptor, demonstrate an age-associated decline. Direct assessment of the properties of the presumed beta adrenergic receptor of cardiac muscle has only recently been possible. Studies are underway to examine this receptor directly. The nature of the digitalis receptor responsible for the inotropic is unclear at present. It should be emphasized, though, that the apparent age change in inotropic response to these agents may be due to change in the receptor or any mediator or intracellular effector mechanism, which ultimately results in the inotropic effect perhaps by increasing calcium entry.

Energy availability

Rakusan and Poupa (1964) initially suggested that aging is characterized by a progressive obliteration of capillaries within the heart of the rat. These investigators found a decrease in the capillary–fibre ratio. The diffusion distance for oxygen was increased to a somewhat greater extent by virtue of myocardial cell hypertrophy. Tomanek (1969) later repeated similar investigations, but studied both exercised and non-exercised rats. Again, there was a lower capillary–fibre ratio and a decreased capillary density in senile rats. After exercise, rats from both age groups had a higher capillary–fibre ratio. Furthermore, following exercise, the capillary–fibre ratio of the senile rats increased to a level equal to the level of the non-exercised adult rats. This increase in capillary–fibre ratio was associated with an increased capillary density. Thus, these studies suggest that the hearts of animals in the oldest group are not limited with regard to their ability to increase capillarity with increasing demands.

Hypoxia, either on the basis of decreased myocardial capillarity or on the basis of altered diffusion characteristics for oxygen (Sobel, Masserman, and Parsa 1964), has been suggested as an important mechanism of age changes in myocardial function. To examine this hypothesis from a functional point of view, the capacity of the coronary vascular bed to delivery oxygen was examined in isolated non-blood perfused rat heart preparations from 12-, 24-, and 27-month-old rat hearts (Weisteldt, Wright, Shreiner, Lakatta, and Shock 1971). Coronary flow for the adult and senile rat under conditions of maximal hypoxic stimulation to coronary vasodilation was determined. The total maximal coronary flow per heart did not differ significantly between animals of these two age groups. When coronary flow was normalized for dry heart weight, there was a small but statistically significant difference in coronary flow. The hearts from the oldest age group had a maximal coronary flow per gram dry heart weight that was 8.5 per cent less than hearts from the adult group. The total weight of hearts from the older group was 7.3 per cent higher than the adult group. Thus, these data suggest that there is some hypertrophy of the myocardium associated with age and that this hypertrophy is not accompanied by a concomitant increase in the size of the coronary vascular bed in the absence of exercise. The total decrease is small. Oxygen extraction was measured in the same hearts. No difference was found. Thus, these observations do not support the notion that there is a major age change in the delivery of oxygen or essential nutrients to the myocardial cell in association with aging.

At present, there is conflicting evidence with regard to alterations in myocardial oxidative phosphorylation with age. Gold, Gee, and Strehler (1968) found no significant difference in terms of efficiency and respiratory control, or in phosphorylation rates in mitochondria isolated from hearts of senile rats. In the hamster, Inamdar, Person, Kohnen, Duncan, and Mackler (1974) again found no significant difference. In contrast, Chen, Warshaw, and Sanadi (1972) found that state-3 (ADP-stimulated) respiration of myocardial mitochondria declined in rats after the age of 20 months, and Frolkis and Bogatskaya (1968) found higher P/O ratios and less mitochondrial content. Future studies examining functional and other metabolic correlates of alterations in mictochondrial respiratory function will be important in assessing the physiological significance of this observation. At present, it is difficult to conclude that alterations in the coronary vasculature, oxygen extraction ability, or oxidative phosphorylation account for major functional changes in the heart with age.

Thus, we have stressed the role of increased stiffness, prolonged relaxation, decreased contractile ability, and receptor mediated inotropic response in describing the age changes in cardiac muscle.

Addendum

Since the time of presentation of the original material, a number of aspects of aging in cardiac muscle have been further clarified. The studies of Spurgeon, Thorne, Yin, Shock, and Weisfeldt (1977) document that there is an age-associated increase in stiffness of left ventricular trabeculae carneae in muscles taken from the left ventricle of senescent rats. The final data dealing with age-associated changes in diastolic stiffness in the intact beagle heart from old and young dogs has also been presented and shows a very clear-cut age related increase in left ventricular stiffness (Templeton, Platt, Willerson, and Weisfeldt 1979). This increase in left ventricular stiffness was noted as being present both during diastole and systole. It remains unclear what the mechanisms of age-associated increase in stiffness are, though it seems that since the changes are systolic as well as diastolic there are changes in either series elastic stiffness or contractile protein stiffness as well as changes in elements contributing to diastolic left ventricular or cardiac muscle stiffness.

With regard to the age-associated prolongation of relaxation, such prolongation of relaxation was also noted in the aging beagle dog hearts (Templeton, Platt, Willerson, and Weisfeldt 1979). In terms of the mechanism of the age-associated prolongation of relaxation studies in rat hearts, studies have been completed in which an age-associated decrease in the rate of calcium uptake by microsomal preparations was apparent (Froehlich, Lakatta, Beard, Spurgeon, Weisfeldt, and Gerstenblith 1978). Thus, one possible mechanism for the prolongation of relaxation is a delay or a prolonged time course of re-uptake of calcium during the time of relaxation following cardiac muscle contraction. Studies in man (Yin, Raizes, Guarnieri, Spurgeon, Lakatta, Fortuin, and Weisfeldt 1978) utilizing one-dimensional M-mode echocardiography in a normal aging population have tended to confirm the studies in isolated cardiac tissue and intact animal models in terms of age changes in the physiological variables of cardiac function. The initial study of increase in left ventricular wall thickness suggested strongly that there is an age-associated increase in left ventricular mass in association with aging in non-hypertensive subjects. Also, there was a decrease in the mitral valve closing velocity suggesting an age-associated alteration in relaxation and/or left ventricular stiffness. Importantly, there was no age-associated change in left ventricular cavity size or shortening fraction (that is estimated ejection fraction). These studies were pursued further by Yin and associates (Gerstenblith, Spurgeon, Froehlich, Weisteldt, and Lakatta, in press) who examined left ventricular function during haemodynamic stress with and without beta-adrenergic blockade using M-mode echo-cardiography in man. In this cross-sectional study no age-associated change in indices of left ventricular function were apparent at rest or in the presence of beta-blockade without stress. With infusion of phenylephrine after beta-adrenergic blockade, aged subjects showed significantly greater dilatation of the left ventricle as estimated by cavity dimension at end-diastole. This observation suggested that in the presence of beta-adrenergic blockade the aging heart could deal with the haemodynamic stress only with increased use of the Frank–Starling mechanism. The over-all picture of these studies is quite similar to that in the aging animal models where left ventricular contractile function is well-preserved in the aged individuals.

Studies showing an age-associated decrease in the inotropic response to the digitalis glycoside, ouabain, have been completed utilizing the rat model. In this same model and in the same preparations there was no age-associated decrease in the inotropic response to paired electrical pacing. These data support the notion that there is an age-associated decrease in the inotropic response to agents whose inotropic effect is mediated through a cell membrane receptor mechanism, whereas there is no apparent age-associated decrease in the inotropic response to agents which do not require such receptors. The age-associated decrease in inotropic response to digitalis glycosides has been confirmed and extended in the beagle dog by Guarnieri, Spurgeon, Weisfeldt, and Lakatta (1978). These studies demonstrated that the dose–response relationship for toxicity in old animals was not significantly different from that of young animals, but the inotropic response was significantly diminished.

Acknowledgements

I would like to acknowledge the substantial contribution of Drs Edward Lakatta, Harold Spurgeon, Gary Gerstenblith, and Nathan W. Shock in the performance and interpretation of these studies.

References

ALPERT, N. R., GALE, H. H., and TAYLOR, N. (1967). The effect of age on contractile protein ATPase activity and the velocity of shortening. In *Factors influencing myocardial contractility* (eds. K. Kavaler, R. D. Tanz, and J. Roberts), pp. 127–33. Academic Press, New York.

BERG, B. N. and HARMISON, C. R. (1955). Blood pressure and heart size in aging rats. *J. Gerontol.*, **10**, 416–19.

CHEN, J. C., WARSHAW, J. B. and SANADI, D. R. (1972). Regulation of mitochondrial respiration in senescence. *J. cell. Physiol.*, **80**, 141–8.

FROEHLICH, J. P., LAKATTA, E. G., BEARD, E., SPURGEON, H. A., WEISFELDT, M. L., and GERSTENBLITH, G. (1978). Studies of sarcoplasmic reticulum function and contraction duration in young adult and aged rat myocardium. *J. mol. cell. Cardiol.*, **10**, 427–38.

FROLKIS, V. V. and BOGATSKAYA, L. N. (1968). The energy metabolism of myocardium and its regulation in animals of various age. *Exp. Gerontol.*, **3**, 199–210.

——, BEZRUKOV, V. V., BOGATSKAYA, L. N., VERKHRATSKY, N. S., ZAMOSTIAN, V. P., SHEVTCHUK, V. G., and SHTCHEGOLEVA, I. V. (1970). Catecholamines in the metabolism and functions regation in aging. *Gerontologia*, **16**, 129–40.

GERSTENBLITH, G., LAKATTA, E. G., SPURGEON, H., SHOCK, N. W., and WEISFELDT, M.L. (1975). Diminished ouabain sensitivity in aged myocardium. *Fed. Proc.*, **34**, 827.

——, SPURGEON, H. A., FROEHLICH, J. P., WEISFELDT, M. L., and LAKATTA, E. G. 1979). Diminished inotropic responsiveness to ouabain in aged rat myocardium. *Circulation Res.* (In press.)

GEY, K. F., BURKARD, W. P., and PLETSCHER, A. (1965). Variation of the norepinephrine metabolism of the rat heart with age. *Gerontologia*, **11**, 1–11.

GOLD, P. H., GEE, M. V., and STREHLER, B. L. (1968). Effect of age on oxidative phosphorylation in the rat. *J. Gerontol.*, **23**, 509–12.

GUARNIERI, T., SPURGEON, H. A., WEISFELDT, M. L., and LAKATTA, E. G. (1978). Unaltered toxicity but decreased inotropic response to acetylstrophanthidin (ACS) in senescence. (Abstract) *Circulation*, **58** (Suppl. II), 11–573.

HERBENER, G. H. and TIEU MINH THU (1971). Quantitation of mitochondrial compartment size and composition in heart and liver of very old mice. *Anat. Rec.*, **169**, 339.

INAMDAR, A. R., PERSON, R., KOHNEN, P., DUNCAN, H., and MACKLER, B. (1974). Effect of age on oxidative phosphorylation in tissues of hamsters. *J. Gerontol.*, **29**, 638–42.

KRUEGER, J. W. and POLLACK, G. H. (1975). Myocardial sarcomere dynamics during isometric contraction. *J. Physiol.*, **251**, 627–43.

LAKATTA, E. G., GERSTENBLITH, G., ANGELL, C. S., SHOCK, N. W., and WEISFELDT, M. L. (1975a). Diminished inotropic response of aged myocardium to catecholamines. *Circulation Res.*, **36**, 262–9.

——, ——, ——, ——, and —— (1975b). Prolonged contraction duration in aged myocardium. *J. clin. Invest.*, **55**, 61–8.

LEE, J. C., KARPELES, L. M., and DOWNING, S. E. (1972). Age-related changes of cardiac performance in male rats. *Amer. J. Physiol.*, **222**, 432–8.

LEE, S. L., MAINWOOD, G. W., and KORECKY, B. (1970). The electrical and mechanical response of rat papillary muscle to paired pulse stimulation. *Can. J. Physiol. Pharmacol.*, **48**, 216–25.

RAKUSAN, K. and POUPA, O. (1964). Capillaries and muscle fibres in the heart of the old rats. *Gerontologia*, **9**, 107–12.

ROLETT, E. L. (1974). Adrenergic mechanisms in mammalian myocardium. In *The mammalian myocardium* (ed. G. A. Langer and J. Brady), pp. 219–50. J. Wiley and Sons, New York.

ROTHBAUM, D. A., SHAW, D. J., ANGELL, C. S., and SHOCK, N. W. (1973). Cardiac performance in the unanesthetized senescent male rat. *J. Gerontol.*, **28**, 287–92.

SHREINER, D. P., WEISFELDT, M. L., and Shock, N. W. (1969). Effects of age, sex, and breeding status on the rat heart. *Amer. J. Physiol.*, **217**, 176–80.

SOBEL, H., MASSERMAN, R., and PARSA, K. (1964). Effect of age on the transvascular passage of I^{131} labelled albumin in hearts of dogs. *J. Gerontol.*, **19**, 501–4.

SPURGEON, H. A., THORNE, P., YIN, P., WEISFELDT, M. L., and SHOCK, N. W. (1976). Changes in dynamic stiffness of aged rat myocardium. *Fed. Proc.*, **35**, 2251.

——, ——, ——, SHOCK, N. W., and WEISFELDT, M. L. (1977). Increased dynamic stiffness of trabeculae carneae from the senescent rat. *Amer. J. Physiol.*, **1**, H373–80.

TEMPLETON, G. H., ECKER, R. R., and MITCHELL, J. H. (1972). Left ventricular stiffness during diastole and systole: the influence of changes in volume and inotropic state. *Cardiovasc. Res*, **6**, 95–100.

——, ADCOCK, R. C., and WILLERSON, J. T. (1973). Influence of hypoxia on isolated papillary muscle stiffness and its elastic and viscous components. *Circulation* (Suppl. IV), **48**, 67 (abs).

——, WILDENTHAL, K., WILLERSON, J. T., and REARDON, W. C. (1974). Influence of temperature on the mechanical properties of cardiac muscle. *Circulation Res.*, **34**, 624–34.

——, PLATT, M. R., WILLERSON, J. T., and WEISFELDT, M. L. (1979). Influence of aging on left ventricular hemodynamics and stiffness in beagles. *Circulation Res.*, **44**, 189–94.

TOMANEK, R. J. (1969). Effects of age and exercise on the extent of the myocardial capillary bed. *Anat. Rec.*, **167**, 55–62.

——, and KARLSSON, U. L. (1973). Myocardial ultrastructure of young and senescent rats. *Ultrastruc. Res.*, **42**, 201–20.

TRAVIS, D. F. and TRAVIS, A. (1972). Ultrastructural changes in left ventricular rat myocardial cells with age. *J. Ultrastruc. Res.*, **39**, 124–48.

WEISFELDT, M. L., LOEVEN, W. A., and SHOCK, N. W. (1971). Resting and active mechanical properties of trabeculae carneae from aged male rats. *Amer. J. Physiol.* **220**, 1921–7.

——, WRIGHT, J. R., SHREINER, D. P., LAKATTA, E., and SHOCK, N. W. (1971). Coronary flow and oxygen extraction in the perfused heart of senescent male rats. *J. appl. Physiol.*, **30**, 44–9.

——, ARMSTRONG, P., SCULLY, H. E., SANDERS, C. A., and DAGGETT, W. M. (1974). Incomplete relaxation between beats after myocardial hypoxia and ischaemia. *J. clin. Invest.*, **53**, 1626–36.

WILENS, S. L. and SPROUL, E. E. (1938). Spontaneous cardiovascular disease in the rat. *Amer. J. Pathol.*, **14**, 177–216.

YIN, F. C., SPURGEON, H. A. RAIZES, G. S., GREENE, H. L., WEISFELDT, M. L., and SHOCK, N. W. (1976). Age associated decrease in chronotropic response to isoproterenol. *Circulation*, **54**, 651.

——, RAIZES, G. S., GUARNIERI, T., SPURGEON, H. A., LAKATTA, E. G., FORTUIN, N. J., and WEISFELDT, M. L. (1978). Age associated decrease in ventricular response to hemodynamic stress during beta; adrenergic blockade. *Brit. Heart J.*, **40**, 1349–55.

Human plasma lipoproteins: implications of genetic variants for the metabolic roles of the lipoprotein Herbert J. Kayden

Introduction

In the past three to four decades remarkable advances have been made in understanding the chemical and physical composition of plasma lipoproteins in man. Sophisticated methodology and instrumentation have been of great help to the many investigators who have been interested in defining the composition of the lipoproteins as an important step in learning the precise metabolic role of these lipoproteins. Much of the published data on lipoproteins are descriptive, and our assumptions about synthesis, metabolism, and specific functions is inferred from experiments in other species. But neither lower mammals, nor fish, amphibia, reptiles, and birds, when studied in their natural state, have lipoprotein particles resembling the lipoproteins found in man. But manipulations of the diet, administration of drugs, and changes in the environment of these experimental animals, have permitted investigators to alter the lipoprotein particles (both in content and composition) toward the pattern that is associated with disease in humans. These studies are of great importance and have provided the best models for the study and the treatment of atherosclerosis.

There is another approach to the study of human plasma lipoproteins that has been extremely fruitful: this is the study of genetic mutations in humans, and it is from the study of these unusual individuals that so much knowledge about lipoproteins has been accumulated. In this chapter, I have selected a number of genetic disorders of lipoproteins—some characterized by an absence or striking diminution in one class of lipoproteins, and others by an excess of a group of lipoproteins. These abnormalities of lipoproteins are accompanied by a particular series of signs and symptoms: the dependence of the latter upon the lipoprotein disorder is the essential challenge to the investigator. Since this has been a special interest of mine, I have selected disorders and studies with which I am most familiar. One additional comment relates to the interrelations between lipoprotein distribution and longevity—there is considerable published evidence that these may be related, and this material will be referred to subsequently.

Classes of lipoprotein

There are several techniques for separating the lipoproteins, but the most widely used system since 1955 is ultracentrifugation (Havel, Eder, and Bragdon 1955). This method involves successive sequential ultracentrifugation of plasma or serum in increasing densities for periods of 20 to 40 hours, leading to the isolation of three major classes of lipoprotein which float to the top of the tubes, and are drawn off for chemical, physical, and electron microscopic studies. The three classes are designated: very low density lipoproteins (VLDL); low density lipoproteins (LDL); and high density lipoproteins (HDL). Table 1 lists the chemical and physical characteristics of the three classes of lipoprotein. Studies

Table 1   Chemical composition of human plasma lipoproteins

	Density (g/ml)[†]	Electro-phoretic mobility [‡]	Per cent protein (by weight)	Per cent of the total lipid (by weight)		
				Chol.[(a)]	Trig.[(b)]	Phos.[(c)]
Chylomicrons	0.95	Remains at origin	1–2	2–12	80–95	3–15
Very low density lipoproteins (VLDL)	0.95–1.006	Pre-beta §	10	9–24	50–80	10–25
Low density lipoproteins (LDL)	1.006–1.063	Beta §	25	57	13	30
High density lipoproteins (HDL)	1.063–1.210	Alpha §	50	30	10	60

†Used to separate and classify lipoproteins in the preparative or analytical ultracentrifuges.
‡On paper or agarose gel.
§As compared to the globulins.
[(a)]Chol. = Cholesterol.
[(b)]Trig. = Triglycerides.
[(c)]Phos. = Phospholipid.

in the past 10 years have concentrated upon the composition of the apoproteins of the individual lipoproteins; Table 2 presents our current description of the apoproteins of the lipoproteins. It should be noted that the 'C' apoproteins are represented in both VLDL and in HDL. The composition of the B apoprotein has not been characterized at the present time, despite the efforts of many laboratories. It is widely held that synthesis of VLDL and HDL takes place by the liver cell, the hepatocyte, and that transfer of the 'C' peptides from VLDL to HDL occurs in the plasma, and that LDL is derived from VLDL and is almost exclusively formed as *plasma* lipoprotein (Hamilton and Kayden 1975).

Table 2 Current lipoprotein terminologies

Lipo-protein	Apolipo-proteins	Lipoprotein families	Polypeptides
VLDL	Apo VLDL	LP-B	Apo B
		LP-C	Apo C-I
			Apo C-II
			Apo C-III-1
			Apo C-III-2
LDL	Apo LDL	LP-B	Apo B
HDL	Apo HDL	LP-A	Apo A-I
			Apo A-II
		LP-C	Apo C-I
			Apo C-II
			Apo C-III-1
			Apo C-III-2

Abetalipoproteinaemia

The genetic disorder, abetalipoproteinaemia, was first described in 1950 and fewer than fifty patients have been described in the world's literature. The disease is believed to be transmitted as an autosomal recessive and is associated with evidences of fat malabsorption, neurologic abnormalities, acanthocytosis (abnormal red blood cells), retinitis pigmentosa, and the complete absence in the plasma of chylomicrons, VLDL, and LDL, and some abnormalities in the composition of HDL. Review articles have appeared which describe this disorder in detail (Kayden 1972; Frederickson, Gotto, and Levy 1972a). The disorder has been viewed by one group as the consequences of the absence of B lipoproteins (or B apoprotein), and erythrocyte, retinal, and neural tissues are abnormal due to this deficiency. Another group of investigators believes that malabsorption of vitamins or other trace components is responsible for subsequent abnormalities in other systems of the body. There is insufficient evidence to establish conclusively which point of view is correct, if indeed these are the only explanations, and if they are mutually exclusive. Proponents of the nutritional deficiency theory have been treating patients with this disorder at a much earlier age than originally, since our diagnostic skills are better, and the severity of the symptoms appears now to be ameliorated.

What is striking, however, is that the absence of several classes of lipoprotein is not incompatible with near normal development of the human organism. In our clinic, two of our patients, a young man of 23, and a young woman of 20, are well developed and intelligent, and it would take a skilled observer to detect any abnormalities in their ordinary functions. The certainty that plasma lipoproteins are essential to the integrity of cell membranes or to the delivery of triglycerides and cholesterol to the tissues can be questioned when one examines certain patients with abetalipoproteinemia. I shall refer several times during this paper to the insecurity of studying solely the *plasma* lipoproteins in connection with *whole body* metabolism of lipids and lipoproteins. There is the obvious constraint that the extrapolations we make concerning human metabolism from patients with abetalipoproteinaemia are inappropriate, and that these patients are merely examples of a highly adaptive state to the genetic abnormality. But I suggest that the intensive study of these patients has been and continues to be rewarding for our evaluation of the interrelationships of plasma lipoproteins and metabolism of lipids in the human subject. It will take many years of additional studies to establish what the consequences of 'B protein' deficiency in plasma lipoproteins are; we have not as yet been able to make any statements about atherosclerosis in these patients, but it is an area of intensive study. No animal model approaches the usefulness of these patients for this whole area. I do not propose to review the disorder labelled hypobetalipoproteinaemia, though its genetic mode of transmission as an autosomal dominant, and the development of abetalipoproteinaemia in the offspring of parents who are heterozygous for hypobetalipoproteinaemia make it a fascinating genetic mutation to study (Cottrill, Glueck, Leuba, Millett, Puppione, and Brown 1974; Biemer and McCammon 1975).

Tangier disease

The complete absence or striking deficiency of high density lipoproteins (HDL) in human plasma has been known since 1960, and the disease has been labelled Tangier Disease, after the island in the Chesapeake Bay near Virginia, USA, where the first cases were identified. Studies in more than a dozen patients have established that the plasma lipoprotein abnormalities, and deposition of cholesteryl esters in the tissues of the body (spleen, liver, lymph nodes, tonsils, cornea, intestinal mucosa, thymus, etc.) and neurological abnormalities are the cardinal features of this genetic disorder, which is probably due to a mutant autosomal recessive gene affecting the synthesis of HDL. I do not plan to give an elaborate review of the metabolic abnormalities and studies of this disorder; two references are supplied (Fredrickson, Gotto, and Levy 1972b; Assmann, Smootz, Adler, Capurso, and Oette 1977). To the investigator who is concerned with defining the metabolic activities of the lipoproteins, the abnormal accumulation of cholesteryl esters in tissues is a challenging observation. Some investigators believe that excessive amounts of free cholesterol within cells are possibly injurious to the integrity of the cell, and therefore, the cells promptly esterify cholesterol to its less polar form as the ester. Is Tangier Disease an example of the failure of the usual transport system of excess cholesterol from the tissue cells back to the liver for appropriate catabolism? Should there not be evidence of exuberant atherosclerosis at a very early age, similar to what we observe in homozygous familial hypercholesterolaemia? Once again, it is apparent that we need to continue to observe these patients carefully in an effort to identify precisely the metabolic consequences of their lipoprotein abnormality.

Disorders characterized by deficiencies in enzyme activities

The disorders which have been discussed so far are concerned with low or absent concentrations of certain plasma lipoproteins. Before discussing genetically determined abnormal states characterized by elevations in plasma lipoproteins, I should like to refer to two disorders which are characterized by deficiencies in enzyme activities involving lipid metabolism. As we shall see, in both of these disorders, although the metabolic pathways are markedly disturbed, accommodation to the lack of these enzyme activities can occur.

The first disorder is called familial hyperchylomicronaemia with deficiency of lipoprotein lipase (Fredrickson and Levy 1972). This latter enzyme is present in the endothelial capillary linings of adipose tissue, and can be measured in the plasma following an appropriate stimulus (intravenously administered heparin) whereupon the enzyme is released into the circulating blood. The enzyme is responsible for liberating fatty acids from the triglycerides and thereby is essential to initiating the conversion of chylomicrons and very low density lipoproteins to smaller moieties. Absence or impaired function of this enzyme results in continued circulation of the large particles, and, under certain circumstances, clinical syndromes involving inflammation of the pancreas. But the disorder is not characterized by premature or accelerated atherosclerosis, and with appropriate dietary modification these patients appear to have a satisfactory nutritional state and normal adipose tissue metabolism. The other enzymatic deficiency concerns an enzyme secreted by the liver, but which is active in the plasma and is responsible for esterifying the hydroxyl group of cholesterol with a fatty acid derived from circulating phospholipids. This enzyme is called lecithin: cholesterol acyl transferase and is abbreviated LCAT (Norum, Glomset, and Gjone 1972). The characteristic plasma lipoprotein abnormality is reflected in a change in the percentage of ester cholesterol of the total cholesterol—from usual levels of 72 per cent of esterified cholesterol to a level below 10 per cent—and elevation of the triglyceride content evidenced by an increase in VLDL. The clinical syndrome associated with LCAT deficiency includes corneal scarring and disease of the kidney leading to kidney failure in some patients in the fourth and fifth decades. But normal development, good nutritional state, and non-acceleration of atherosclerosis are features of the small number (fewer than twelve) of patients with this genetic disorder. The circulating lipoproteins have a different morphology as seen in the electron microscope, but cell development does not seem impaired. This disorder again raises the question of whether we have overemphasized the importance of the structure of human plasma lipoproteins.

Familial hypercholesterolaemia

Of all the genetically determined disorders of human plasma lipoproteins, the most widely distributed, best recognized, and intensively studied is the disease familial hypercholesterolaemia (or hyperbetalipoproteinaemia). The disorder is transmitted as an autosomal dominant, and the clinical syndrome includes tendon and skin manifestations, and most importantly, atherosclerosis is strikingly accelerated. In the homozygous state, familial hyperbetalipoproteinemia can be suspected by analysis of cord blood, and occlusive disease of the coronary arteries may occur in the first decade of life. The lethal effects of this genetic disorder have been well documented in family studies and in the rarity of adult survivors of the homozygous state. The study of the plasma lipoproteins in such subjects has usually shown only a marked increase in the concentration of LDL, and despite many efforts, no qualitative abnormality in the LDL has been consistently identified. The content as well as the percentage of HDL is reduced. Clinical experience had taught us that many patients with this disorder appeared to have almost 'fixed' levels of LDL, and they were most resistant to all forms of treatment and manipulations of diet. Other patients, with what appeared to be an indistinguishable biochemical and clinical state, had lipoprotein levels that were not quite so resistant to treatment, and vigorous therapy could modify plasma LDL concentrations.

A significant advance in our knowledge of the basic abnormality in familial hypercholesterolaemia has been made by the studies of M. Brown and J. Goldstein (1974a, b; 1976). In an elegantly conceived and executed series of experiments, they have shown that fibroblasts grown in tissue culture from skin biopsies of patients with familial hypercholesterolaemia exhibit different responses to changes in the composition of the nutrient medium from fibroblasts obtained from normal subjects and correspondingly treated. It has been known for many years that cells require cholesterol for membrane synthesis for division and repair, and that this cholesterol is preferentially taken up by the cells from the medium. If the medium is deprived of lipid, the cells begin to synthesize cholesterol from 2 carbon elements. Brown and Goldstein (1974a) showed that when the synthesizing system was operating at a high level of activity, due to substitution of lipoprotein deficient serum for normal medium, the restoration of lipid (sterol) to the medium suppressed the high rate of activity in normal cells, but was ineffective in cells from homozygous hypercholesterolaemic patients. Extending their studies, they documented that cells from normal subjects regulated the amount of specific lipoprotein (LDL) to be taken into the cell by adjusting the number of receptors for LDL to be synthesized by the cell and to function at the cell surface for the uptake of LDL. Cells from patients with the genetic abnormality homozygous hypercholesterolaemia were completely deficient or showed a striking reduction in the number of receptors that developed during the manipulation of nutrient medium. This study of peripheral tissues (as opposed to intestine and liver) suggests that cells at the periphery may have an important catabolic role in the metabolism of LDL. We have confirmed the findings by Brown and Goldstein, and have demonstrated that lymphocytes in culture exhibit similar qualitative responses to those of the fibroblasts—and that lymphoid cells from homozygous hypercholesterolaemic patients also demonstrate abnormal responses to culture medium manipulation; studies on fresh lymphocytes in short-term culture have similar characteristics (Kayden, Hatam, and Beratis 1976; Ho, Brown, Kayden, and Goldstein 1976; Ho, Brown, Bilheimer, and Goldstein 1976). These studies focus attention on the tissues, and raise questions about the primacy of the plasma lipoprotein abnormalities, both quantitatively and perhaps qualitatively. We appear to be severely handicapped if we restrict our studies to measurements of plasma lipoproteins. Further evidence of the virtual immutability of plasma LDL concentrations in certain patients with familial homozygous hypercholesterolaemia is provided by the studies of Deckelbaum, Lees, Small, Hedberg, and Grundy (1977). In two patients with this disorder, complete bile diversion was accomplished by ligation of the common bile duct and external drainage of all the bile. Calculations of the amount of sterol lost by this route was 560 g over 14 months in one patient and 400 g over 10 months in the other, equivalent to 14 and 5 total body cholesterol pools respectively. Despite this massive drainage, the plasma levels showed no change in cholesterol level, and there was no evident effect upon the tissue stores. In these patients it is apparent that sterol synthesis had merely increased to equal the maximum rate of cholesterol catabolism that can be achieved. Our approach to therapy must be directed toward the control of synthesis of LDL or of a change in the tissue—perfusing directed levels of LDL.

Hyperalphalipoproteinaemia

In the past 2–3 years, attention has been focused on the concentration of HDL in plasma, and kindreds have been described in whom 'hyperalphalipoprotein-aemia' exists. It is not apparent that the elevation in this fraction of the plasma lipoprotein is due to a genetic role controlling HDL synthesis. What is striking, however, is that the life span of individuals in the kindreds was longer than for control populations as determined by life tables, and that the incidence of myocardial infarction (as a reflection of atherosclerosis) was considerably lower than in control populations. What extrapolations can be made from this data on hyperalphalipoproteinaemia, which admittedly is difficult to classify as a genetic disorder? A number of studies have documented that individuals in certain populations who are apparently free of coronary disease have higher HDL concentrations than affected individuals matched for age and sex in the same geographical region. Investigators studying populations where longevity is common have reported that the concentration of HDL is higher than in other populations where the life span is not as long. For this volume on aging, I should perhaps have altered the order of discussion of the various lipoprotein disorders, placing hyperalphalipoproteinaemia first. But the evidence of genetic control of HDL concentration in these individuals is not strong, and it may be possible to document that the influence is more precisely demonstrable as certain cellular phenomena (as in homozygous hypercholesterolaemia), and that the plasma manifestation is merely representative of the genetic activity.

Relationship between HDL concentration and atherosclerosis

The observation of varying concentrations of HDL and LDL as a function of age and sex has been known for more than 25 years (Barr, Russ, and Eder 1951). In the ensuing years, many analyses have been made in individuals who have sustained a myocardial infarction, and the impression that higher levels of LDL are associated with ischaemic heart disease was accepted. But the newer emphasis upon the absolute concentrations of HDL, stimulated by the writing of Miller and Miller (1975), have suggested that a reduction in HDL concentration may accelerate the development of atherosclerosis—and correspondingly, the question is posed whether increasing HDL concentration may not be beneficial. As indicative of the interest this has generated, I wish to cite only a few studies. The distribution of plasma lipoproteins in middle-aged male runners was measured and compared to a matched control group in California: the former had higher HDL concentrations than the latter (Wood, Haskell, Klein, Lewis, Stern, and Farquhar 1976). Vigorous exercise along with weight reduction increased the HDL concentration in mildly obese women over a four-month period.

From a large body of experimental data, the hypothesis has been derived that HDL serves to transport free cholesterol from the tissues to the liver for catabolism and excretion. In the studies employing tissue culture experiments on fibroblast and lymphoid lines, HDL was a poor inhibitor of LDL uptake by the cells, suggesting specificity for a receptor for LDL. Studies by others using arterial smooth-muscle cultures from swine have suggested that HDL does partially inhibit the uptake and degradation of LDL, and this results in some suppression of the net increment in sterol content of the cells induced by LDL (Carew, Hayes, Koschinsky, and Steinberg 1976). This area of investigation is presently one of the most exciting and active fields currently pursued by laboratories interested in the interrelation between lipoproteins, cellular metabolism, and atherogenesis.

Summary

In summary, I have attempted to stress the important contributions that studies of human diseases due to genetic mutations, reflected in abnormal or unusual plasma lipoprotein concentrations, have made to our understanding of the metabolic role of the lipoproteins and to the disease atherosclerosis. It is apparent that we do not have sufficient information about the synthesis or catabolism of lipoproteins to understand what regulates plasma levels of the individual lipoproteins. In familial homozygous hypercholesterolaemia it would appear that the primary abnormality is manifested at the cellular level, and the elevated circulating lipoproteins may be a consequence, rather than the initiating event. In a book on aging it is most appropriate to indicate that one lipoprotein, HDL, is associated with longevity and a decreased incidence of atherosclerosis and ischaemic heart disease. We must continue our efforts to understand lipoprotein chemistry and metabolism. Perhaps learning how to increase HDL in humans will lengthen our lives and protect us from atherosclerosis.

References

ASSMANN, G., SMOOTZ, E., ADLER, K., CAPURSO, A., and ODETTE, K. (1977). *J. clin. invest.*, **59**, 565.

BARR, D. P., RUSS, E. M., and EDER, H. A. (1951). *Amer. J. Med.*, **11**, 480.

BIEMER, J. J. and McCAMMON, R. E. (1975). *J. lab. clin. Med.*, **85**, 556.

BROWN, M. S. and GOLDSTEIN, J. L. (1974a). *Proc. Nat. Acat. Sci.*, **71**, 788.
—— and —— (1974b). *Biol. Chem.*, **249**, 7306.
—— and —— (1976). *Science, N.Y.* **191**, 150.
CAREW, T. E., HAYES, S. B., KOSCHINSKI, T., and STEINBERG, D. (1976). *Lancet*. 1315.
COTTRILL, C., GLUECK C. J., LEUBA, V., MILLETT, F., PUPPIONE, D., and BROWN, V. W. (1974). *Metabolism*, **23**, 779
DECKELBAUM, R. J., LEES, R. S., SMALL, D. M., HEDBERG, S. E., and GRUNDY, S. M. (1977). *New Engl. J. Med.*, **296**, 465.
FREDRICKSON, D. S. and LEVY, R. I. (1972). In *The metabolic basis of inherited disease* (eds. J. B. Stanbury, J. B. Wyngaarden, and D. S. Fredrickson) p. 51. McGraw-Hill, New York.
——, GOTTO, A. M., and LEVY, R. I. (1972a). In *The metabolic basis of inherited disease* (eds. J. B. Stanbury, J. B. Wyngaarden, and D. S. Fredrickson) p. 493. McGraw-Hill, New York.
——, ——, ——, (1972b). In *The metabolic basis of inherited disease* (eds. J. B. Stanbury, J. B. Wyngaarden and D. S. Frederickson, p. 513. McGraw-Hill, New York.
HAMILTON, R. L. and KAYDEN, H. J. (1975). In *The liver, normal and abnormal functions* (ed. F. F. Becker), p. 351. Marcel Dekker, New York.
HAVEL, R. J., EDER, H. A., and BRAGDON, J. H. (1955). *J. clin. Invest.*, **34**, 1345.
HO, Y. K., BROWN, M. S., KAYDEN, H. J., and GOLDSTEIN, J. L. (1976). *J. exp. Med.*, **144**, 444.
——, ——, BILHEIMER, D. W., and GOLDSTEIN, J. L. (1976). *J. clin. Invest.*, **58**, 1465.
KAYDEN, H. J. (1972). *Ann. Rev. Med.*, **22**, 285.
——, HATAM, L., and BERATIS, N. G. (1976). *Biochemistry*, **15**, 521.
MILLER, G. J. and MILLER, N. E. (1975). *Lancet*, **i**.
NORUM, K. R., GLOMSET, J. A., and Gjone, E. (1972). In *The metabolic basis of inherited disease* (eds. J. B. Stanbury, J. B. Wyngaarden, and D. S. Frederickson), p. 531. McGraw-Hill, New York.
WOOD, P., HASKELL, W., KLEIN, H., LEWIS, S., STERN, M. P., and FARQUHAR, J. W. (1976). *Metabolism*, **25**, 1249.

Session 4

Cellular aspects of atherogenesis

Cellular aspects of atherogenesis Russell Ross

Introduction

Atherosclerosis is the chief cause of death in the Western World (National Heart and Lung Institute 1971). Despite its widespread nature, we have only recently begun to understand the underlying mechanisms associated with the aetiology and pathogenesis of this disease. During the past 20 years most research has focused upon the increased accumulation of lipids within the artery wall (National Heart and Lung Institute 1971), and only recently has attention been focused upon the fact that the lesions of atherosclerosis result from the focal proliferation of smooth muscle cells within the intima of affected sites within the artery wall (National Heart and Lung Institute 1971; Ross and Glomset 1973, 1976; Wissler 1974; Geer and Haust 1972). To understand the mechanisms involved in this intimal smooth muscle proliferative response, it is necessary to understand the factors that maintain the integrity of the lining endothelial cells, and of the intimal and medial smooth muscle cells, and their relationship to both cellular and humoral elements within the blood.

Even though there is now general agreement that the lesions of atherosclerosis are focal proliferative lesions, the factors responsible for the genesis of these lesions are only beginning to be understood. At least three biological phenomena are fundamental to the formation of these lesions. Each of these must be taken into account if we are to understand how this multifactorial disease comes about. These phenomena include:

(1) proliferation of smooth muscle cells within the intima of the affected region;
(2) marked increase in the formation by these cells of connective tissue matrix constituents, including collagen, elastic fibre proteins, and proteoglycans;
(3) deposition of both intracellular and extracellular lipid.

One could go so far as to suggest that if there were no intimal smooth muscle proliferation, there would be no lesions of atherosclerosis.

The 'response to injury' hypothesis

John Glomset and Laurence Harker, my colleagues from the University of Washington, and I have proposed that the lesions of atherosclerosis result as a response to 'injury' of the lining endothelial cells. This proposal represents a modification and unification of the earlier hypotheses proposed by Rudolph Virchow and by J. B. Duguid. Virchow (1856) suggested that when sites in the artery wall are injured, they develop an inflammatory response that is subsequently associated with the proliferation of intimal smooth muscle cells. Duguid (1949) went on to modify this notion by suggesting that platelet thrombi would adhere to these sites of injury and become incorporated into the lesion. Subsequently, French (1966), Mustard and Packham (1975), and ourselves (Ross and Glomset 1973, 1976) have modified this hypothesis to take into account many aspects of the behaviour of arterial cells as they respond to mitogens, lipoproteins, and other substances.

The 'response to injury' hypothesis suggests that the lesions of atherosclerosis result from 'injury' to the lining endothelial cells. This 'injury' leads to alterations in endothelial cell–cell and endothelial cell–connective tissue attachment. These alterations in the endothelium could make them susceptible to the shearing stresses of the normal flow of blood in the artery, resulting in focal sites of altered endothelium or in actual desquamation of the endothelium leading to exposure of the subendothelial connective tissue. At these sites, platelets from the circulation could adhere, aggregate, and release factors normally present within the thrombocytes into the underlying artery wall. At the same time, plasma constituents such as lipoproteins would have free access into the artery wall at the sites where the endothelial barrier had been removed.

The hypothesis suggests that these phenomena precede focal intimal smooth muscle cell proliferation, formation by these cells of connective tissue proteins, and, in the presence of hyperlipidemia, the deposition of lipids. Furthermore, if the endothelial injury is represented by a single occurrence, then the proliferative lesions could be reversible (as may occur in anyone from time to time) and regress. Should the insult be repetitive on a chronic basis, after many years the lesion could become slowly progressive until the proliferative response becomes sufficiently extensive to produce thrombosis and clinical sequelae.

In vivo experiments

The investigations in our laboratories have been aimed at understanding the factors associated with smooth muscle cell proliferation and with the maintenance of endothelial cell integrity. Control of connective tissue synthesis by endothelium and smooth muscle and the factors that regulate lipid metabolism also continue to be objects of research by our group.

Together with Michael Stemerman (Stemerman and Ross 1972), we were able to demonstrate that by using the method of Baumgartner (Baumgartner and Studer 1966), one passage through the internal iliac artery and the aorta with a balloon catheter results in the local removal of the endothelial cells. This event is immediately followed by the adherence of platelets at the sites of exposed subendothelial connective tissue together with focal degranulation of these platelets. This occurs within 10 minutes to 48 hours after de-endothelialization. Within 5–7 days smooth muscle cells were observed migrating through fenestrae in the internal elastic laminae into the intima and proliferating within the intima. Within 30 days after de-endothelialization, the intima contained as many as 20–30 layers of newly proliferated smooth muscle cells surrounded by newly-formed connective tissue matrix. In normo-lipidemic monkeys, these lesions regress after another 3 months (a total of 6 months after injury) so that the intima contains only 2–4 cell layers.

In sharp contrast, if the same experiments are performed in hypercholestero-laemic monkeys (Ross and Harker 1976; Ross and Glomset 1974), (serum cholesterol 250–350 mg per cent), the lesions are no longer reversible. In fact, in addition to interfering with regression, chronic hypercholesterolaemia results in deposition of lipids within the smooth muscle cells as well as in the connective tissue matrix surrounding them.

The observation that platelet adherence aggregation and release is an early event following injury to the endothelium correlated in an interesting manner with a series of studies of arterial smooth muscle cells in culture that were probing for factors important in the proliferation of these cells.

In vitro studies

As with other diploid cells, it is possible to demonstrate that primate arterial smooth muscle cells require serum for proliferation in culture. Studies of the serum requirement by these cells demonstrated that if the serum was made from platelet-free plasma (MPS) rather than from whole blood (MBS) that such platelet-free plasma derived serum (MPS) lacked the capacity to support the growth of the cells in culture. We were further able to demonstrate that all of the mitogenic capacity of whole blood serum (MBS) missing in MPS could be restored to the latter either by adding a purified preparation of platelets to the plasma at the time it was calcified to form serum, or by adding a supernatant derived from exposure of purified platelets to thrombin to the MPS (Ross, Glomset, Kariya, and Harker 1974). The results of these experiments taken together with those by others (Kohler and Lipton 1974; Westermark and Wasteson 1976) conclusively demonstrated that the principal mitogenic capacity of whole blood serum is derived from a factor released from platelets during the process of serum formation.

This platelet-derived factor has been semi-purified and can be demonstrated to be a relatively low molecular weight (10 000–23 000 daltons), basic, relatively heat-stable protein. It has many similarities to a factor isolated from serum by Antoniades, Stathakos, and Scher (1975) and to a factor derived from the pituitary by Gospodarowiscz and Moran (1975) both of which will stimulate the growth of cells in culture. The relationship between these two mitogens and the one derived from the platelet are under continuing investigation.

These studies demonstrated that it is possible to keep diploid cells, such as arterial smooth muscle cells, in a situation of relatively true quiescence in the presence of adequate amounts of nutrients (such as 5 per cent MPS), analogous to the quiescence in which these cells are to be found in the intact artery wall where they would be exposed to filtrates of plasma, rather than serum. (Serum is to be defined under these circumstances as the result of the process of blood coagulation, and exposure of platelets to thrombin during this process.)

In fact, normal cells *in vivo* never 'see' serum unless there is injury accompanied by blood coagulation. These observations, taken together with the *in vivo* studies of endothelial desquamation with a balloon catheter suggest a role for platelets in the process of atherogenesis.

The role of platelets in atherogenesis

To determine whether the adherence, aggregation, and release by platelets at sites of exposure of subendothelial connective tissue were of significance, .we investigated their role in two disease processes associated with atherosclerosis, chronic homocystinaemia, and hypercholesterolaemia. We were able to demonstrate that chronically homocystinaemic baboons have shortened platelet survival similar to that observed in individuals who are homocystinuric (Harker, Slichter, Scott, and Ross 1974) or in some hypercholesterolaemic patients who have clinical evidence of atherosclerosis. There is a direct correlation between the decrease in platelet survival and the loss of endothelium in segments of the artery wall (unpublished observations). We studied these phenomena in the homocystinaemic baboon and after six days of chronic homocystinaemia the baboons were missing approximately 10 per cent of the endothelium from their aorta, while platelet survival was half normal levels (Harker *et al.* 1974). Ninety days of chronic homocystinaemia led to the development at these sites of classical fibromusculoelastic lesions characteristic of preatherosclerotic lesions in man (Harker, Ross, Slichter, and Scott 1976; National Heart and Lung Institute 1971). These intimal proliferative smooth muscle lesions could be prevented if platelet function was inhibited with the agent dipyridemol. Under these circumstances the amount of endothelial injury remained unchanged, whereas platelet survival returned to normal levels. When platelet function was inhibited in this way, even though endothelial injury remained, there were essentially no intimal smooth muscle proliferative lesions (Harker *et al.* 1976). Thus it seems that for smooth muscle proliferation to occur platelets must be able to adhere, aggregate, and release their constituents at sites of arterial injury.

These findings have been confirmed by Moore, Friedman, Singal, Gauldie, and Blajchman (1976) in rabbits in which lesions have been induced with a balloon catheter or with an indwelling catheter. The lesions in these animals were prevented if the rabbits were made thrombocytopenic with an antiplatelet serum prior to ballooning.

Subsequently Ross and Harker (1976) demonstrated decreased platelet survival similar to that observed in the homocystinaemic baboons, in monkeys that were chronically hypercholesterolaemic. When these chronic hypercholesterolaemic monkeys were sacrificed, it was possible to demonstrate that they were missing approximately 5 per cent of the endothelium of their aorta, in similar fashion to the homocystinaemic baboons. There appears to be a relationship bɔtween the different phenomena of chronic hypercholesterolaemia, endothelial injury, decreased platelet survival (as a manifestation of focal platelet adherence, aggregation, and release), and an associated intimal smooth muscle proliferation.

Summary

Cell culture studies of growth properties of arterial smooth muscle cells and of the significance of platelet factors in a culture medium for arterial smooth muscle proliferation have been correlated in an investigation of the importance of these phenomena *in vivo*. Studies in hypercholesterolaemic monkeys and homocystinaemic baboons have supported the notion that focal sites of endothelial injury are accompanied by adherence of platelets and release of platelet constituents together with the ingress of plasma factors into the artery wall at the sites of injury. These are followed by intimal smooth muscle proliferation, formation of new connective tissue proteins by the smooth muscle cells, and, in instances of chronic hyperlipidemia, by the deposition of lipids. Further investigations concerning the nature of the platelet factor and its effect upon cells should enhance our understanding of the nature of the intimal smooth muscle proliferative response. At the same time studies of endothelial cells, and factors necessary for maintenance of endothelial cell integrity should provide further insight into means of lesion prevention.

Acknowledgements

This research was supported in part by grants from USPHS AM 13970 and HL 18645, and the R. J. Reynolds Industries, Inc.

References

ANTIONADES, H. N., STATHAKOS, D., and SCHER, C. D. (1975). Isolation of a cationic polypeptide from human serum that stimulates proliferation of 3T3 cells. *Proc. Nat. Acad. Sci. USA*, **72**, 2635–9.

BAUMGARTNER, VON H. B., and STUDER, A. (1966). Folgen des Gefasskatheterismus am Normo- und Hyperscholesterinaemischen Kaninchen, *Pathol. Microbiol. (Basel)*, **29**, 393–405.

DUGUID, J. B. (1949). Pathogenesis of artiosclerosis. *Lancet*, **ii**, 925–7.

FRENCH, J. E. (1966). Atherosclerosis in relation to the structure and function of the arterial intima, with special reference to the endothelium. *Int. Rev. exp. Pathol.*, **5**, 253–353.

GEER, J. C. and HAUST, M. D. (1972). Smooth muscle cells in atherosclerosis. *Monogr. Atheroscler.*, **2**, 1–88.

GOSPODAROWICZ, D. and MORAN, J. S. (1975). Mitogenic effect of fibroblast growth factor on early passage cultures of human and murine fibroblasts. *J. Cell Biol.*, **66**, 451–7.

HARKER, L. A., SLICHTER, S. H., SCOTT, C. R., and ROSS, R. (1974). Homocystinemia: vascular injury and arterial thrombosis. *New Engl. J. Med.*, **291**, 537–43.

——, Ross, R., Slichter, S., and Scott, C. R. (1976). Homocystine-induced arterio-sclerosis: the role of endothelial cell injury and platelet response in its genesis. *J. clin. Invest.*, **58**, 731–41.

Kohler, N. and Lipton, A. (1974). Platelets as a source of fibroblast growth-promoting activity. *Exp. Cell Res.*, **87**, 297–301.

Moore, S., Friedman, J. R., Singsl, D. P., Gauldie, J., and Blajchman, M. (1976). Inhibition of injury induced thromboatherosclerotic lesions by antiplatelet serum in rabbits. *Thromb. Diath. Haemorrh.*, **36**, 70–81.

Mustard, J. F. and Packham, M. A. (1975). The role of blood and platelets in athero-sclerosis and the complication of atherosclerosis. *Thromb. Diath. Haemorrh.*, **33**, 444–56.

National Heart and Lung Institute (1971). *Arteriosclerosis: a report by the National Heart and Lung Institute* Task Force on Arteriosclerosis. (DHEW Publication No. (NIH) 72-219), Vol. 2. Government Printing Office, Washington D.C.

Ross, R. and Harker, L. (1976). Hyperlipidemia and atherosclerosis. *Science, N. Y.* **193**, 1094–100.

—— and Glomset, J. A. (1973). Atherosclerosis and the arterial smooth muscle cell. *Science, N. Y.* **180**, 1332–9.

—— and —— (1974). In *Studies of primate arterial smooth muscle cells in relation to atherosclerosis, arterial mesenchyme and arteriosclerosis*, (eds. W. D. Wagner and T. B. Clarkson), pp. 265–79. Plenum Press, New York.

—— and —— (1976). The pathogenesis of atherosclerosis. *New Engl. J. Med.*, **295**, 369–77, 420–5.

——, ——, Kariya, B., and Harker, L. (1974). A platelet-dependent serum factor that stimulates the proliferation of arterial smooth muscle cells *in vitro*. *Proc. Nat. Acad. Sci., USA*, **71**, 1207–10.

Stemerman, M. B. and Ross, R. (1972). Experimental arteriosclerosis. I. Fibrous plaque formation in primates, an electron microscope study. *J. exp. Med.*, **136**, 769–89.

Virchow, R. (1856). *Phlogose und Thrombose im Gefassystem, gesammelte Abhand-lungen zur wissenschaftlichen Medicin*, p. 458. Meidinger Sohn and Company, Frankfurt-am-Main.

Westmark, B. and Wasteson, A. (1976). A platelet factor stimulating human normal glial cells. *Exp. Cell Res.*, **98**, 170–4.

Wissler, R. W. (1974). In *Development of the atherosclerotic plaque. The myocardium, failure and infarction* (ed. E. Braunwald), pp. 155–66. H. P. Publishing Company, New York.

Concerning the biological basis of atherosclerosis
Theodore H. Spaet

Introduction

Although many factors contribute to the aging process, perhaps foremost among these are the ones that affect the cardio-vascular system. Arteriosclerosis and atherosclerosis are changes in arteries that progress to a stage where they may ultimately close, thereby cutting off blood to the organs they supply. Although almost any organ may thus be deprived of its lifelines, those most dramatically affected are the heart, the brain, and the kidneys. A man may be said to be as aged as his arteries.

The normal artery consists of three layers. Innermost, defined as closest to the lumen where the blood is transported, is the *intima*. This layer is lined by specialized cells called endothelium; these cells carefully regulate the passage of blood components through the arterial wall, and in doing so show great selectivity. Thus, the materials that reach the deeper layers of the vessel wall are those required for the health of the vessel cells, or those which can be disposed of efficiently. The endothelial cells reside on a bed of connective tissue, but in many human arteries the intima is augmented by several layers of smooth muscle cells, each of which has its associated connective tissue. The intima is separated from the deeper arterial layers by a sheath of connective tissue, the 'internal elastic lamina'.

The middle arterial layer is called the *media*, and in normal vessels this is thickest of the three. It consists of multiple layers of smooth muscle cells sandwiched between various connective tissues. In arteries with fewer than about 17 cell layers of medial cells, there are no capillaries to nourish the media or to carry off its wastes; therefore these tasks must be accomplished by passage of substances from the vessel lumen and by drainage through deeper layers respectively. In small animals, such as the rat and rabbit, this is the situation that universally prevails. However, in the arteries of man and larger mammals, the outer portion of the media contains 'vasa vasorum', capillaries that provide nourishment and drainage similar to that in other tissues. In any case, the normal vessel wall is provided with a drainage system sufficient for its needs.

The *adventitia* is the outermost vascular layer. It is composed of sparse fibroblasts and collagenous connective tissue, and it also contains capillaries and perhaps lymphatic channels as well. Presumably the adventitia is the drainage area for the rest of the vessel wall.

As with endothelial cells, the smooth muscle cells of the other layers, and the fibroblasts of the adventitia are rarely replaced, and show little proliferative activity.

Experimental atherosclerosis

The conditions and relationships described so far apply only to normal vessels. Complex changes are seen in diseased arteries, which include intimal thickening, and deposits of fatty materials and calcium salts. In man, these changes are often seen at an advanced stage, and the factors that brought them about are usually obscure and probably multiple: it is almost impossible to distinguish between initiating and augmenting events. In contrast, the experimental animal can be used to study the consequences of specific manipulations, and very early effects can be characterized. Since many animal diseases have their counterpart in man, it is hoped that experimental atherosclerosis in animals is also a valid model. Our own experiments have concentrated upon the consequences of removing the endothelial cell barrier in rabbits and rats, and the following remarks will emphasize what we have learned from these studies.

A technique for removing endothelium from large arteries in rabbits was devised by Baumgartner (1963), in which an inflated balloon catheter is passed through the vessel under study. This manipulation removes the endothelial cells virtually completely, without producing detectable damage to the deeper vascular structures. In the studies to be described, we have used this technique in rabbits and rats, and have studied the histological and ultrastructural consequences in a variety of circumstances (Spaet, Stemerman, Vieth, and Lejnieks 1975).

When the endothelium is removed, naked connective tissue is now exposed to blood. At this point, blood platelets enter the picture. Such cells normally function to plug up small blood vessels when these are severed or ruptured, and they serve this function by sticking to exposed connective tissues. Although platelets do not react with intact endothelial cells, they readily stick to the connective tissue of de-endothelialized arteries, to form a platelet layer. If the damage occurs in an already distorted and pathological artery, the platelets may react to form a mass or 'thrombus', which can represent the final step to closure of the vessel. However, in the newly injured artery, the reactions produced by the platelet response have quite different implications, as will be discussed.

Within three days after the balloon vessel injury, a healing response becomes evident. This response has two components. One of these concerns endothelial cells from arterial branches which have escaped injury; these start to multiply, and spread over the injured area. This process is rapid at first but slows progressively. Thus, re-endothelialization of ballooned arteries in rabbits is not complete even six months after injury. The other component concerns the smooth muscle cells of the media. These engage in the dual response of poliferation and migration across the internal elastic lamina, so that the healing intima becomes a structure composed of smooth muscles cells and their connective tissue products. However, healing does not result in restoration of the vessel wall to its original state. Instead, the intimal smooth muscle cells continue to multiply, to produce progressive thickening of this structure, the picture of arteriosclerosis. We have examined ballooned aortas from rabbits up to two years after injury, and persistence of intimal thickening is present in all of them. These studies show that loss of endothelium is followed by pathological changes resembling early arteriosclerotic changes in man. In fact, in some of the rabbits studied at two years, there are the typical lipid-laden lesions of atherosclerosis, with cholesterol deposits, even though the animals have been given no special diets. Moreover, atherosclerosis can be produced more rapidly by repeated balloon injury, again without dietary manipulation (Friedman, Moore, and Singal 1975).

The signals to which the blood vessel cells respond has been the subject of considerable recent study. Endothelial cells evidently multiply when they do not have other similar cells in contact with all their edges, and thereby have a stimulus that causes them to cover the blood vessel surface whenever a gap appears. The messengers for smooth muscle cell migration and proliferation are now being characterized, and they present a more complex picture. Early clues were provided by the pioneering studies of Ross and his associates (Ross and Glomset 1976), whereby a platelet role was established by means of tissue culture experiments. It was found that arterial smooth muscle cells required a 'serum factor' for optimal proliferation, and a low-molecular-weight platelet protein appeared to be the source of this factor. Meanwhile, working in another laboratory, Gospodarowicz and Moran (1975) demonstrated the presence of a protein with similar properties derived from the pituitary gland, which stimulated the growth of fibroblasts in tissue culture. Our studies have attempted to apply these '*in vitro*' observations to animal pathology. We have been able to show that rabbits whose blood platelets have been severely depleted by injections of sheep antiserum to rabbit platelets, fail to develop arteriosclerotic lesions in ballooned arteries (Friedman, Stemerman, Wenz, Moore, Gauldie, Gent, Tiell, and Spaet 1977). Moreover, these lesions are significantly retarded in hypophysectomized rats (Tiell, Stemerman and Spaet 1976). The smooth muscle cell reaction is selectively inhibited: endothelial regrowth proceeds normally. These findings suggests that the different cell strains respond to different proliferative stimuli.

The blood vessel lined with smooth muscle instead of endothelial cells is not only platelet-reactive, it also has increased permeability to many plasma components, and it can no longer regulate the entry of substances into the deeper layers. These are thus flooded with constituents which they can no longer handle. Presumably this is the basis for the development of the atherosclerotic plaque and the more advanced arterial disease. Perhaps this is where diet makes its major contribution, since a high cholesterol intake will add a correspondingly additional burden to the disposal problem. The literature on this topic is enormous (Wissler and Geer 1972).

Implications for human disease

If the animal experiments constitute a valid model for man, the question is immediately raised as to how human endothelium is damaged so as to leave exposed subendothelial tissues. The possibilities for such damage are numerous indeed. Infection with certain bacteria or viruses, immune reactions, hypertension, diabetes, ingestion of toxins, and many other adverse environmental conditions are all potential offenders. Endothelial cells have been found circulating in the blood in many disorders, and their presence in this abnormal location indicates that they have become detached from vessel walls (Bouvier, Gaynor, Cintron, Bernhardt, and Spaet 1970).

Finally, what can be done to use our understanding of these reactions in the prevention of heart disease, stroke, and the other consequences of advanced atherosclerosis? Unfortunately, our state of knowledge in this field is still relatively primitive. The technology is not yet at hand which will enable us to make dramatic inroads into the inexorable progress of atherosclerosis. True, certain patients can be helped considerably, as has been shown in the modern control of high blood-pressure where heart attacks and strokes can be greatly reduced. True, promising results have been obtained when drugs that depress platelet function have been used to prevent arterial thrombosis; and restriction of dietary fat and weight loss have proved to be of benefit in high-risk patients.

Vascular disease still represents a major problem in basic biomedical research. It is not presently susceptible to a crash programme, in which known technology can be mobilized to a predictable end. Rather, creative investigation must be encouraged which will serve as fertile soil for new scientific breakthroughs.

References

BAUMGARTNER, H. R. (1963). *Z. Ges. Exp. Med.*, **137**, 227.

BOUVIER, C. A., GAYNOR, E., CINTRON, J. R., BERNHARDT, B., and SPAET, T. H. (1970). *Thromb. Diath. Haem. Suppl.*, **40**, 163.

FRIEDMAN, R. J., MOORE, S., and SINGAL, D. P. (1975). *Lab. Invest.*, **30**, 404.

STEMERMAN, M. B., WENZ, B., MOORE, S., GAULDIE, J., GENT, M., TIELL, M. L., and SPAET, T. H. (1977). The effect of thrombocytopenia on experimental arteriosclerotic lesion formation in rabbits. Smooth muscle cell proliferation and re-endothelialization. *J. clin. Invest.* **60**, 1191.

TIELL, M. L., STEMERMAN, M. B., and SPAET, T. H. (1978). The influence of the pituitary on arterial intimal proliferation in the rat. *Lire, Res.* **42**, 644.

Discussion—Session 4 N. Simionescu

The experimental results reported by Drs Ross and Spaet indicate that the endothelial injury in animals is followed by modifications of the intima which are similar to those observed in atherosclerosis in humans. However, the understanding of the intimate mechanisms of the endothelium involvement in atherogenesis largely depends on the concomitant progress made in the knowledge of the molecular and cellular characteristics of the normal endothelium and its age-associated changes.

Therefore, four lines of investigation should be promoted in parallel:

1. *The molecular and cellular biology of the arterial endothelium*, revealing the molecular organization which accounts for its normal metabolic and boundary characteristics.

2. *The aging (chronobiology) of the arterial endothelium* defined as mechanisms of changes which characterize the 'aged' endothelium, and its possible relationships with atherosclerosis.

3. *The clinical pathology of the arterial endothelium*, giving estimates on the early perturbations associated with the initiation of the atheromatous plaques in humans.

4. *Experimental pathology*, exploring the endothelial injury as atherogenetic mechanisms.

Very little is known about the first three aspects. I want to focus my discussion on some promising trends in one of them, the molecular and cellular biology of arterial endothelium. On this issue, there are three basic aspects we have to know a little more about:

(a) the metabolic activities of the endothelium;
(b) its molecular microenvironment;
(c) its characteristics as a semi-permeable barrier monitoring the nutrition and the house-cleaning of the vascular wall.

Metabolic activities. The endothelium contributes to the balance between the coagulant and anticoagulant systems by producing the tissue factor, the anti-haemophilic factor, (VIII) the plasminogen activator, prostacyclin, etc. It also interferes in the metabolism of the circulating vaso-active substances which are potentially aggressive for the integrity of the endothelial lining. The latter secretes enzymes which inactivate the norepenephrine, serotonin, and bradykinin. and convert angiotensin I in angiotensin II by the angiotensin converting enzyme. It also produces prostaglandins. The activities so far detected vary largely from one vascular bed to another and it remains to be established which are the metabolic peculiarities of the arterial endothelium and how their perturbations are or are not associated with atherogenesis.

Arterial endothelium as a semi-permeable barrier. Despite its apparent uniformity, when examined in detail the vascular endothelium shows a certain degree of heterogeneity. This involves all features which are potentially instrumental in permeability such as the vesicles, the transendothelial channels, and the intercellular junctions. Let us take as example the organization of contacts between endothelial cells. These can be expressed in two terms:

1. Intercellular coupling via gap (communicating) junctions.
2. Intercellular sealings secured by the tight (occluding) junctions.

We found that each vascular segment has its own characteristic organization of the endothelial junctions. In arteries, the coupling via communicating (gap) junctions is extensive, but the sealing through tight junctions is particularly variable not only from one artery to another, but also between regions of the same artery.

Some heterogeneity involves the permeability to water-soluble molecules and the size limit of the permeant molecules remains to be determined. Moreover, there is not convincing information as to whether and how the lipids and lipoproteins can cross the arterial endothelium. This raises the crucial question whether the lipid deposition of the atheromatous plaque is of a blood origin or represents the product of an abnormal local synthesis.

The molecular environment of the endothelium. The cell coat of the blood front of the endothelium is made up of two layers:

1. A movable layer formed by plasma proteins among which the presence of fibrinogen is still uncertain—the α-macroglobulin detected here seems to defend the endothelium against proteolysis.

2. A fixed layer consisting of the saccharide portions of the cell membrane glycoproteins.

Introducing a very useful tool, the cationic ferritin, Danon and co-workers have demonstrated the existence on both fronts of the endothelium of high-density anionic sites, and stressed their possible role in thrombogenesis. There are data suggesting the existence of some specific receptors (e.g. for angiotensin II) on the endothelial cell membrane. The blood front is not attractive for the blood cells, and does not activate the coagulation systems; that makes the blood-endothelial interface highly compatible. On the contrary, the subendothelial structures are attractive for the blood cells and are thrombogenic.

Using lectins coupled with electron-dense markers (isotopes, horseradish peroxidase, ferritin, etc.), recent investigations show that the endothelial cell membrane displays on both its fronts α-mannose, δ-galactose, N-acetylgalactosamine, and N-acetylglucosamine residues. There is a high density of mannose and galactose residues in the basal lamina. These saccharides so far detected are located on plasmalemma and vesicles and are absent at the level of junctions. These oligosaccharides may play a role as recognition sites for molecules to be transported by an active process across the endothelium.

Such investigations are just beginning and it is going to be a long, but promising, way before we learn more about the molecular mapping of the endothelial surface and the nature of these disturbances which may mark the early stages in the endothelium involvement in atherogenesis.

CHAPTER II

Session 9

Assessment of cell populations

Introduction Leonard Hayflick

Introduction

It is now fifteen years since we published our observation on the finite lifetime of cultured normal human cells and interpreted this finding as a manifestation of aging at the cellular level. That hypothesis was put forward with some trepidation since we realized that it was based on evidence that had previously been interpreted very differently. I think that it is a tribute to many cytogerontologists, some of whom are here today, that the further investigation of the Phase III phenomenon has now made its interpretation as a phenomenon of aging a very tenable hypothesis. We will hear more evidence on this point by the contributors to this session.

Oxygen tension and vitamin E: effects on cellular senescence in vitro Vincent J. Cristofalo and Arthur K. Balin

Introduction

Although oxygen is usually thought of as being primarily involved in cellular respiration, it has been implicated as influencing many fundamental cellular processes. For example, Warburg (1956), in the 1930s, proposed that hypoxia, or any aerobic respiratory injury leading to a decreased utilization of oxygen and an increase in glycolysis, would cause cancer, a theory that still has adherents (Goldblatt et al. 1973). On the other hand, the free radicals induced by oxygen, by analogy to the known carcinogenicity of the free radicals induced by radiation (Gerschman et al. 1954), have been implicated in the aetiology of cancer (Harman 1962).

Cellular differentiation can also be influenced by oxygen tension. For example, chick limb mesodermal cells will differentiate into muscle cells when exposed to high oxygen tensions and into cartilage cells when exposed to low oxygen tensions (Caplan and Koutroupas 1973).

Oxygen effects have also been implicated in the changes that occur during biological aging (Harman 1962; Pryor 1971). For example, oxygen-induced peroxidation of polyunsaturated lipids causes cellular damage through its free radical intermediates (Tappel 1965). According to the free radical theory of aging, normal cellular function is ultimately limited by peroxidative damage to highly labile lipids of the cell membrane (Packer *et al.* 1967). Free radical intermediates resulting from peroxidation of polyunsaturated fatty acids are thought to react with proteins (Roubal and Tappel 1966) leading to polymerization of macromolecules, inactivation of enzymes (Tappel 1973), and possibly, cross-linking of DNA (Bjorksten 1974).

Human diploid cell cultures represent an ideal model system in which to investigate the characteristics and mechanisms of action of oxygen at different partial pressures on cell growth, metabolism, and aging. These cells can be serially subcultivated many times, but, after a period of time, the proliferative capacity begins to decline, debris accumulates, the culture degenerates, and eventually is lost (Hayflick and Moorhead 1961; Hayflick 1965).

The degeneration of the culture has been interpreted as a manifestation of aging at the cellular level (Hayflick 1965; Cristofalo 1972). This interpretation is supported by several lines of evidence. For example, the length of the life span of cells in culture is inversely correlated with the age of the donor (Hayflick and Moorhead 1961; Martin *et al.* 1970; LeGuilly *et al.* 1973; Schneider and Mitsui 1976). Also, cells taken from individuals with conditions characterized by symptoms of premature senescence (such as Werner's syndrome and progeria have a markedly shortened life span *in vitro* (Goldstein 1969; Martin *et al.* 1970).

A number of morphologic and biochemical changes occur over the population life span including changes in DNA synthetic capacity, macromolecular content, and lipid content (Cristofalo *et al.* 1970; Cristofalo 1976). In addition, as cultures of human diploid cells age, the number of lysosomes and amorphous insoluble deposits increases (Robbins *et al.* 1970; Lipetz and Cristofalo 1972) and intracellular fluorescent deposits associated with the lysosomes and most pronounced in the non-dividing cells accumulate (Deamer and Gonzales 1974). These deposits have been interpreted as being analogous to lipofuscin accumulated in the cells of aging mammals (Tappel 1973; Deamer and Gonzales 1974).

The results of studies purporting to demonstrate animal life span extension after the addition of dietary anti-oxidants have been equivocal (Comfort, Youhotsk–Gore, and Panhmanathan 1971; Comfort 1974). Usually these studies have shown a maximal mean life span extension of 10–25 per cent, but they have not extended the maximum recorded life span of the species (Harman 1961, 1968; Comfort *et al.* 1971; Epstein and Gershon 1972). Furthermore, this extension is less than that resulting from calorie restriction (McCay *et al.* 1943) and may be due, in part, to an anorexic effect (Harman 1968; Comfort *et al.* 1971) rather than an anti-oxidant effect (Comfort 1974). However, Packer and Smith have reported that the addition of 10 μg/ml or 100 μg/ml of the anti-oxidant d-1-α-tocopherol extended the population doublings of WI-38 cells from 65 to 115 (Packer and Smith 1974). Consistent with this result is the findings of Pereira *et al.* (1976) which show that anti-oxidants such as d-1-α-tocopherol protected WI-38 cells from light damage. Thus, using the diploid cell system, many aspects of the relationships between oxygen, anti-oxidants, and metabolism and aging can be investigated.

We have studied aspects of the effects of oxygen tension on cell growth and division, cell metabolism, and cell aging including the effects of vitamin E on aging. The results of our study comprise the basis for this report.

Materials and methods

The human diploid cell line WI-38 (Hayflick 1965) was obtained from Dr. L. Hayflick of Stanford University. Cells were grown in a modification of auto-clavable Eagle's minimal essential medium (MEM) (Eagle 1959) as previously described (Cristofalo and Sharf 1973). Cultures were monitored routinely for mycoplasma contamination by the method of Levine (1972).

Cell population doublings were calculated by comparing cell counts per vessel at seeding with counts at confluency.

Per cent labelled nuclei was determined autoradiographically by the method of Cristofalo and Sharf (1973).

The following gas mixtures were obtained in analysed certified standard mixtures from Matheson Gas Products (East Rutherford, New Jersey): 5 per cent CO_2, balance N_2; 5 per cent O_2, 5 per cent CO_2, balance N_2; 20 per cent O_2, 5 per cent CO_2, balance N_2; 53 per cent O_2, 5 per cent CO_2, balance N_2; 95 per cent O_2 and 5 per cent CO_2. The growth vessels were gassed to equilibrium both before and after the cells were seeded.

The cultures were kept stationary for the first 24 hours post-inoculation to allow the cells to attach. They were then transferred (unless indicated) to a horizontally moving platform on a water bath shaker adjusted to move through a 4-cm excursion cycle in 9 seconds.

Media P_{O_2}, P_{CO_2}, and pH measurements were performed immediately upon withdrawal of the media sample through a closed system at 37 °C in an Instrumentation Laboratory Model 113 Blood Gas analyser (Instrumentation Laboratories, Lexington, Massachusetts). At an atmospheric pressure of 760 mm Hg, a 5 per cent CO_2, 20 per cent O_2, 75 per cent N_2 gas mixture equilibrated in a flask with media at 37 °C would give a P_{H_2O} of 47 mm Hg, P_{CO_2} 35.6 of mm Hg, P_{O_2} of 142.6 mm Hg, and P_{N_2} of 534.8 mm Hg.

Glucose and lactate content of the media were determined on frozen aliquots utilizing a Beckman Glucose Analyser (Beckman Instruments, Inc., Fullerton, California) or the Glucostat Special Reagent Kit (Worthington Biochemical Corp., Freehold, New Jersey) and a pyridine nucleotide coupled spectrophotometric lactate assay (Sigma Chemical Co., St. Louis, Missouri). Cell viability was monitored by the ability to exclude erythrocin B dye (Phillips 1973). Cultures were photographed using an inverted Nikon model Ms phase contrast microscope with photographic attachment. Cellular protein content was determined by the method of Lowry *et al.* (1951).

For the studies with vitamin E, at each weekly subcultivation, freshly prepared vitamin E homogenate was added to culture media at a concentration of either

10 or 100 μg/ml. Equivalent aliquots of homogenized media without vitamin E were added to culture media to control for homogenized media effects. Because of the slightly reduced attachment of cells initially exposed to vitamin E, all cultures were incubated without shaking.

For cytophotometric studies, the cells were inoculated at 1×10^4 cells/cm^2 in 2.0-ml media into each chamber of two chamber Labtek vessels (Labtech, Inc., Westmont, Illinois, 5.29 cm^2/well). The media height was 5 mm above the cell surface. The vessels were either placed in a humidified 5 per cent CO$_2$: air incubator at 37 °C or in desiccators containing 3–5 cm of water to maintain humidity and equilibrated with 5 per cent CO$_2$, 50 per cent O$_2$, 45 per cent N$_2$ or 5 per cent CO$_2$, 95 per cent O$_2$ (Matheson Gas Products, East Rutherford, New Jersey). The desiccators were placed in an incubator at 37 °C.

The cells were grown for various time intervals, as indicated in the text. One hour before harvest, ^{3}H-thymidine was added to the vessels to a final concentration of 2.5 μCi/ml (2 Ci/mMol, New England Nuclear, Boston, Massachusetts). At the indicated times, the chambers were disassembled, the slides rinsed three times in 37 °C phosphate-buffered saline, fixed for 30 min in 3 : 1 CH$_3$OH : CH$_3$CO$_2$H followed by 5 min in CH$_3$OH, and allowed to air dry. At the completion of the experiment, all slides were simultaneously hydrolysed for 45 minutes in 5 N HCl at 25 °C (DeCosse and Aiello 1966), were stained with Schiff's reagent for 2 hours, were washed three times in freshly prepared bleach (0.4 g Na$_2$S$_2$O$_5$, 1.0 ml conc. HCl, 100 ml H$_2$O), rinsed in water, and dehydrated through a graded ethanol series. They were then air dried, and processed through autoradiography as described by Cristofalo and Sharf (1973). After the slides were developed, they were dehydrated through a graded ethanol–xylene series as described by Grove and Mitchell (1974), and coverslips were mounted with Harleco synthetic resin (Harleco, Philadelphia, Pennsylvania).

The percentage of labelled cells was determined by counting 500 nuclei at random (5 grains per nucleus over background). The DNA content of the unlabelled interphase nuclei was determined on a randomly selected population ($N > 100$ $\lambda = 565$ nm) with a Vickers M85 scanning microdensitometer (Vickers Instruments, York, England) as described by Goldstein (1970, 1971).

The percentage of mitotic cells was determined by counting > 1000 nuclei at random, and the numbers accurately reflect mid–late prophase through telophase. The DNA content of mitotic figures provided an internal 4C DNA standard. In some experiments, peripheral red blood cells of a 15-month-old white leghorn hen (2.4 pg DNA/cell) (Altman and Dittmer 1972) were processed with the experimental slides to provide an external DNA standard that could be used to define the diploid DNA content in cases where no mitotic figures could be found.

The relative grain intensity of the labelled nuclei was determined on a randomly selected population ($N > 75$) using the scanning microdensitometer at a ($\lambda = 460$ nm) where the absorption due to the Feulgen stained DNA was small.

To illustrate morphology, some slides were processed differently. Instead of the ^{3}H-thymidine pulse, they were fixed for 5 min in CH$_3$OH, stained with

May–Grunwald–Giemsa reagent (5 min), dehydrated, and mounted as described above. These slides were photographed through a Leitz Orthoplan microscope on Kodak photomicrography colour film no. 2483 with a Kodak 8 A filter over a tungsten light source.

Statistical significance was determined (unless otherwise indicated) by unpaired *t*-test analysis using a separate variance formula with the *t* value for a given level of significance determined by averaging *t* values for $n_1 - 1$ and $n_2 - 1$ degrees of freedom (Popham 1967).

Results

Effects of changing ambient oxygen tension on cell growth

Growth under normal atmospheric oxygen tension (P_{O_2} 131 ± 15 mm Hg) is illustrated in Fig. 1. During the first 24 hours following inoculation, 25–50 per cent of the inoculated cells failed to survive. Exponential growth began approximately 24 hours after inoculation and continued for 3 to 4 days yielding 10^7 cells

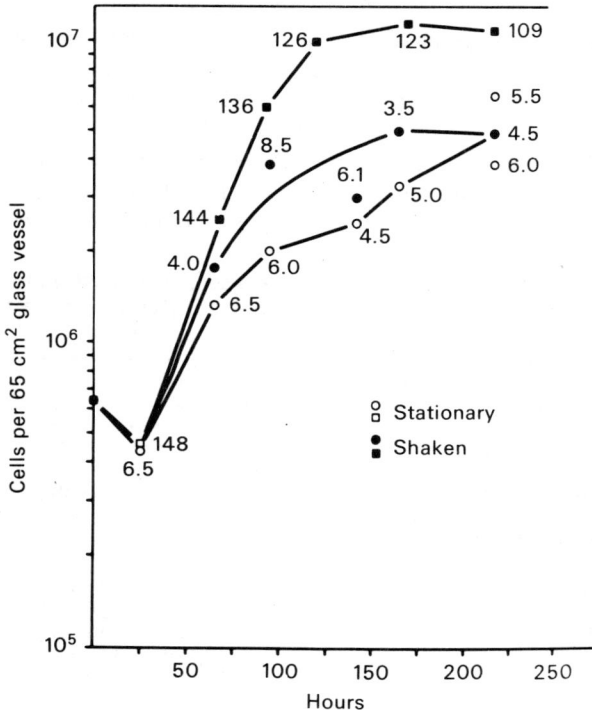

FIG. 1. The growth of WI-38 cells incubated shaken and stationary under $P_{O_2} = 5.6 \pm 1.3$ mm Hg and shaken under $P_{O_2} = 131 \pm 15$ mm Hg. The numbers associated with each point represent the measured P_{O_2} (in mm Hg) of the media at harvest. The cells in glass flasks (65 cm²) were incubated stationary for 24 hours and then placed on a slow shaker (●, ■) or left stationary (○). (From Balin *et al.* 1976.)

per vessel or about 1.5×10^5 cells/cm². When glass vessels were equilibrated with an analysed mixture of 5 per cent CO_2, balance N_2, a small amount of oxygen ($P_{O_2} = 7.8 \pm 3.5$ mm Hg, $N = 50$) remained in the media. Comparison of cell growth at $P_{O_2} = 44 \pm 7$ mm Hg or $P_{O_2} = 134 \pm 11$ mm Hg shows significant ($p < 0.001$) inhibition of growth in vessels incubated under $P_{O_2} = 7.8$ mm Hg. Furthermore, the population doubling time of the cells grown under $P_{O_2} = 7.8$ mm Hg was significantly longer (21.8 hours vs. 16.6 hours, $p < 0.001$) than that of cells grown under $P_{O_2} = 44$ mm Hg. Additionally, the growth inhibition at $P_{O_2} = 7.8$ mm Hg was reversible, since flasks re-equilibrated with $P_{O_2} = 134$ mm Hg, without changing the medium after 115 hours, recovered and achieved saturation densities near those grown entirely at $P_{O_2} = 134$ mm Hg (data not shown).

Fig. 1 also shows the results of an experiment designed to test whether shaking was detrimental to growth. Our cultures were incubated on a slowly-moving horizontal platform to insure that oxygen diffusion gradients would be minimized in the media. A paired t-test analysis at each specific time point in the growth curve of four shaken versus stationary experiments under $P_{O_2} = 7.8$ mm Hg demonstrated significantly better growth ($p < 0.02$) in the shaken cultures.

There were no significant differences in the initial growth rate between the shaken and stationary cells grown in glass vessels under $P_{O_2} = 7.8$ mm Hg, or $P_{O_2} = 37$ mm Hg, or in polystyrene flasks under a $P_{O_2} = 26$ mm Hg (data not shown).

Cells incubated at P_{O_2}s between 26 and 50 ± 5 mm Hg displayed similar growth kinetics and confluent saturation densities (Table 1). In this range, the population doubling time during exponential growth was 16.5 hours. Although

Table 1 The population-doubling time and cell yield of WI-38 cells incubated under various partial pressures of oxygen (Taken from Balin, Goodman, Rasmussen, and Cristofalo (1976))

P_{O_2}	Population-doubling time in hours		Stationary phase cells $\times 10^4$ cm²
7.8 ± 3.5†	21.8 ± 2.9 (8)‡	stationary	6.5 ± 2.4 (17)
		shaken	7.3 ± 1.9 (16)
26 ± 4	16.2 ± 1.7 (6)		15.9 ± 1.6 (10)
44 ± 7	16.6 ± 2.0 (14)		15.2 ± 2.3 (30)
134 ± 11	19.4 ± 1.7 (6)		14.9 ± 2.4 (18)
291 ± 25	72 ± 20 (5)		2.3 ± 1.2 (12)
$291 \rightarrow 50$§	28.7 ± 5.4 (3)		8.0 ± 1.5 (8)
389 ± 11	N.G.* (5)		0.83 ± 0.05 (5)
560 ± 38	N.G.* (10)		0.33 ± 0.14 (12)
$560 \rightarrow 50$§	27.8 ± 9.5 (3)		11.5 ± 3.2 (4)
692 ± 19	N.G.* (3)		0.33 ± 0.26 (4)

Results of representative experiments with cells of passage 20–27 (> 90 per cent labelled nuclei). P_{O_2} measured in the media of each flask at harvest. Results obtained using glass and polystyrene vessels were similar and were combined by oxygen tension.
† ± standard deviation.
‡(N)—number of determinations.
§Re-equilibrated at 55 hours.
*N.G.—no gain in cell number.

the doubling time increased to 19.4 hours at a P_{O_2} of 134 mm Hg (16.6 hours vs. 19.4 hours, $p < 0.02$), there were no differences in the saturation densities achieved when cells were grown under various oxygen tensions ranging from 25 to 134 mm Hg.

Striking effects upon cell growth and metabolism were observed when the P_{O_2} was increased to 291 mm Hg. The percentage of cells attached after 24 hours was identical to that obtained at lower oxygen tensions; however, with a P_{O_2} of 291 mm Hg, the maximum cell number was only 10–20 per cent ($p < 0.001$) of that achieved when cells were grown under P_{O_2}s from 25–140 mm Hg. This effect of increased P_{O_2} on cell growth was reversible, at least in part, since cells exposed to a P_O of 291 mm Hg for 55 hours and then re-exposed to a P_{O_2} of 50 mm Hg entered a period of logarithmic growth that ceased after the cell sheet became confluent. The population at confluence was somewhat less ($p < 0.001$) than that achieved by control cells grown entirely under a P_{O_2} of 50 mm Hg.

At $P_{O_2} = 291$ mm Hg, the doubling time was increased to 72 hours ($p < 0.001$), and at $P_{O_2} = 389$, $P_{O_2} = 560$, or $P_{O_2} = 692$ mm Hg the cell number did not increase.

Cells that were seeded at a P_{O_2} of 560 mm Hg attached normally but did not proliferate. Cell growth resumed, however, in flasks that were re-equilibrated with a P_{O_2} of 50 mm Hg at 55 hours. After a 24–48-hour lag period, the cell number increased exponentially until the cell sheet achieved confluence. The population at confluence was somewhat less than that achieved by control cells grown entirely under a P_{O_2} of 50 mm Hg. Although there was no apparent growth under a P_{O_2} of 560 mm Hg, 55–70 per cent of these cells excluded erythrocin B after 168 hours. Furthermore, cultures that were exposed to a P_{O_2} of 560 mm Hg for 168–192 hours and were then refed with fresh media and re-equilibrated with a P_{O_2} of 134 mm Hg gradually recovered, became confluent, and could be subcultivated weekly.

To test whether growth inhibition by oxygen was due to an effect on the media or an effect on the cells, flasks were incubated without cells at 37°C for 200 hours under 5 per cent CO_2 95 per cent N_2 or 5 per cent CO_2 95 per cent O_2. After this incubation, fresh glutamine was added (2 mM) and the atmosphere and media equilibrated with 5 per cent CO_2 5 per cent O_2 90 per cent N_2 to a P_{O_2} of 50 ± 5 mm Hg. Cells were then seeded and subsequently, over the next 250 hours, displayed no difference in growth kinetics, saturation densities, or measured metabolic parameters when compared with cells growth on fresh media under P_{O_2} 50 ± 5 mm Hg (data not shown). Additionally, media from flasks in which cells were inhibited by elevated oxygen tensions supported the growth of cells seeded at a P_{O_2} of 134 mm Hg (data not shown).

To exclude the possibility that the inhibition of growth was due either to glucose depletion or to lactate accumulation (see below), cells that had grown under a P_{O_2} of 291 mm Hg for 200 hours were subcultivated into fresh medium at the usual seeding density of 1×10^4 cells/cm². Incubated under a P_{O_2} of 134 mm Hg, these cells grew to confluence and could be split weekly; incubated under a P_{O_2} of 290 mm Hg they did not proliferate, even after 3 weeks of weekly refeeding of fresh media. There was no difference in cell attachment at 24 hours between these conditions.

Effects of oxygen tension on cell morphology
The morphology of the cells whose growth has been detailed above is shown in Fig. 2. At a P_{O_2} of 28 mm Hg (Fig. 2(a)), where growth was maximal, the cells appeared to be no different from WI-38 cells cultured under room air (P_{O_2} 128, Fig. 2(b)). However, under a P_{O_2} of 315 mm Hg the cells appeared larger, had lost their discrete spindle shape, and had acquired a coarser granularity. At a P_{O_2} of 565 mm Hg (Fig. 2(d)), the cells appeared shrivelled with less cytoplasm than cells grown at 315 mm Hg.

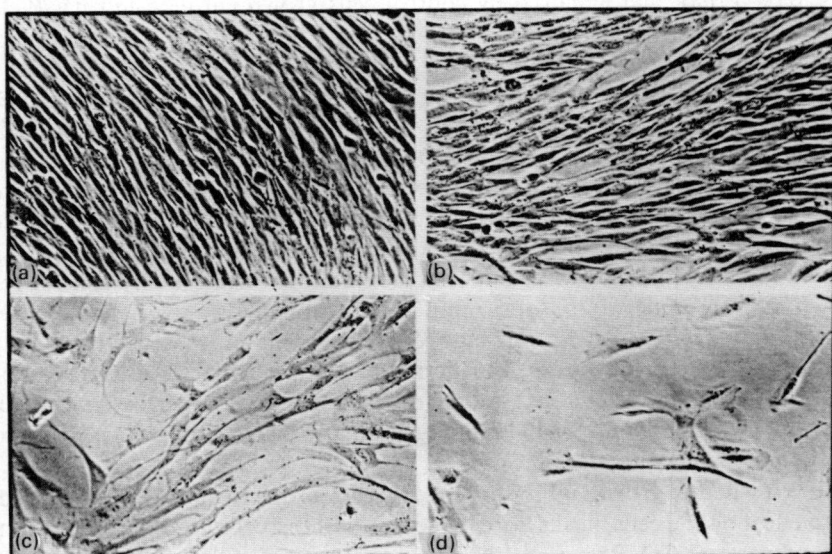

FIG. 2. The morphology of WI-38 cells incubated under various oxygen tensions after 100 hours of growth. (A) P_{O_2} = 28 mm Hg; (B) P_{O_2} = 128 mm Hg; (C) P_{O_2} = 315 mm Hg; (D) P_{O_2} = 565 mm Hg. The bar in D is 100 μm. (From Balin *et al.* 1976.)

Metabolic effects of altered oxygen tension
The effect of oxygen tension on the time course of glucose consumption and lactate production is illustrated in Table 2. The respiratory rate during exponential phase was similar at P_{O_2}s of 44 and 134 mm Hg and averaged 46 and 54 mM/(hour × 10⁶ cells), respectively. At P_{O_2} = 7.8 mm Hg, oxygen consumption was severely reduced to about one-fourth that at atmosphere pressure of O_2.

Cellular oxygen consumption during stationary phase when growth was suppressed by a P_{O_2} of 4.7 mm Hg was negligible. During stationary phase at a

Table 2 The effect of oxygen tension on glucose and oxygen consumption and lactate production during growth of WI-38 cells.

Po_2	O_2 consumed (μm/(hour $\times$ 10^6 cells))	Glucose consumed (μm/(hour $\times$ 10^6 cells))	Lactate produced (μm/(hour $\times$ 10^6 cells))
7.8 $\pm$ 3.5†	0.13 $\pm$ 0.19 (8)‡	0.42 $\pm$ 0.08 (8)	0.72 $\pm$ 0.13 (8)
26 $\pm$ 4		0.31 $\pm$ 0.02 (4)	0.53 $\pm$ 0.09 (4)
44 $\pm$ 7	0.46 $\pm$ 0.14 (7)	0.31 $\pm$ 0.05 (13)	0.52 $\pm$ 0.10 (13)
134 $\pm$ 11	0.54 $\pm$ 0.10 (4)	0.23 $\pm$ 0.09 (7)	0.38 $\pm$ 0.16 (7)
291 $\pm$ 25		1.47 $\pm$ 0.47 (4)	2.12 $\pm$ 0.78 (4)
291 $\rightarrow$ 50		0.60 $\pm$ 0.17 (3)	0.94 $\pm$ 0.27 (3)
389 $\pm$ 11		0.94 $\pm$ 0.10 (3)	1.33 $\pm$ 0.20 (3)
560 $\pm$ 38		1.62 $\pm$ 0.21 (2)	1.73 $\pm$ 0.11 (2)
560 $\rightarrow$ 50§		0.38 $\pm$ 0.03 (2)	0.50 $\pm$ 0.13 (2)

Results of representative experiments with cells of passage 20–27 (> 90 per cent labelled nuclei). Average rate of various growth parameters were calculated from 24 hours after seeding to confluency. The average number of cells was determined by the area under an arithmetically plotted growth curve. Po_2 was measured in the media of each flask at harvest. Results obtained using glass and polystyrene vessels were similar and were combined by oxygen tension. Oxygen consumption was not determined in polystyrene flasks because of the complications introduced by gas diffusion. The calculations for cells that did not become confluent were made over the same interval that was required for cells that were exposed to lower oxygen tensions to become confluent.
† $\pm$ Standard deviation.
‡ (N)—number of determinations.
§ Re-equilibrated at 55 hours.

P_{O_2} of 134 mm Hg, cellular oxygen consumption was 0.17 ± 0.05 μM/(hour $\times$ 10^6 cells). Thus the oxygen utilization of exponentially growing cells at atmosphere oxygen pressure was three times greater than that of stationary cells at the same oxygen tension.

When we averaged eight experiments conducted at $P_{O_2} = 7.8$ mm Hg, we found 88 per cent of the initial glucose was present at 70 hours, 72 per cent of the initial glucose was present at 100 hours, and 40 per cent of the initial glucose was present at 150 hours. During log growth the cells incubated under $P_{O_2} = 7.8$ mm Hg consumed more glucose ($p < 0.01$) and produced more lactate ($p < 0.01$) per cell than cells incubated under $P_{O_2} = 44$ mm Hg. No significant differences occurred in glucose consumption or lactate production per cell among cells grown under $P_{O_2} = 26, 44, 134$ mm Hg.

Additionally, despite severely reduced growth at elevated oxygen tensions, both the cell population exposed only to a P_{O_2} of 291 mm Hg and the cell population whose atmosphere was changed from a P_{O_2} of 291 to a P_{O_2} of 50 mm Hg at 55 hours utilized the available glucose and produced lactate. In fact, cells exposed to a P_{O_2} of 291 mm Hg consumed four to six times more glucose ($p < 0.01$) and produced four to six times more lactate ($p < 0.01$) per cell than cells grown entirely at $P_{O_2} = 130$ mm Hg (Table 2), despite the reduced growth. Cells incubated under $P_{O_2} = 389$ or 560 mm Hg showed four to six times the metabolic activity of cells incubated under $P_{O_2} = 134$ mm Hg. Cells exposed to a P_{O_2} of 560 mm Hg and then re-equilibrated with a P_{O_2} of 50 mm Hg at 55 hours consumed glucose and produced lactate at the same rates respectively as cells grown entirely under a P_{O_2} of 50 mm Hg.

Table 3 The effect of oxygen tension on protein content of WI-38 cells†

P_{O_2} (mm Hg) Exponential growth‡	μg protein/10^6 cells
24 ± 7§	221 ± 40 (12)‖
49 ± 6	222 ± 47 (12)
137 ± 9	286 ± 42 (12)
314 ± 34	519 ± 61 (12)
Confluent¶	
137 ± 9	184 ± 17 (19)

†Cells passage 20–7 (> 90 per cent labelled nuclei).
‡Exponential growth cells were harvested at 96 hours. These cultures were re-fed with ½ volume of fresh media 24 hours before harvesting.
§Standard deviation.
‖No. of determinations.
¶Confluent cells were harvested at 168 hours. These cultures were not re-fed with fresh media before harvesting.

Effect of oxygen tension on cellular protein content
The effect of oxygen on cellular protein content is summarized in Table 3. During exponential growth of young cells at a P_{O_2} of 24 or 49 mm Hg, protein content is similar to 220 μg/10^6 cells. At a P_{O_2} of 137 mm Hg, cellular protein content increased slightly to 286 μg/10^6 cells ($p < 0.01$). When cells were grown at a P_{O_2} of 314 mm Hg, multiplication was inhibited, but the protein content per cell nearly doubled to 519 μg/10^6 cells ($p < 0.001$).

At a P_{O_2} of 137 mm Hg, cells contained more protein during exponential growth than at confluence ($p < 0.001$). Thus, if growth inhibition is induced by contact inhibition rather than elevated oxygen tension, cellular protein content is not increased.

Life span studies
The effect of varying oxygen tension on the life span of WI-38 cells is shown in Fig. 3. Cells serially subcultivated at P_{O_2}s of 24, 49, or 137 mm Hg grew similarly and phased out after a similar number of population doublings, here 67–71. Cells incubated at P_{O_2}s of 341 and 608 mm Hg did not proliferate.

As mentioned above, at a P_{O_2} of 7.8 mm Hg, growth of WI-38 cells was reversibly inhibited. To determine the effect of very low oxygen tensions on life span, a series of cultures were grown in sealed glass vessels that were kept stationary to maximize any oxygen diffusion gradients. Under these conditions of minimal oxygen, the cultures phased out after about 20 per cent fewer population doublings than control cells.

Recovery after exposure to elevated oxygen tensions
Cells incubated at a P_{O_2} of 341 mm Hg for 1 week and then subsequently exposed to a P_{O_2} of 137 mm Hg recovered and were subcultured for nearly as long as control cells. Some cell populations exposed to a P_{O_2} of 341 mm Hg for periods ranging from 2–7 weeks also retained recoverability.

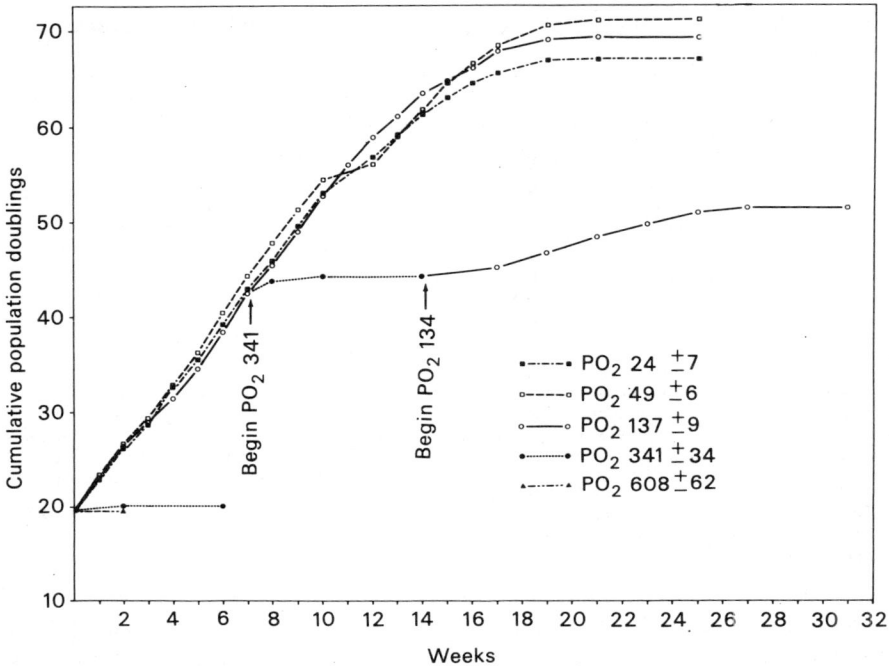

FIG. 3. The effect of oxygen tension on the life span of human diploid cells. Cells were serially subcultivated as described in Materials and methods at the indicated oxygen tension. (From Balin *et al.* 1977.)

However, recovery of the cell population from prolonged exposure to elevated partial pressures of oxygen was sharply limited if the cells were exposed to a P_{O_2} of 341 mm Hg for more than 2 weeks. Furthermore, the life spans of the cell populations that did recover were shorter than sister cultures never exposed to this elevated oxygen tension.

Cells that had 95 per cent labelled nuclei prior to a 7-day exposure to $P_{O_2} = 341$ mm Hg were found to have 29 ± 12 per cent ($N = 17$) labelled nuclei 24 hours after this exposure. However, if these cells were allowed to recover at a P_{O_2} of 137 mm Hg for 7 days and were then subcultivated weekly, the percentage labelled nuclei increased to a plateau at about 77 ± 7 per cent labelled nuclei ($N = 18$) for weeks 2–4, and then gradually decreased over many subsequent weeks of growth as previously described by Cristofalo and Sharf (1973).

The fraction of the cell population capable of initiating DNA synthesis after a 96-hour exposure to elevated oxygen tension is shown in Table 4. From the decline in microscope fields/1000 cells, it is evident that cell doubling occurred during recovery after exposure to $P_{O_2} = 375$ mm Hg. Less cell growth was obtained when 0.1 μCi/ml ^{3}H-thymidine was added to the culture for the entire 72-hour recovery period than when it was only for the last 24 hours of the period, probably due to radiation damage (Cristofalo 1976).

Table 4 Cell recovery at $P_{O_2} = 137$ mm Hg after a 96-hour exposure to elevated oxygen tension†

P_{O_2} hours 0–96	Hours of continuous label‡	³H-thymidine (μCi/ml)	Microscope field 1000 cells	Labelled nuclei§ (per cent)
375 mm Hg	96–120	0.1	87 ± 24¶	37 ± 8
	120–144	0.1	47 ± 17	68 ± 6
	144–168	0.1	29 ± 3	71 ± 5
	96–168	0.1	64 ± 11	77 ± 6
	96–168	2.5	97 ± 5	63 ± 6
640 mm Hg	96–120	0.1	112 ± 16	2 ± 0.5
	120–144	0.1	97 ± 9	23 ± 5
	144–168	0.1	85 ± 19	53 ± 3
	96–168	0.1	136 ± 31	34 ± 4
	96–168	2.5	127 ± 21	34 ± 3

†Three or four experiments in each category; 1000–2000 cells counted for each experiment.
‡Cells were exposed to the elevated oxygen tension for 96 hours before the atmosphere was changed to a P_{O_2} of 137 mm Hg to allow recovery. The cell media was not changed. A continuous label of ³H-thymidine was added at the indicated hour of the recovery period. The slides were fixed at the end of the labelling period. Thus, not all slides recovered for 72 hours.
§Cells in this experiment had completed 40 per cent of their life span and had 88 per cent labelled nuclei by the Cristofalo index (Cristofalo and Sharf 1973).
¶Standard deviation.

The last column of Table 4 shows the per cent-labelled nuclei obtained from continuous labelling with ³H-thymidine. During the first 24 hours of recovery only 37 per cent of the cells became labelled. The two subsequent 24-hour periods yielded 68 and 71 per cent. Labelling for the entire 72-hour recovery period gave 77 per cent labelled nuclei. Estimates of the percentage of cells able to recover, obtained from long labelling periods with ³H-thymidine, are probably high since many of the labelled cells will divide during the labelling period. However, when 2.5 μCi/ml ³H-thymidine was added for the entire 72-hour period, the cells did not proliferate (the 97 ± 5 fields/1000 cells is similar to that obtained from control cultures after 97 hours of exposure to $P_{O_2} = 375$ mm Hg and fixed before recovery was allowed). Thus, 63 ± 6 per cent of the cells in this population were capable of initiating DNA synthesis as compared to 88 per cent for cells never exposed to elevated oxygen. Similarly, after 96 hours' exposure to 640 mm Hg, 34 per cent (control 88 per cent) of the cells were capable of initiating DNA synthesis in the first 72 hours of recovery. Note that in this experiment the radiation damage induced by 0.1 μCi/ml of ³H-thymidine, in conjunction with the effect of 96 hours of a P_{O_2} of 640 mm Hg, was also sufficient to prevent the cells from dividing.

That substantial portions of the population were able to initiate DNA synthesis after exposure to elevated oxygen tensions suggests that we were not simply selecting a few resistant clones of cells.

Effect of vitamin E and oxygen tension on cell life span
Vitamin E (d-1-α-tocopherol), an agent known to trap free radicals, has been reported to extend the life span of WI-38 cells in culture (Packer and Smith

Table 5 The effect of vitamin E and oxygen tension on the life span of WI-38 cells. (Taken from Balin, Goodman, Rasmussen, and Cristofalo 1977)

Media supplement	Expt. 1 P_{O_2}† = 24 mm Hg PDL		Expt. 2 P_{O_2} = 49 ± 6 mm Hg‡ PDL		Expt. 3 P_{O_2} = 137 ± 9 mm Hg PDL		Expt. 4 P_{O_2} = 341 ± 34 mm Hg PDL	
	Begin	Phase-out§	Begin	Phase-out	Begin	Phase-out	Begin	Phase-out
—	18	67	19	61	19	63	16.0	17.5
4 ml homogenized media	27	69	37	64	35	65	16.0	17.5
10 µg DL-α-tocopherol/ml	24	66	37	63	35	64	16.0	17.3
100 µg DL-α-tocopherol/ml	18	67	33	64	33	67	16.0	17.1

The cells were serially subcultivated at the indicated oxygen tension and grown without shaking as described in Methods. The media supplement was freshly prepared and added at each weekly subcultivation. For each experiment, the supplemented cells were derived from the unsupplemented cultures in that experiment, at the indicated PDL (begin). Experiment 1 was performed under our routine 5 per cent CO_2 : room air atmosphere.
†Average P_{O_2} during growth period.
‡Standard deviation.
§Phase-out was defined as the inability to achieve confluence after four feedings over a 4-week period.

1974). In our experiments, when vitamin E was first placed in the media, about 14 per cent (60 ± 11 vs. 74 ± 7 per cent, $N = 9$, paired t-test $p < 0.02$) fewer cells attached at 20 hours in the vitamin E flasks than in controls that had an equivalent amount of homogenized media added. This slightly decreased attachment was associated with a slight decrease in cell yield during the few weeks of cultivation under these conditions. However, cell attachment and cell yield equalized after 6–8 weeks of subcultivation under the two conditions.

Table 5 summarizes representative experiments that show the effects of d-1-α-tocopherol on the life span of WI-38 cells at various oxygen tensions. Under our routine 5 per cent CO_2 : room air atmosphere, sister cultures carried serially in unsupplemented media, or 10 μg, or 100 μg d-1-α-tocopherol per ml showed no differences in life span. Similarly, cells carried serially under a P_{O_2} of 49 or 137 mm Hg showed no differences in the population-doubling level at phase-out with or without vitamin E. Cells grown under a P_{O_2} of 341 ± 34 mm Hg were not protected by the addition of the antioxidant. Thus, in this series of experiments, vitamin E did not alter the life span of WI-38 cells in culture.

Growth inhibition of human diploid cells in cultures by elevated oxygen tensions in relation to the cell cycle

We have shown above that growth and life span of human diploid cells is reversibly inhibited by elevated oxygen tensions. It was of interest, therefore, to explore the biological basis of this oxygen-induced inhibition by determining whether oxygen inhibits randomly or at some particular stage of the cell cycle.

Fig. 4 summarizes the results of a typical set of experiments in which the relative DNA content of individual cells was determined. Cells grown for 72 hours at a P_{O_2} of 138 mm Hg were actively proliferating with 45 per cent of the population undergoing DNA synthesis from hour 71–72 and 2.5 per cent of the population undergoing mitosis (Fig. 4(a)). The DNA content of the unlabelled interphase nuclei fell into two populations, with 40 per cent of the population containing a 2C DNA content. Occasionally, at all oxygen tensions, a few cells (< 2 per cent) were encountered with an 8C content of DNA.

As shown previously, cells exposed to a P_{O_2} of 373 mm Hg for 72 hours grew very slowly. The data show a striking accumulation of cells with a 4C content of DNA (47 per cent by 72 hours) (Fig. 4(b)) which was accompanied by two decreases in the percentage of the population undergoing mitosis (0.1 per cent at 72 hours) and engaged in DNA synthesis (13 per cent during hour 71–72). Cells exposed to a P_{O_2} of 640 mm Hg did not proliferate; after 72 hours, 70 per cent of the population contained a 2C complement of DNA and only 10 per cent a 4C DNA complement (Fig. 4(c)). Less than 0.1 per cent of the population was undergoing mitosis. This was accompanied by 1 per cent of the cells engaged in DNA synthesis from hour 71–72, and the appearance of 19 per cent of the population with an intermediate (3C) content of DNA.

To clarify these findings, the time course of the change in population distribution during growth under the various oxygen tensions was investigated.

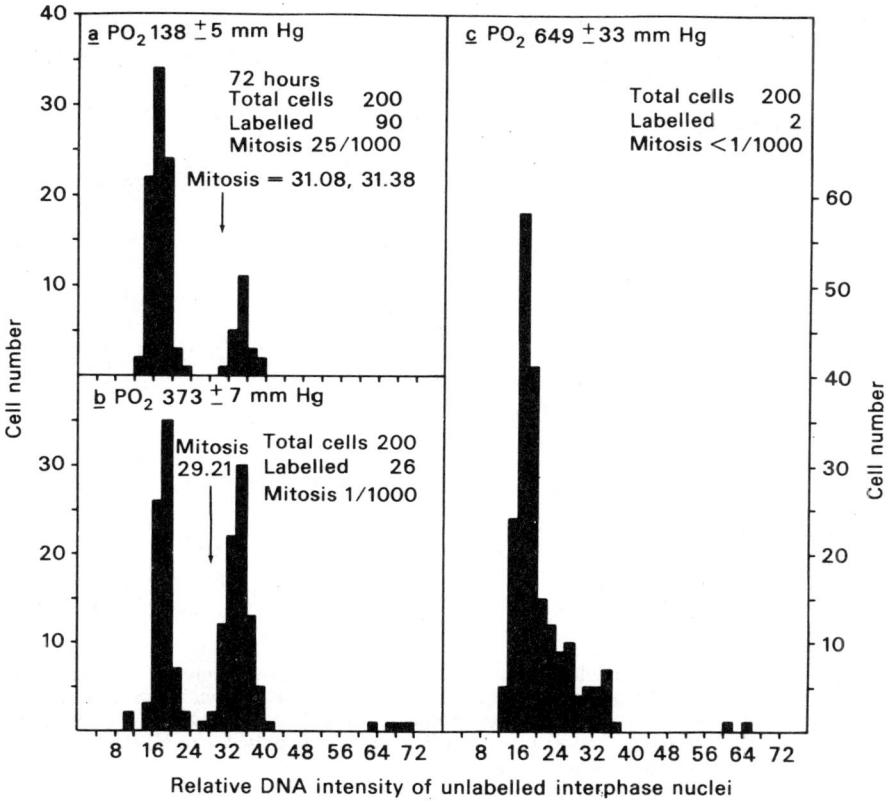

FIG. 4. A representative histogram showing the cell cycle distribution of a cell population grown at various oxygen tensions for 72 hours. The scanning microdensitometer was used to determine the relative DNA content of the unlabelled interphase nuclei. Young confluent WI-38 cells were subcultivated and incubated at the indicated oxygen tensions at hour 0, pulsed with [³H]thymidine from hour 71 to 72, fixed at hour 72, and then Feulgen-stained and processed through autoradiography as described in Methods. 200 cells were selected randomly and scored as labelled (5 grains over background) or mitotic cells. The relative DNA content of the unlabelled interphase nuclei is plotted in the histogram. Metaphase mitotic figures are used to define the 4-C DNA content. Note that the condensed chromosomes of the mataphase mitotic cells usually fall at the lower end of the 4-C distribution. (From Balin *et al.* 1978.)

Immediately after a confluent population was subcultivated (time 0), the population distribution was approximately 93 per cent 2C, 5 per cent 4C, 2 per cent labelled < 0.1 per cent mitosis (Fig. 5), and the DNA content was 7.69 ± 1.9 μg DNA/ 10^6 cells ($N = 19$). The cells retained this distribution for 14–18 hours before the percentage of the population undergoing DNA synthesis began to increase. The population was parasynchronous for the first 36 hours at a P_{O_2} of 138 mm Hg, but became random by 48 hours (data not shown). A larger percentage of the population initiated DNA synthesis by 24 hours when cells were grown at a P_{O_2} of 138 mm Hg (57 per cent) (Fig. 5(a)) than at a P_{O_2} of 365 mm Hg (45 per cent) (Fig. 5(b)) indicating that the G_0, G_1 transition to S is slightly delayed at

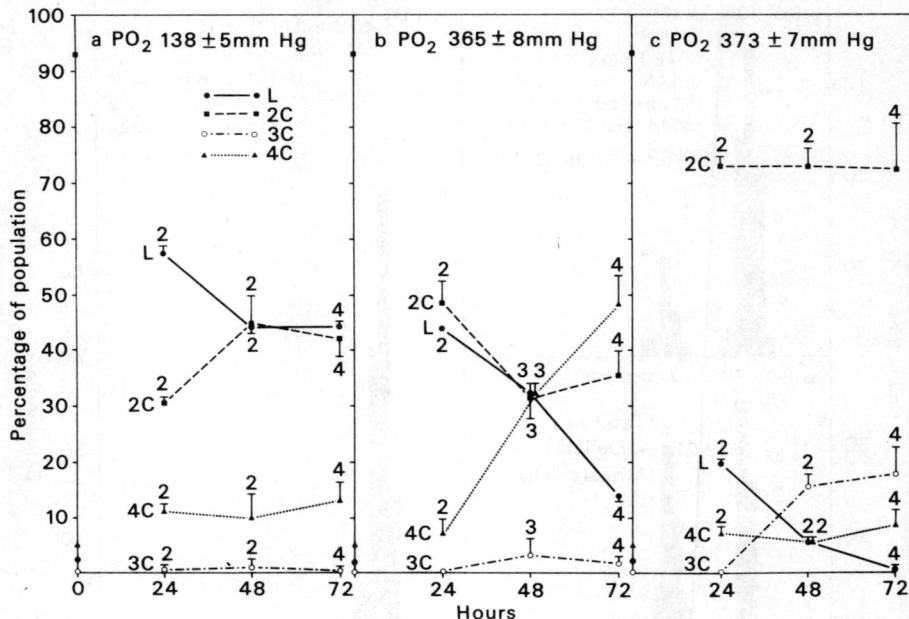

FIG. 5. A representative experiment illustrating the time course of the change in the interphase population distribution during the growth of young WI-38 cells exposed to various oxygen tensions at seeding. Cells were seeded from confluent cultures and exposed to the indicated oxygen tension immediately upon subcultivation. The slides were pulsed with ³H-thymidine for 1 hour immediately prior to fixation (see Methods).

The per cent labelled nuclei was determined from 500 randomly selected cells, and the interphase cell distribution was determined from > 100 random measurements. Cells with other DNA contents such as 8C represented < 2 per cent of the population and are not plotted on these graphs. The number associated with each point is the number of replicate slides counted; error bars indicate standard deviation. The population distribution at time zero is the distribution of young confluent WI-38 cells for the first 14–18 hours immediately after subcultivation (see text). (From Balin *et al.* 1978.)

the higher oxygen tension. Additionally, the data reveal that cells exposed to a P_{O_2} of 365 mm Hg manifest a decreasing percentage of the population engaged in DNA synthesis declining from 45 per cent at hour 24 to 13 per cent by hour 72 (Fig. 5(b)). This suggests that the delay in initiation of DNA synthesis at a P_{O_2} of 365 mm Hg became more pronounced with increasing time of exposure to the elevated oxygen tension. The most striking finding during the 72-hour incubation at a P_{O_2} of 365 mm Hg was the increasing proportion of the population found to have a 4C DNA content (Fig. 5(b)), while no increase in the number of mitotic figures was observed. Thus, the population exposed to a P_{O_2} of 365 mm Hg was primarily delayed after completion of DNA synthesis but before mitosis.

The cell population exposed to a P_{O_2} of 590 mm Hg immediately after subcultivation manifested a marked delay in the initiation of DNA synthesis, since

73 per cent of the cells contained a 2C content of DNA and 20 per cent incorporated ^{3}H-thymidine from hour 23–24 (as compared to 35 per cent containing a 2C content of DNA and 58 per cent incorporating ^{3}H-thymidine when exposed to a P_{O_2} of 138 mm Hg) (Fig. 5(c)). With continued exposure to a P_{O_2} of 590 mm Hg, there was no further initiation of DNA synthesis, as evidenced by 70 per cent of the population retaining a 2C DNA content at hours 48 and 72 and no increase in cell number. Furthermore, the 20 per cent of the population that was capable of initiating DNA synthesis aborted before completion, as shown by the progressive decline in the proportion of the population incorporating ^{3}H-thymidine and the corresponding increase in unlabelled 3C cells. Unlabelled cells did not move through the cell cycle since there was no increase in 4C interphase cells or mitotic cells. Thus, when confluent cells were subcultivated and were exposed to a P_{O_2} of 590 mm Hg, initiation of DNA synthesis was inhibited.

Analysis of the relative grain intensity of labelled cells also indicates that elevated oxygen tensions may decrease the rate of DNA synthesis. A histogram of the relative grain intensity of the labelled cells after a 48-hour exposure to oxygen is portrayed in Fig. 6. The relative grain intensity of the labelled cells

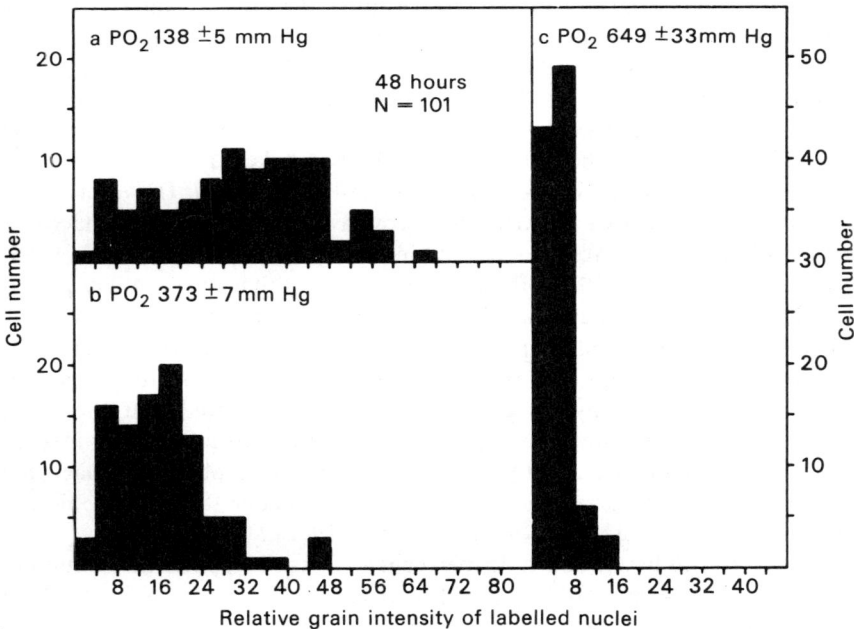

FIG. 6. Representative histogram showing the relative grain intensity of the population of labelled nuclei after a 48-hour exposure to various oxygen tensions as measured by the scanning microdensitometer. Labelled nuclei had 5 grains per nucleus over background. Young confluent WI-38 cells were subcultivated and incubated at the indicated oxygen tensions immediately upon subcultivation. The slides were pulsed with ^{3}H-thymidine from hours 47–8, fixed at hour 48, then Feulgen-stained and processed through autoradiography as described in Methods. 101 randomly selected labelled nuclei were counted. Unlabelled nuclei have a relative intensity of 1.9 ± 2.0 ($N > 100$). (From Balin *et al.* 1978.)

after a 48-hour exposure to oxygen reflects the amount of ^{3}H-thymidine incorporated into DNA during the 1-hour pulse period. It is evident that there is an inverse correlation between the rate of ^{3}H-thymidine incorporation and the oxygen tension in these cells (Fig. 6). Furthermore, the decrease in the rate of ^{3}H-thymidine incorporation began shortly (by 5 hours) after exposure to the elevated oxygen tension and was greatest at the P_{O_2} of 592 mm Hg (data not shown).

The average grain intensity of the labelled nuclei of cells incubated at $P_{O_2} = 353$ or 592 mm Hg tended to remain constant or decrease over a 72-hour incubation, although it tended to increase after 48 hours at $P_{O_2} = 138$ mm Hg (data not shown). The explanation for the increase in average grain intensity between hours 48 and 72 is not certain; however, it is possible that, after 48 hours, cell growth at $P_{O_2} = 138$ mm Hg was sufficient to reduce the thymidine concentration contributed by the serum.

Discussion

The reversible depression in cellular growth under $P_{O_2} = 7.8$ mm Hg demonstrates that WI-38 cell proliferation can be retarded by insufficient oxygen.

Kilburn *et al.* (1969) reported a depression of growth in mouse LS cells grown in suspension culture at very low P_{O_2}s (1.2 mm Hg). Others have found an inhibition of growth accompanied by an increased glycolytic rate under anaerobic conditions (Dales and Fisher 1959; Dales 1960; Rueckert and Mueller 1960; Clark 1964; Sanford and Westfall 1969; Sanford *et al.* 1970). However, some investigators have reported equally good growth under aerobic and anaerobic conditions (Pomerat and Willmer 1939; Jones and Bonting 1956; Harris 1956; Pace *et al.* 1962). Harris (1956), for example, reported that over a 4-day period with daily changes of medium the growth rate and final population density was the same for cells grown under 5 per cent CO_2 95 per cent N_2 and 5 per cent CO_2 95 per cent O_2. He noted, using an oxygen electrode, that the medium was not entirely freed of oxygen by his gassing procedure but stated that the small amount of oxygen remaining was rapidly consumed by the cells. Other investigators who have reported equally good growth under aerobic and anaerobic conditions have not reported the P_{O_2} of the media under their anaerobic environments (Jones and Bonting 1956; Pace *et al.* 1962).

Although our study showed a 15 per cent increase in population-doubling time at a P_{O_2} of 134 mm Hg compared to that at a P_{O_2} of 44 mm Hg, there were no differences in the saturation density achieved or cellular rates of glucose consumption, oxygen utilization, or lactate production during exponential growth. This illustrates the broad range of oxygen tensions that can support normal growth; results that are in agreement with data obtained from widely different cell lines (Pace *et al.* 1962; Kilburn *et al.* 1969). Furthermore, as noted earlier, other investigators have noted a more rapid doubling time when the percent of oxygen was decreased below that present in room air (Cooper, Burt, and Wilson 1958; Cooper, Wilson, and Burt 1959; Zwartouw and Westwood 1958; Pace *et al.* 1962).

Cristofalo and Kritchevsky (1966) have reported that the oxygen consumption by a suspension of trypsinized WI-38 cells under room air was independent of the glucose concentration of the incubation medium from 0 to 7.7 mM, and averaged about 0.14 ± 0.05 μmol/(hour $\times 10^6$ cells). Our present results, at P_{O_2}s 119 mm Hg (0.17 ± 0.05 μmol/(hour $\times 10^6$ cells), agree with this previous measurement. However, as expected, we found a threefold greater oxygen consumption during exponential growth of cells under P_{O_2}s of 44–134 mm Hg (about 0.5 μmol/(hour $\times 10^6$ cells) (Table 2)).

The present results for glucose utilization and lactate production under a P_{O_2} of 134 mm Hg are similar to those obtained previously by Cristofalo and Kritchevsky (1965) and by Kruse and Miedema (1965).

With the characterization of the reversible inhibition of cell proliferation at $P_{O_2} \geq 290$ mm Hg, we have extended the findings of previous investigators (Rueckert and Mueller 1960; Brosemer and Rutter 1961; Drew *et al.* 1964) who have used transformed cell lines to demonstrate an oxygen-dependent inhibition of cell proliferation.

The markedly increased glucose consumption and lactate production per cell at $P_{O_2} = 291$ and 560 mm Hg at a time when cell proliferation is inhibited make it unlikely that the sulfhydryl groups in key glycolytic enzymes, e.g. glyceralde-hyde-3-phosphate dehydrogenase, are oxidized and the enzymes inactivated. Thus, in these intact cells, failure of cell proliferation is not due simply to an inhibition of energy metabolism. These results are in agreement with those of Rueckert and Mueller (1960) using HeLa cells, Kilburn *et al.* (1969) using mouse LS cells, and Allen, Goodman, Besarab, and Rasmussen (1973) using the toad bladder.

The contrast between a depressed rate of cellular proliferation and an increased rate of glycolysis may be an important clue to the mechanisms of growth inhibition. It is possible, for example, that the energy and reducing equivalents necessary for cell divisions are diverted and consumed in an attempt to compensate for increased oxidation of cellular components, particularly membrane lipids as proposed by Allen *et al.* (1973).

The fact that the life span of WI-38 cells *in vitro* is not extended by serial cultivation at P_{O_2}s of 5.6, 26, or 50 mm Hg, suggests that neither oxygen toxicity nor free radical reactions play a significant role in limiting the life span of human diploid WI-38 cells *in vitro* under ambient oxygen tensions. This conclusion is supported by the results showing that the addition of the free radical trapping agent d-1-α-tocopherol at each subcultivation did not prolong life span. Furthermore, recovery after growth arrest resulting from exposure to elevated partial pressures of oxygen suggests that oxygen inhibits growth by a mechanism different from that responsible for the ultimate limitation on the proliferative capacity of the cell population. If accumulated peroxidative damage played a significant role in limiting the life span of human diploid cells in culture, one would need to explain why similar damage does not limit the life span of tumour cell populations. It seems unlikely that the unlimited life span of HeLa or mouse LS cells could be due to a more efficient scavenging of free radicals since growth of these tumour cells is also very sensitive to inhibition by elevated partial pressures of oxygen (Rueckert and Mueller 1960; Kilburn *et al.* 1969).

Packer and Smith (1974) reported that the addition of 10 or 100 μg/ml d-1-α-tocopherol to WI-38 cells at each subcultivation extended the *in vitro* life span of the cells from 65 population-doubling level (PDL) to 115 PDL. Furthermore, they reported that a brief exposure to d-1-α-tocopherol (from the 45th to 73rd PDL) conferred the same effect as continual exposure. Using methodology similar to theirs, we have been unable to reproduce this result. Packer and Smith used a single substrain of WI-38 cells; we used multiple substrains of WI-38 cells and repeated the experiment over 15 times. More recently, Packer and Smith (1974) have indicated that there may have been some unique property of the one serum lot they used, which explains their results in that set of experiments.

Other investigators have found either no effect or a mild inhibitory effect of d-1-α-tocopherol on fibroblast growth *in vitro* (Chinese hamster fibroblasts, V79 lung fibroblasts) grown on medium containing glucose (Corwin and Humphrey 1972). In rats, antioxidant compounds provide partial protection from the toxicity of a P_{O_2} of 4560 mm Hg but did not protect against the toxicity of the more moderate P_{O_2} of 760 mm Hg (Gerschman *et al.* 1954).

We have discussed above the conflicting reports in the literature concerning the lowest oxygen tension that could sustain cell growth. We demonstrated that at a P_{O_2} of 7.8 ± 3.5 mm Hg, WI-38 cell growth was markedly inhibited. Serial cultivation of these cells at a P_{O_2} of 5.6 ± 1.4 mm Hg demonstrated some variability in the PDL at phase out, but in no case did the life span equal or exceed that of control cells. These observations are of interest since Warburg (1956) hypothesized that hypoxia or any respiratory injury sufficient to decrease oxygen consumption and increase glycolytic metabolism was the basis of the aetiology of neoplasia. Although controversial (Weinhouse *et al.* 1956), this point of view has been proposed by others such as Goldblatt and Cameron (1953) who reported transformation of rat fibroblasts upon intermittent exposure to low oxygen tensions (for example, exposure to 15 minutes of N_2 every 12 hours for 3 days, repeated every few months until transformation occurs). In a subsequent publication dealing with the malignant transformation of fibroblasts and epithelial cells exposed to hypoxic conditions, both the cultures intermittently exposed to N_2 and the control cultures transformed (Goldblatt *et al.* 1973). Goldblatt *et al.* (1973) explained this by postulating that the control cells, which had free access to oxygen, transformed because of inadequate diffusion of atmospheric oxygen into the liquid medium of the stationary flask. More recently, Goldblatt and Friedman (1974) reported inhibition of spontaneous transformation of rat fibroblasts when 1 per cent human haemoglobin was included in the culture medium. However, Sanford was unable to induce malignant transformation of cells *in vitro* by intermittent anaerobiosis (Sanford 1965). Thus, it is worthwhile to point out that WI-38 cells serially carried at a P_{O_2} of 5.6 mm Hg where oxygen consumption is minimal and glycolytic metabolism is markedly increased retain their limited life span *in vitro*.

At the other end of the spectrum, cell proliferation is very sensitive to increased partial pressures of oxygen. However, the cells have an extraordinary ability to recover from exposure to elevated oxygen tensions. Much of this population, not simply a few resistant clones, is capable of initiating DNA synthesis in the first 72 hours following a 96-hour exposure to a P_{O_2} of 375 mm Hg (72 per cent) or 640 mm Hg (40 per cent). The life span of a population exposed to a P_{O_2} of 341 mm Hg for 1 week appears to be the same as the life span of a culture never exposed to the elevated oxygen tension. However, prolonged exposure (5–7 weeks) to elevated oxygen tensions prevents most cultures from recovering. Interestingly, the life span of the cell populations that did recover was shorter than control cells.

The cytophotometric–autoradiographic data show that exposure to a P_{O_2} of 350 mm Hg primarily delays cells after DNA synthesis but before mitosis. This indicates that the step most sensitive to oxygen causes a G_2 (or early prophase) delay. Another step, somewhat less sensitive to oxygen inhibition, delayed resting (G_0) cells from initiating DNA synthesis. A third step sensitive to oxygen inhibition reduced the rate of ³H-thymidine incorporation into the DNA of cells that were exposed to elevated oxygen tensions during DNA synthesis either by decreasing the rate of DNA synthesis or by decreasing thymidine transport and/or utilization. From our results, these few alternatives cannot be completely resolved. However, oxygen did not block thymidine transport and utilization completely (independent of the effect which slows the rate of DNA synthesis to zero) because there were no cells synthesizing DNA and traversing the cell cycle but not incorporating ³H-thymidine. This was shown by the lack of 3C cells and the absence of any increase in 4C cells. On the other hand, the rate of DNA synthesis was slowed to zero for most cells exposed to a P_{O_2} of 592 mm Hg for 72 hours. It should be noted that the cell cycle stage in which oxygen inhibited cells accumulate is not necessarily the cell cycle stage in which the oxygen-sensitive steps are located.

Drew *et al.* (1964) reported that 95 per cent O_2 inhibited DNA synthesis of exponentially growing HeLa cells. He and his associates monitored DNA synthesis by determining the relative grain intensity of autoradiographs prepared by pulse-labelling exponentially-growing HeLa cells with ³H-thymidine or ¹³¹I-deoxyuridine. They also estimated, on the basis of the per cent of labelled nuclei, that G_2 was prolonged by 1 hour. In contrast, both confluency and aging in WI-38 cell populations are associated with an accumulation of cells with a 2C content of DNA (Grove 1974; Grove and Mitchell 1974; Yanishevsky *et al.* 1974).

In general, cells are exposed to a broad range of oxygen tensions *in vivo*. For example, ambient air has a P_{O_2} of 158; tracheal air in the human a P_{O_2} of 149; alveolar air of a P_{O_2} of 100; arterial blood a P_{O_2} of 95; and mixed venous blood overestimates the tissue P_{O_2} because gradients on the order of tens of mm Hg probably exist between the blood in the capillary systems and the sites of O_2

reduction (Forster 1965). Moreover, the rat continues breathing until the intracellular P_{O_2} in its brain falls below 0.2 mm Hg (Chance, Cohen, Jobis, and Schoener 1962).

From our *in vitro* studies as well, there appears to be a broad range of oxygen tensions in which cells can live and divide normally in culture, and higher limit of this range is probably well above the P_{O_2} to which cells are normally exposed *in situ*. Our results do not seem to support the free radical theory of aging.

Summary

In this study we have characterized the effect of oxygen on human diploid celf growth, metabolism, and life span in culture. In addition, the biological basis of the oxygen-induced growth inhibition was explored by determining where in the cell cycle cells exposed to elevated oxygen tensions were delayed.

Cells grown under a P_{O_2} of 7.8 mm Hg had a significantly slower growth rate, lower saturation densities, and higher rates of glucose consumption and lactate production than did cells grown under a P_{O_2} of 44 mm Hg. There were no significant differences in saturation density or the rates of glucose consumption or lactate production between cells grown under $P_{O_2} = 26$, 44, or 134 mm Hg. Population-doubling time was slightly prolonged at a P_{O_2} of 134 mm Hg compared to a P_{O_2} of 44 mm Hg. Cells grown under a P_{O_2} of 291 mm Hg showed only 20–30 per cent of the growth rate and 10–20 per cent of the saturation density of cells grown under a P_{O_2} of 134 mm Hg. Despite this reduced growth, cells grown under a P_{O_2} of 291 mm Hg consumed four to six times as much glucose and produced four to six times as much lactate per cell as cells grown at a P_{O_2} of 134 mm Hg. Cells grown under a P_{O_2} of 560 mm Hg attached but did not proliferate. This toxic effect of oxygen on cell proliferation was reversible and was not due to an effect of oxygen on the media.

When human diploid cells (WI-38) were serially subcultivated, at a $P_{O_2}^-$ of 5.6 mm Hg the number of doublings to phase out was less than that of control cells at a P_{O_2} of 137 mm Hg. Cultures grown at P_{O_2}s of 24, 49, or 137 mm Hg phased out after a similar number of population doublings. Population life span was markedly shortened by chronic exposure to elevated P_{O_2}s, a phenomenon that was, in part, reversible.

d-1-α-Tocopherol (10 or 100 μg/ml) homogenized into the media at each weekly subcultivation did not extend the life span of cells at reduced, ambient, or elevated oxygen tensions.

A combined cytospectrophotometric–autoradiographic analysis showed that when confluent cells were exposed to a P_{O_2} of 350 mm Hg, they were primarily delayed after DNA synthesis but before mitosis; at a P_{O_2} of 600 mm Hg, they were inhibited from initiating DNA synthesis, and those cells that did initiate DNA synthesis aborted before completion. The rate of ^{3}H-thymidine incorporation into DNA was inversely correlated with the oxygen tension at P_{O_2}s of 140 mm Hg. The most sensitive step to inhibition by elevated oxygen tension caused cells to be delayed within a 4C content of DNA.

Acknowledgements

This work was supported by USPHS grants CA14345 from the National cancer Institute, and AG00378 from the National Institute of Aging, and NR205–005 from the Office of Naval Research.

References

ALLEN, J. E., GOODMAN, D. B. P., BESARAB, A., and RASMUSSEN, H. (1973). Studies on the biochemical basis of oxygen toxicity. *Biochim. Biophys. Acta*, **320**, 708–28.

ALTMAN, P. L. and DITTMER, D. S. (1972). *Biology data handbook*, 2nd edn, Vol. VI, p. 390. Fed. Am. Soc. Exp. Biol., Bethesda, Maryland.

BALIN, A. K., GOODMAN, D. G., RASMUSSEN, H., and CRISTOFALO, V. J. (1976). The effect of oxygen tension on the growth and metabolism of WI-38 cells. *J. Cell. Physiol.*, **89**, 235–50.

——, ——, ——, and —— (1977). The effect of oxygen and vitamin E on the *in vitro* life-span of human diploid cells. *J. Cell Biol.*, **74**, 58–67.

——, ——, ——, and —— (1978). Oxygen-sensitive stages of the cell cycle of human diploid cells. *J. Cell. Biol.*, **78**, 390–400.

BJORKSTEN, J. (1974). Cross linkage and the aging process. In *Theoretical aspects of aging* (ed. M. Rockstein), pp. 43–59. Academic Press, New York.

BROSEMER, R. W. and RUTTER, W. J. (1961). The effect of oxygen tension on the growth and metabolism of a mammalian cell. *Exp. Cell Res.*, **25**, 101–13.

CAPLAN, A. I., and KOUTROUPAS, S. (1973). The control of muscle and cartilage development in the chick limb: the role of differential vascularization. *J. Embryol. exp. Morph.*, **29**, 571–83.

CHANCE, B., COHEN, P., JOBIS, F., and SCHOENER, B. (1962). Intracellular oxidation-reduction states *in vivo. Science, N.Y.*, **137**, 499–508.

CLARK, M. E. (1964). Growth and morphology of adult mouse fibroblasts under anaerobic conditions and at limiting oxygen tensions. *Exp. Cell Res.*, **36**, 548–60.

COMFORT, A. (1974). The position of aging studies. *Mech. Age. Dev.*, 3, 1–31.

——, YOUHOTSKY-GORE, I., and PATHMANATHAN, K. (1971). Effect of ethoxyquin on the longevity of C3H mice. *Nature, Lond.*, **229**, 254–5.

COOPER, P. D., BURT, A. M., and WILSON, J. N. (1958). Critical effect of oxygen tension on rate of growth of animal cells in continuous suspended culture. *Nature, Lond.*, **182**, 1508–9.

——, WILSON, J. N., and BURT, A. M. (1959). The bulk growth of animal cells in continuous suspension culture. *J. Gen. Microbiol.*, **21**, 702–20.

CORWIN, L. M. and HUMPHREY, L. P. (1972). Vitamin E: substrate dependent growth effect on cells in culture. *Proc. Soc. exp. Biol. Med.*, **141**, 609–12.

CRISTOFALO, V. J. (1972). Animal cell cultures as a model system for the study of aging. In *Advances in Gerontological Research* (ed. B. L. Strehler), Vol. 4, pp. 45–79. Academic Press, New York.

—— (1976). Thymidine labelling index as a criterion of aging *in vitro. Gerontology*, **22**, 9–27.

—— and KRITCHEVSKY, D. (1965). Growth and glycolysis in the human diploid cell strain WI-38. *Proc. Soc. exp. Biol. Med.*, **118**, 1109–13.

—— and —— (1966). Respiration and glycolysis in the human diploid cell strain WI-38. *J. Cell. Physiol.*, **67**, 125–32.

—— and SHARF, B. B. (1973). Cellular senescence and DNA synthesis. *Exp. Cell Res.*, **76**, 419–27.

——, HOWARD, B. V., and KRITCHEVSKY, D. (1970). The biochemistry of human cells in culture. In *Research progress in organic, biological and medicinal chemistry*, Vol. 2, pp. 95–146. North-Holland, Amsterdam.

DALES, S. (1960). Effects of anaerobiosis on the rates of multiplication of mammalian cells cultures *in vitro. Can. J. Biochem. Physiol.*, **38**, 871–8.

—— and FISHER, K. C. (1959). The effect of carbon monoxide on oxygen consumption, glucose utilization, and growth in mammalian cells *in vitro. Can. J. Biochem. Physiol.*, **37**, 623–38.

DEAMER, D. W. and GONZALES, J. (1974). Autofluorescent structures in cultured WI-38 cells. *Arch. Biochem. Biophys.*, **165**, 421–6.

DeCOSSE, J. J. and AIELLO, N. (1966). Feulgan hydrolysis: effect of acid and temperature. *J. Histochem. Cytochem.*, **14**, 601–4.

DREW, R. M., PAINTER, R. B., and FEINENDEGEN, L. E. (1964). Oxygen inhibition of nucleic acid synthesis in HeLa S3 cells. *Exp. Cell Res.*, **36**, 297–309.

EAGLE, H. (1959). Amino acid metabolism in mammalian cell cultures. *Science, N.Y.*, **130**, 432–7.

EPSTEIN, J. and GERSHON, D. (1972). Studies on aging in menatodes. IV. The effect of antioxidants on cellular damage and lifespan. *Mech. Age. Dev.*, **1**, 257–64.

FORSTER, R. E. (1965). Oxygenation of the tissue cell. *Ann. N.Y. Acad. Sci.*, **117**, 730–5.

GERSCHMAN, R., GILBERT, D. L., NYE, S. W., DWYER, P., and FENN, W. O. (1954). Oxygen poisoning and X-irradiation: a mechanism in common. *Science, N.Y.*, **119**, 623–6.

GOLDBLATT, H. and CAMERON, G. (1953). Induced malignancy in cells from rat myo·cardium subjected to intermittent anaerobiosis during long propagation *in vitro. J. Exp. Med.*, **97**, 525–52.

—— and FRIEDMAN, L. (1974). Prevention of malignant change in mammalian cells during prolonged culture *in vitro. Proc. Natl. Acad. Sci. USA*, **71**, 1780–2.

——, ——, and CECHNER, R. L. (1973). On the malignant transformation of cells during prolonged culture under hypoxic conditions *in vitro. Biochem. Med.*, **7**, 241–52.

GOLDSTEIN, D. J. (1970). Aspects of scanning microdensitometry. I. Stray light (giare). *J. Micros.*, **92**, 1–16.

—— (1971). Aspects of scanning microdensitometry. II. Spot size, focus, resolution. *J. Micros.*, **93**, 15–42.

GOLDSTEIN, S. (1969). Lifespan of cultured cells in progeria. *Lancet*, **i**, 424.

GROVE, G. L. (1974). A cytophotometric analysis of nuclear DNA contents of cultured human diploid cells in log and in plateau phases of growth. *Exp. Cell Res.*, **87**, 386–7.

—— and MITCHELL, R. B. (1974). DNA microdensitometry as a measure of cycling-non-cycling activity in aged human diploid cells in culture. *Mech. Age. Dev.*, **3**, 235–40.

HARMAN, D. (1956). Aging: a theory based on free radical and radiation chemistry. *J. Gerontol.*, **11**, 298–300.

—— (1961). Prolongation of the normal lifespan and inhibition of spontaneous cancer by antioxidants. *J. Gerontol.*, **16**, 247–54.

—— (1962). Role of free radicals in mutation, cancer, aging, and the maintenance of life. *Radiat. Res.*, **16**, 753–63.

—— (1968). Free radical theory of aging: effect of free radical reaction inhibitors on the mortality rate of male LAF₁ mice. *J. Gerontol.*, **23**, 476–82.

—— (1969). Prolongation of life: role of free radical reactions in aging. *J. Am. Geriatr. Soc.*, **17**, 721–35.

HARRIS, H. (1956). The relationship between the respiration and multiplication of rat connective tissue cells *in vitro*. *Br. J. Exp. Pathol.*, **37**, 512–17.

HAYFLICK, L. (1965). The limited *in vitro* lifetime of human diploid cell strains. *Exp. Cell Res.*, **37**, 614–36.

—— and MOORHEAD, P. S. (1961). The serial cultivation of human diploid cell strains. *Exp. Cell Res.*, **25**, 585–621.

JONES, M. and BONTING, S. L. (1956). Some relationships between growth and carbohydrate metabolism in tissue cultures. *Exp. Cell Res.*, **10**, 631–9.

KILBURN, D. G., LILLY, M. D., SELF, D. A., and WEBB, F. C. (1969). The effect of dissolved oxygen partial pressure on the growth and carbohydrate metabolism of mouse *LS* cells. *J. Cell Sci.*, **4**, 25–37.

KRUSE, P. F. Jr. and MIEDEMA, E. (1965). Glucose uptake related to proliferation of animal cells *in vitro*. *Proc. Soc. Exp. Biol. Med.*, **119**, 1110–12.

LeGUILLY, Y., SIMON, M., LENOIR, P., and BOUREL, M. (1973). Long term culture of human adult liver cells: morphological changes related to *in vitro* senescence and effect of donor's age on growth potential. *Gerontologia*, **19**, 303–13.

LEVINE, E. M. (1972). Mycoplasma contamination of animal cell cultures: a simple, rapid detection method. *Exp. Cell Res.*, **74**, 99–109.

LIPETZ, J. and CRISTOFALO, V. J. (1972). Ultrastructural changes accompanying the aging of human diploid cells in culture. *J. Ultra. Res.*, **39**, 43–56.

LOWRY, O. H., ROSEBROUGH, N. J., FARR, A. L., and RANDALL, R. J. (1951). Protein measurement with the Folin phenol reagent. *J. Biol. Chem.*, **193**, 265–75.

McCAY, C. M., SPERLING, G., and BARNES, L. L. (1943). Growth, ageing, chronic diseases, and lifespan in rats. *Arch. Biochem.*, **2**, 469–79.

MARTIN, G. M., SPRAGUE, C. A., and EPSTEIN, C. J. (1970). Replicative lifespan of cultivated human cells. *Lab. Invest.*, **23**, 86–92.

PACE, D. M., THOMPSON, J. R., and VAN CAMP, W. A. (1962). Effects of oxygen on growth in several established cell lines. *J. Nat. Cancer Inst.*, **28**, 897–909.

PACKER, L. and SMITH, J. R. (1974). Extension of the lifespan of cultured normal human cells by Vitamin E. *Proc. Natl. Acad. Sci. USA*, **71**, 4763–7.

——, DEAMER, D. W., and HEATH, R. L. (1967). Regulation and deterioration of structure in membranes. *Adv. Geront. Res.*, **2**, 77–120.

PEREIRA, O., SMITH, J. R., and PACKER, L. (1976). Photosentitization of human diploid cell cultures by intracellular flavins and protection by anti-oxidants. *Photochem. Photobiol.*, **24**, 237–42.

PHILLIPS, H. (1973). Dye exclusion tests for cell viability in tissue culture. In *Tissue culture: methods and applications*, (eds. P. Kruse, Jr and M. K. Patterson), pp. 406–8. Academic Press, New York.

POMERAT, C. M. and WILLMER, E. N. (1939). Studies on the growth of tissues *in vitro*. VII. Carbohydrate metabolism and mitosis. *J. Exp. Biol.*, **16**, 232–49.

POPHAM, W. T. (1967). *Educational statistics: use and interpretation*, pp. 129–63. Harper and Row, New York.

PRYOR, W. A. (1971). Free radical pathology. *Chem. Eng. News*, **49**, 34–51.

ROBBINS, E., LEVINE, E. M., and EAGLE, H. (1970). Morphological changes accompanying senescence of cultured human diploid cells. *J. Exp. Med.*, **131**, 1211–22.

ROUBAL, W. T. and TAPPEL, A. L. (1966). Polymerization of proteins induced by free-radical lipid peroxidation. *Arch. Biochem. Biophys.*, **113**, 150–5.

RUECKERT, R. R. and MUELLER, G. C. (1960). Effect of oxygen tension on HeLa cell growth. *Cancer Res.*, **20**, 944–9.

SANFORD, K. K. (1965). An attempt to induce malignant transformation of cells *in vitro* by intermittent anaerobiosis. *J. Nat. Cancer Inst.*, **35**, 719–25.

—— and WESTFALL, B. B. (1969). Growth and glucose metabolism of high and low tumour-producing clones under aerobic and anaerobic conditions *in vitro*. *J. Nat. Cancer Inst.*, **42**, 953–9.

——, ——, and JACKSON, J. L. (1970). Glycolysis during culture of neoplastic and non-neoplastic murine cell lines under aerobic and anaerobic conditions. *J. Nat. Cancer Inst.*, **44**, 611–14.

SCHNEIDER, E. L. and MITSUI, Y. (1976). Examination of the relationship between *in vitro* cellular aging and *in vivo* human age. Personal communication.

TAPPEL, A. L. (1965). Free radical lipid peroxidation damage and its inhibition by vitamin E and selenium. *Fed. Proc.*, **24**, 73–83.

—— (1973). Lipid peroxidation damage to cell components. *Fed. Proc.*, **32**, 1870–4.

WARBURG, O. (1956). On the origin of cancer cells. Science, **123**, 309–14.

WEINHOUSE, S., WARBURG, O., BURK, D., and SCHADE, A. C. (1956). On respiratory impairment in cancer cells. *Science*, **124**, 267–72.

YANISHEVSKY, R., MENDELSOHN, M. L., MAYALL, B. H., and CRISTOFALO, V. J. (1974). Proliferative capacity and DNA content of aging human diploid cells in culture: a cytophotometric and autoradiographic analysis. *J. Cell. Physiol.*, **84**, 165–70.

ZWARTOUW, H. T. and WESTWOOD, J. C. N. (1958). Factors affecting growth and glycolysis in tissue culture. *Br. J. Exp. Pathol.*, **39**, 529–39.

Effects of age on cell division capacity George M. Martin, Charles E. Ogburn, and Curtis A. Sprague

Introduction

In 1961, Hayflick and Moorhead (1961) proposed that the limited replicative life span of cultivated human diploid somatic cells might serve as a model for the study of cellular aging. The single most important piece of evidence which has been cited in support of this idea is the observation of an inverse relationship between the age of the donor and culture longevity (Martin, Sprague, and Epstein 1970; LeGuilly, Simon, Lenoir, and Bourel 1973). This claim has been refuted by Kohn (1975) for the case of the age range 20–100 years and by Goldstein (1977) for the case of non-diabetic subjects. In this chapter we review critically the evidence and the various interpretations of that evidence. We conclude that there is in fact a strong statistical support for a negative regression of culture longevity upon donor age, for at least some cell-types, whether or not one excludes data from the pre-maturational age groups. However, in the case of human dermis, the tissue most intensively studied from this point of view, the extent of the regression is low and the variance extremely high. Moreover, it

remains to be demonstrated that the phenomenon has significance for the pathogenesis of age-related declines in the structure and function of that tissue.
Probably of greater significance are comparable studies, only recently undertaken, in which other cell-types are investigated, notably those originating from
the blood vessels. We urge our colleagues to turn their attention to the analysis
of these and other systems in which:

(1) Markers exist for a more reliable identification of the cultivated cell types,
therefore permitting correlations of cellular alterations *in vitro* with those
observed *in vivo*.
(2) There is reason to believe that a limited replicative potential may be an
important ingredient to the pathogenesis of the major age-related disorders.

We shall also draw attention to the little appreciated and poorly understood
paradox of multi-focal cellular proliferation which characterizes the pathology of
aging of mammalian organisms (Martin 1977).

Methods

Details of the culture media, culture procedures, and other methodology
employed for the studies on skin and aorta have been published (Martin *et al.*
1970; Martin and Sprague 1973; Martin, Ogburn, and Sprague 1975). Supple-
mentary information is given in the body of the text and in the captions to the
tables and figures.

As these studies have been underway for many years, it has not been possible
to utilize a single lot of serum; many dozens of different batches of newborn
calf serum have been utilized, undoubtedly with substantial differences in mitogenic activities. In all cases, the sera were heat-inactivated (100-ml bottles in a
water bath at 56° for 30 min) and used at final concentrations of 9 per cent in
Waymouth's medium.

Results

Growth potential of 'fibroblast' cultures from human skin
*Estimates of the variance of the method and the influence of the site of
biopsy.* Table 1 summarizes the results of an experiment in which two
series of replicate explant cultures were established at autopsy (4-h post-mortem
time) from the same individual, a 44-year-old male with rheumatic heart disease
who died following open-heart surgery. In one series, five Leighton tube (Bellco,
Vineland, N.J. #1904–19105) cultures were established from the left mid-upper
mesial arm (two 1-mm³ explants of dermis + epidermis per Leighton tube) and
in another series, seven comparable explant cultures were set up from the
left-mid-anterior forearm. Each culture was split at the second passage and these
pairs were then individually passaged in 6-ounce prescription bottles until
senescence. Thus, a total of 10 cultures from the upper arm and 14 from the
forearm were independently 'aged'. It is apparent from Table 1 that the growth

Table 1 Growth potential (cumulative population doublings) of replicate cultures of diploid human skin fibroblast-like cells derived from two different biopsy sites from the same autopsied subject, a 44-year-old male who died of the complications of rheumatic heart disease. A one-cm ellipse of epidermis and dermis was aseptically removed from either the mesial aspect of the mid-left upper arm (UA) or from the volar aspect of the mid-left forearm (FA). The specimens were diced into 1-mm cubes, pairs of which were chosen at random as explants to be placed in each of a series of Leighton tubes (LT). Cultures from each Leighton tube were split in half (A and B) after the second passage via trypsinization and all of the resulting individual cultures were independently 'aged' via serial passaging and cell counts

	FA	UA
LT 1 A	46.6	25.3
B	48.3	25.6
LT 2 A	50.7	25.2
B	47.7	24.6
LT 3 A	41.9	27.9
B	44.7	25.3
LT 4 A	41.9	25.9
B	40.4	26.0
LT 5 A	36.9	21.6
B	33.2	22.2
LT 6 A	42.0	
B	43.3	
LT 7 A	32.2	
B	31.4	

potential of cultures from the forearm is in all instances greater than those derived from the upper arm. The mean value for the forearm cultures is 40 per cent greater than the mean value for the upper arm cultures. The difference between these means is highly significant ($[P(t \geq 8.23) < 0.001]$). Table 1 also illustrates, especially in the case of the forearm cultures, that there is less variation between pairs of cultures derived from the same Leighton tube than there is among cultures derived from different Leighton tubes. In the latter case, cultures were initiated from independent skin explants from neighbouring regions of skin while in the former case, the pairs of cultures were derived from the same explants following their establishment. This conclusion was confirmed by an additional set of experiments in which duplicate cultures were followed from each of two Leighton tubes. As in the previous experiment, pairs of 1-mm^3 explants were used in each Leighton tube, the individual explants deriving from different areas of the same biopsy. Table 2 shows a clear trend towards greater inter-pair variance (Leighton tube 1 vs. 2) than *intra*-pair variance (subculture A vs. B).

In terms of our interest in the relationship between age of donor and growth potential of culture, we can draw two important lessons from these various data:

(1) It is essential to standardize the site of biopsy;
(2) It is important either to set up multiple independent explant cultures from the same individual (replicates derived from a single established mother

Table 2 Growth potential (cumulative population doublings) of duplicate cultures of diploid human skin fibroblast-like cells. One cm ellipses of epidermis and dermis were aseptically removed from the mesial aspects of the mid-upper arms at autopsy from different individuals. The specimens were diced into 1 mm cubes. Four segments were selected at random from each subject, two of them placed in each of two Leighton tubes as explants. Cultures from each Leighton tube were split in half (A and B) after the second passage via trypsinization and all four resulting cultures were independently 'aged' via serial passaging and cell counts. LT1 – Leighton tube no. 1; LT2 – Leighton tube no. 2. See Martin, Sprague and Epstein (1970) for further methodological details

| Age (y) | LT1 | | LT2 | | X |
	A	B	A	B	
13	42.9	39.9	26.0	25.5	33.6
29	46.6	42.3	36.1	37.4	40.6
36	46.0	43.0	47.0	47.0	45.8
47	27.7	34.5	35.7	32.9	32.8
55	25.9	21.4	22.0	20.0	22.3
58	33.7	30.0	32.9	29.9	31.7
63	32.4	30.2	16.8	16.0	23.9
67	32.1	31.6	31.1	30.2	31.3
68	30.9	35.0	27.9	26.6	30.1
74	34.0	31.4	18.6	16.3	25.1
81	18.2	17.7	23.0	23.4	20.6
89	15.9	18.5	25.3	26.4	21.6

culture would not suffice) or else, if one is restricted to single small biopsies (as is usually the case), one must examine comparatively large numbers of individuals and carry out a statistical analysis.

Effects of age of donor. Fig. 1 is reproduced from a previous publication (Martin *et al.* 1970) in which we calculated a linear regression line for a group of subjects aged 0–90; the regression coefficient was -0.20 ± 0.05 standard deviation cell doublings per year with a correlation coefficient of -0.50. Data from patients with three alleged premature aging syndromes, Werner's syndrome, progeria (Hutchinson–Gilforsd syndrome), and Rothmund's syndrome were excluded from the regression calculation.

Figure 2 gives a preliminary summary analysis for an overlapping group of 104 subjects, aged 20–90 years. There is a highly significant negative regression ($p = < 0.001$) of proliferative potential upon donor age with a regression coefficient of -0.18 cell doublings/year. However, there is a wide scatter of the points, giving a correlation coefficient of only -0.33. As in the previous figure, the cultures were all derived from a standard biopsy site, the mesial aspect of the mid-upper arm. A few were from normal subjects but the great majority were from patients suffering from a wide variety of non-infectious disorders, most of them derived from autopsy specimens. Statistical analysis fails to reveal any relationship between post-mortem time and culture longevity in the samples examined. A detailed analysis of this data is in progress and will be published elsewhere. For example, it will be important to review all case histories and family histories for evidence of diabetes mellitus as Goldstein, Littlefield, and

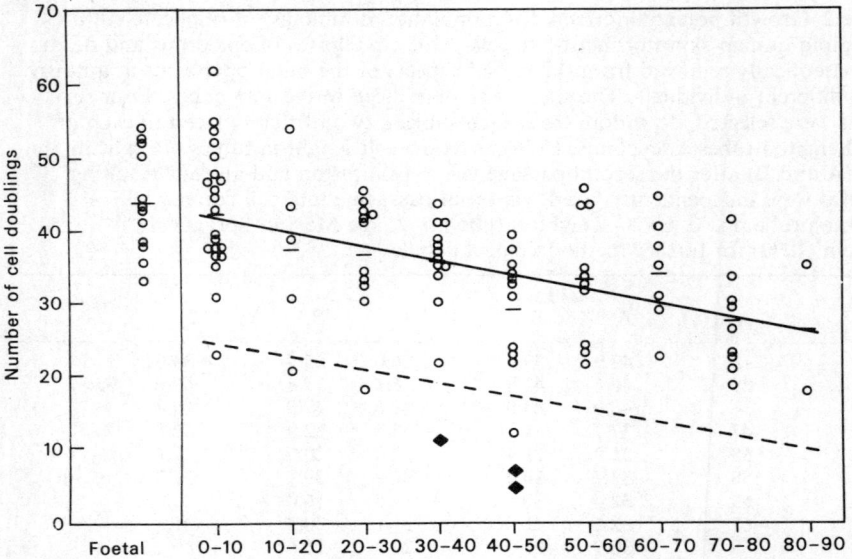

FIG. 1. The replicative life-spans of cultures of human skin fibroblast-like cells, as estimated by the numbers of cumulative population cell doublings, plotted against donor age. The three closed diamonds are the results from patients with Werner's syndrome. The mean for each age group is indicated by a horizontal bar. The solid line is the calculated linear regression and the dashed line is the lower 95 per cent confidence limit for the regressive line. (After Martin, Sprague, and Epstein (1970), which should be consulted for further details.)

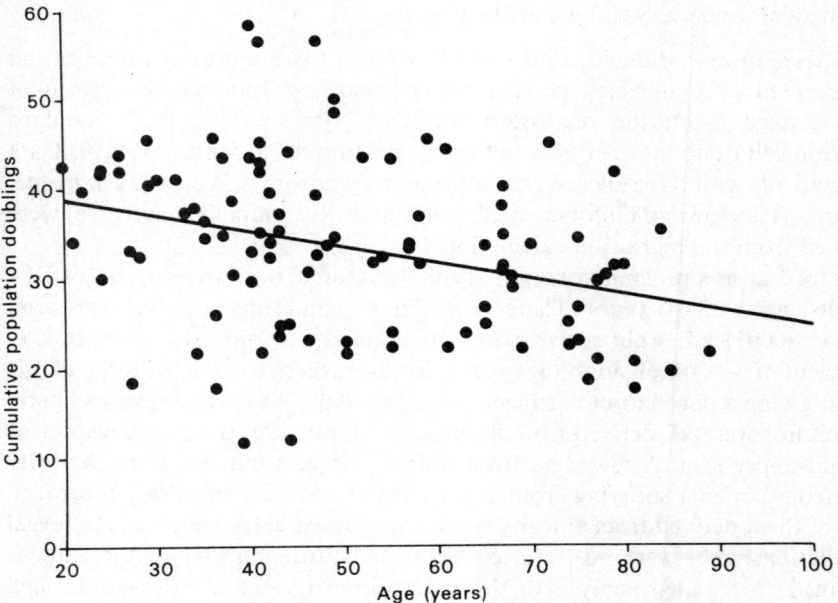

FIG. 2. Cumulative population doublings of human skin fibroblast cultures plotted as a function of donor age (> 20 y). The solid line is the calculated regression (method of least squares), which gives -0.18 cell doublings per year ($p < 0.001$). See text for further details.

Soeldner (1969) and Vracko and Benditt (1975) have reported diminished growth potential of these subjects.

Growth potential of cells from the vascular wall

Experimental animals provide better controlled materials to examine the relationship of growth potential to donor age. Because of our special interest in a potential role of clonal senescence in the pathogenesis of age-related degenerative vascular disorders, we have utilized the aorta for such studies.

Figure 3 summarizes the results of a secondary cloning experiment with the aortas of a randomly bred strain of mice. Details of the methodology and results have been previously published (Martin *et al.* 1975). In brief, cells for cultures were obtained after treatments of aortic segments with elastase. Such treatments yield a great deal of cellular debris and variable clumping, so that precise viable cell counts are not possible and therefore accurate primary cloning efficiencies could not be obtained. After these primary cultures became confluent, however, it was possible to obtain accurate *secondary* cloning efficiencies and these clearly revealed a decline of growth potential as a function of donor age. It was not possible to maintain serial passages of such cultures in order to determine

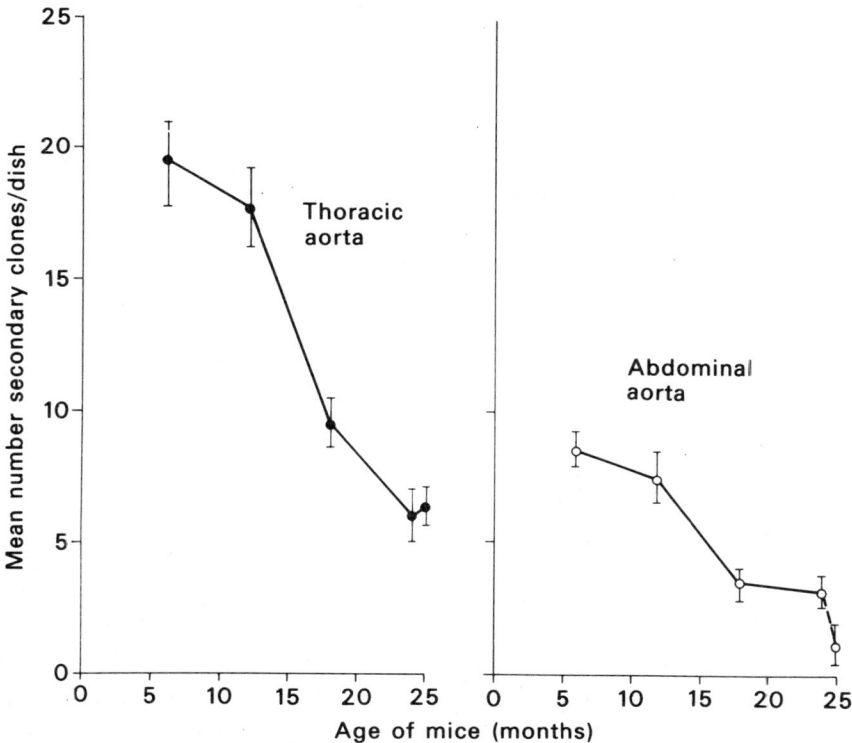

FIG. 3. Mean (±S.E.) number of secondary clones from male mouse aortas (strain ICR) plotted as a function of age. (See Martin, Ogburn, and Sprague (1975) for details.)

cumulative cell doublings, as in the case of the human cultures, since mouse cells readily undergo spontaneous transformation. Such transformation results in what we have termed 'neoplastoid' cell lines (Martin and Sprague 1973) with apparently unlimited growth potential.

Using another set of mouse aortas from the same colony of animals, we used an entirely independent method for assessing the relationship between donor age and replicative potential. Again, the original publication (Martin and Sprague 1973) should be consulted for details of the methods and results. Briefly, we set up organoid cultures of segments of aorta in serum-containing tissue culture medium of a type known to be capable of initiating DNA synthesis (i.e., we did not employ 'maintenance media' designed to minimize cell proliferation). The cultures were given tritiated thymidine at various time intervals as a marker for DNA synthesis. The latter was assessed via autoradiography. This simple but powerful method permits an unambiguous identification of cell type. As can be seen from Fig. 4, there is good evidence for a decline in replicative potential of *all* cell types within the vascular wall. There are anomolous points on some of the curves, which we now believe are attributable to variations of sampling, as

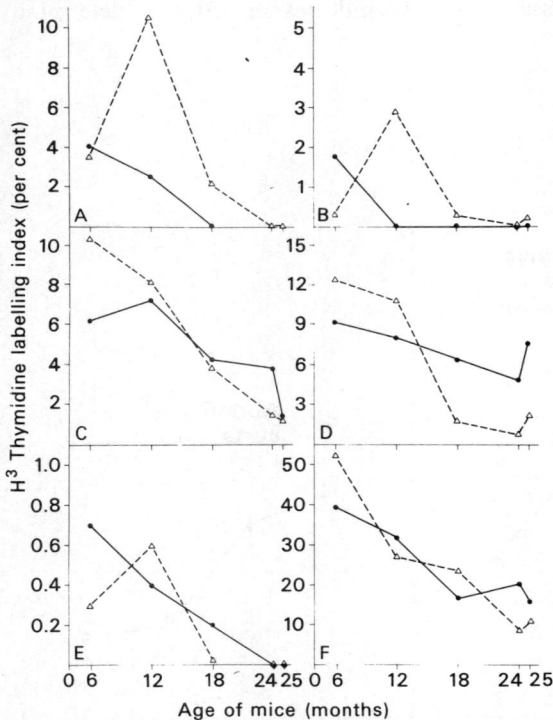

FIG. 4. Tritiated thymidine labelling indices (per cent labelled cells) plotted as a function of donor age from various cell types within thoracic aortas and adventitial tissues of strain ICR male mice: (A) endothelial lining of intima; (B) endothelium of adventitial blood vessels; (C) adventitial fibroblasts; (D) adventitial adipocytes; (E) smooth muscle of media; (F) adventitial mesothelium. (See Martin, Ogburn, and Sprague (1975) for details.)

there is evidence (Schwartz and Benditt 1973) that the distributions of labelled cells (at least in the case of endothelium) is non-random.

Discussion

Human skin fibroblast cultures

The regression coefficient of -0.18 for the presently reported cohort of subjects aged 20–90 (Fig. 2) is very similar to the 1970 study (Fig. 1) which gave a regression coefficient of -0.02 for the age range 0–90. Therefore, it seems to be the case that, on the average, the *older* a human subject, the lower the growth potential of his skin fibroblasts in culture. However, the source of material used for both studies was extremely heterogeneous. Multiple regression analyses will have to be carried out in an effort to sort out possible contributions of disease-type and treatments. For example, there could be a tendency for older patients to have had neoplasms treated by chemotherapy, with resulting decreased cell growth from such subjects. Careful scrutiny of available clinical and family history data must also be carried out for evidence of diabetes mellitus and pre-diabetes, since Goldstein *et al.* (1969) and Vracko and Benditt (1975) have presented evidence that the growth potential of skin fibroblast cultures derived from such subjects is diminished. Goldstein in fact claims that statistically significant negative regressions of growth potential upon donor age can only be demonstrated with his skin biopsy material from diabetics or pre-diabetics (Goldstein 1977). While a negative regression line could be drawn for Goldstein's small ($N = 25$) group of normal subjects, this was not considered to be statistically significant.

On the other hand, Schneider and Mitsui (1976) have reported statistically significant differences in a variety of growth potential parameters between 2 groups of normal donors of skin: young (aged 21–36) and old (aged 63–92).

The differences in growth potentials of skin fibroblast cultures from old vs. young donors which we and others have reported are modest. There are two polar interpretations of this fact:

(1) One can imagine a strong selection by the culture methods in favour of the healthiest and, presumably, 'youngest' cells, and against any cells which may have sustained injury or which may have utilized larger proportions of their growth potentials. Therefore, to find *any* degree of difference *in vitro* may be indicative of more profound deficiencies *in vivo*.

(2) Alternatively, one can conclude that, since the observable differences are so small and since there is so much variability from donor to donor, loss of replicative potential of dermal cells cannot be of great significance to the aging process.

One cannot resolve these different views until more precise information is available concerning the cell type(s) being cultivated, so that *in vivo–in vitro* comparisons can be carried out. There is no compelling evidence that the cells established in culture are derived from dermal fibroblasts. Collagen production is not a sufficient marker, as many cells synthesize collagens of one type or another, or may modulate the collagen type being synthesized during culture (Mayne, Vail, Mayne, and Miller 1976). In any case, the pathobiology of aging skin is probably a much less crucial determinant of life span in man than that of other tissues. Such considerations led us to examine the replicative potential of cells of blood vessels as a function of donor age.

Aortic cultures
Attempts were made to culture various cell types from human aortas arising from post-mortem materials from donors of various ages, but only rarely could cultures be established. Post-mortem changes in these cell types may be more rapid, or there may be many fewer cells capable of proliferating; both situations are likely to be correct. Successful cultures were usually those from neonates or children, in keeping with the general tissue culture experience.

The work with cultures from mice summarized in Figs. 3 and 4 clearly indicates that, the older the animal, the lesser the growth potential of its vascular cells. *All* cell-types seem to be involved in this decline, including those with intrinsically high and those with intrinsically low proliferative potentials. These various declines are clearly *post*-maturational, the youngest group studied (6 months) being well past sexual maturity for a mouse. Comparable autoradiographic studies have recently been applied to the Fischer 344 rat. Non-parametric statistical analysis of the results (to be reported elsewhere) once again show a decrease, as a function of age, in the numbers of endothelial and smooth muscle cells capable of undergoing DNA synthesis.

We have speculated elsewhere (Martin *et al.* 1975) on the potential significance of these studies for degenerative vascular diseases of the aged. With respect to the most important of these disorders, atherosclerosis, a pathogenetic model was proposed based upon a multifocal clonal senescence of vascular cells. We suggested that the myointimal proliferative lesions of atherosclerosis resulted from a release of such cells from local regulatory inhibitory influences. Such apparently paradoxical proliferations are widespread within aging mammals. In the human, these involve cartilage and synovial cells (osteoarthrosis), prostatic epithelial and fibro-muscular cells (benign prostatic hypertrophy), glial cells (C.N.S. gliosis), parenchymal fibrosis (ex., in the thyroid), adipocytes (regional obesity), melanocytes (senile lentigos), epidermal cells (verruca senilis), etc. (Martin 1977). It is possible that such paradoxical proliferations allow the expression of previously initiated neoplastic lesions. Thus, aging may be the most universal promoting agent in the two-stage mechanism of carcinogenesis (Martin 1977).

With respect to the problem of atherogenesis, excellent markers are now available for the identification of endothelial cells and considerable progress has been made towards establishing markers for smooth muscle cells (Martin and Ogburn 1977). Furthermore, it should be possible to harvest essentially pure populations of endothelial cells and smooth muscle cells from their *in vivo* sources from donors of various ages. Thus, one should be in the position of answering the question: are the changes which one finds in the properties of a specific cell-type which is aged *in vitro* similar to those alterations of properties which accompany aging of the same cell type *in vivo*? Only then will we be able to validate the cell culture model as a model for the study of aging.

Other tissues
We are greatly indebted to the pioneering work of Hayflick (1965) in establishing human foetal lung strains, and especially WI-38, as a well-characterized system to study *in vitro* cell senescence. However, we believe that such cultures, like the skin fibroblast model system, suffer from the problem that one cannot identify with certainty the cell-type of origin (although it has been suggested to be of vascular origin) (Franks and Cooper 1972). The histology of foetal lung is vastly different from that of adult lung, and it is quite possible that different cell-types could be preferentially grown from the two different sources. Thus, it is difficult to know the significance of the differences in growth potential which have been reported between foetal vs. adult lung cultures (Hayflick 1965).

The growth potential of a great variety of other tissues have been studied, mainly with explants in which variations in cell outgrowths were followed as a function of damage. Much of this work has been carried out and recently reviewed by Czech workers (Soukupová, Holečková, and Hněvkovský 1970). Of special interest were the differences between adult (8–12 months) and old (21–24 months) rats and the increase in variance as a function of age. The investigators concluded that '. . . the organs of older donors looked like a mosaic of tissue regions with many, few or perhaps no cells capable of life *in vitro*'. This is consistent with the considerable variance which we observed with human skin fibroblast cultures (Figs. 1 and 2). Small biopsies could provide 'hot spots' or 'cold spots' with respect to presence of cells capable of sustained replication.

Soukupová *et al.* carried out experiments with trypsin and collagenase in order to evaluate the role of extracellular materials in the differential rates of cell migration and proliferation as a function of age. The results did not implicate a primal role of such extracellular factors. Our primary and secondary cloning experiments with elastase digestions of mouse aorta (Martin *et al.* 1975) (Fig. 3) also argue against a crucial role of extracellular macromolecules, as isolated cells, free of their extracellular matrices, still revealed differences in growth potentials as a function of donor age.

Surprisingly little data are available on the effects of age on cell division capacity *in vivo*. One of the few careful cell cycle analyses is that of Thrasher (1967), in which a lengthening in G1 was demonstrated in intestinal crypt cells as a function of age. Most of the studies on mitotic indices have also shown that these decline in various tissues as a function of age; these studies are cited in Buetow's review (1971.)

The best transplantation studies of proliferative capacity as a function of donor age are those with haematopoietic cells (Harrison 1973, 1975; Micklem and Ogden 1976). While there is ultimately a decline in the proliferative potential of such cells when serially passaged, there is no evidence that the proliferative capacity of haematopoietic cells from old donors is less than that from young donors. One could speculate that there has been strong selective pressure towards the creation of a vast proliferative reserve for such tissue because of the common environmental stresses of traumatic haemorrhage, haemolytic parasites, and acute and chronic leukocytotic infections. If this were the case, it might be difficult to demonstrate any differences between old and young animals.

In conclusion, we believe that the bulk of the evidence favours a systematic decline, with age, in the replicative potentials of most cell types. It is beyond the scope of this paper to discuss potential mechanisms for such declines. Suffice it to say that most experiments are guided by one of two major ideas:

(1) The declines are specifically programmed by the genome.
(2) The declines are the results of cell injuries, mutations, or biosynthetic errors, the effects of which are modulated by the genome.

Summary

Cultures of diploid human fibroblasts have finite replicative life spans. It has been suggested that such cultures may serve as models for the study of aging. The most crucial line of experimentation in support of this hypothesis is the relationship between the age of donor and life span of cultures.

New studies from this laboratory are reported which demonstrate the variance of culture life span with replicative assays from the same donor. These studies document substantial differences in life span as a function of site of skin biopsy. It is concluded that a statistical analysis of a large number of specimens from a standard site of biopsy is essential for the investigation of the question of the role of donor age.

Previously published age regression studies involving subjects aged 0–90 were reviewed. New data for the age group 20–90 were presented. The preliminary analysis of the latter indicated a highly significant ($p < 0.001$) negative regression of -0.18 cell doublings per year of donor age, but with a low correlation coefficient ($r = -0.33$). The clinical heterogeneity of the subjects which formed the basis of these studies was emphasized; a multiple regression analysis of the data will be required for definitive analysis.

Previously published data from this laboratory involving aging of vascular cells was also reviewed; two different methods revealed clear evidence of declines in cell division capacities of all cell-types investigated as a function of donor age in post-maturational mice. The importance of such studies for the pathobiology of aging was emphasized, as they could lead to the types of *in vitro–in vivo* correlations essential for the validation of the *in vitro* model of cell senescence.

Finally, brief reference was made to the few extant *in vivo* studies on the effects of age on cell division capacity.

It is concluded that, as an animal ages, there is a decline in the cell division capacities of most cell-types. The significance of such declines for the pathobiology of aging remains to be established. The authors suggest that clonal senescence of somatic cells may lead, via alterations in intercellular regulation, to regional hyperplasias. Such proliferative lesions are fundamental to many of the important age-related disorders.

Acknowledgements

This work was supported by NIH research grants AG 00257, AM 04826, and GM 13543.

References

BUETOW, D. E. (1971). In *Cellular and molecular renewal on the mammalian body. Cellular content and cellular proliferation changes in the tissues and organs of the aging mammal*, (eds. I. L. Cameron and J. D. Thrasher), p. 87. Academic Press, New York.
FRANKS, L. M. and COOPER, T. W. (1972). *Int. J. Cancer*, **9**, 19.
GOLDSTEIN, S. (1979). In *Metabolic basis of endocrinology* (eds. A. Degroot, Martini, Potts, Nelson, Winegrad, C. Odell, Steinberger, and Cahill). Grune and Stratton, New York.
——, LITTLEFIELD, J. W., and SOELDNER, J. S. (1969). *Proc. Nat. Acad. Sci.*, **64**, 155.
HAYFLICK, L. (1965). *Exp. Cell Res.*, **37**, 614.
—— and MOORHEAD, P. S. (1961). *Exp. Cell Res.*, **25**, 585.
HARRISON, D. E. (1973). *Proc. Nat. Acad. Sci.*, **70**, 3184.
—— (1975). *J. Gerontol.*, **30**, 279.
KOHN, R. R. (1975). *Science*, **188**, 203.
LEGUILLY, Y., SIMON, M., LENOIR, P., and BOUREL, M. (1973). *Gerontologia*, **19**, 303.
MARTIN, G. M. (1977). *Amer. J. Path.*, **89**, 484.
—— and SPRAGUE, C. A. (1973). *Exp. mol. Path.*, **18**, 125.
——, ——, and SPRAGUE, C. (1975). *Adv. exp. Med. Biol.*, **61**, 163.
——, ——, and EPSTEIN, C. J. (1970). *Lab Invest.*, **23**, 86.
—— and Ogburn, C. E. (1977). In *Growth, nutrition and metabolism of cells in culture. Cell, tissue and organoid cultures of blood vessels* (eds. G. H. Rothblat and V. J. Cristofalo), Ch. 1, pp. 1–56. Academic Press, New York.
MAYNE, R., VAIL, R. S., MAYNE, P. M., and MILLER, E. J. (1976). *Proc. Nat. Acad. Sci.*, **73**, 1974.
MICKLEM, H. S. and OGDEN, D. A. (1976). In *Stem cells of renewing cell populations. Aging of haematopoietic stem cell populations in the mouse*, (eds. A. B. Cairnie, P. K. Lala, and D. G. Osmond), p. 331. Academic Press, New York.
SCHNEIDER, E. L. and MITSUI, Y. (1976). *Proc. Nat. Acad. Sci.*, **73**, 3584.
SCHWARTZ, S. and BENDITT, E. P. (1973). *Lab Invest.*, **28**, 699.
SOUKUPOVÁ, M., HOLEČKOVÁ, E., and HNĚVSKÝ, P. (1970). In *Aging in cell and tissue culture. Changes of the latent period of explanted tissues during ontogenesis*, (ed. E. Holečková and V. J. Cristofalo), p. 41. Academic Press, New York.
THRASHER, J. D. (1967). *Anat. Res.*, **157**, 621.
VRACKO, R. and BENDITT, E. P. (1975). *Fed. Proc.*, **34**, 68.

Session 10

Information transfer

Possible implications of the reorganization of the cell genome for the transfer of information in dividing cells

A. Macieira-Coelho

Introduction

Aging *in vitro* has been defined as the finite life span of cells measured in terms of the number of population doublings (Hayflick and Moorhead 1961). However, the investigator comparing life span *in vitro* of fibroblast-like cells from different species will have the feeling of going 'through a looking glass' and penetrating into a nonsense world. Chicken embryonic fibroblasts, for instance, will invariably die after a certain number of doublings, and so far no one has obtained a spontaneous permanent cell line from this type of cell (Ponten 1971). On the other hand mouse cells behave exactly opposite and invariably become spontaneous permanent cell lines (Earle 1943). Human fibroblasts from normal donors appear to be intermediate between these extremes, since they are particularly resistant to spontaneous acquisition of an infinite division potential. However, they seem to be more unstable than chicken fibroblasts, since they can easily become established cell lines after infection with SV_{40} (Girardi, Jensen, and Koprowski 1965) or herpes viruses (Geder, Lausch, O'Neill, and Rapp 1976). Other avian cells (quail fibroblasts) do not establish spontaneously but can acquire an infinite life-span after treatment with Rous sarcoma virus (RSV) (Ogura and Friis 1975). Cells from rodents can spontaneously develop permanent cell lines but with a variable frequency; for instance the probability of obtaining a permanent cell line from Syrian hamster fibroblasts is higher than that for rabbit fibroblasts but less than for Chinese hamster or mouse cells (Terzi and Hawkins 1975).

The situation is summarized in Fig. 1 where one finds a gradient-like pattern going from cells where the stability of the life span seems to be almost absolute (chicken fibroblasts) to cells with absolute instability (mouse fibroblasts). It is possible though, that the scale illustrated in Fig. 1 is just the visible part of the 'iceberg' and that eventually one will find a separate scale for each species.

This difference in the probability of yielding a permanent cell line seems to be a crucial property of cells since it is related to two fundamental aspects of cell biology, i.e., aging and cancer. The relationship with the former was first suggested by Hayflick and Moorhead (1961), who found that human fibroblasts

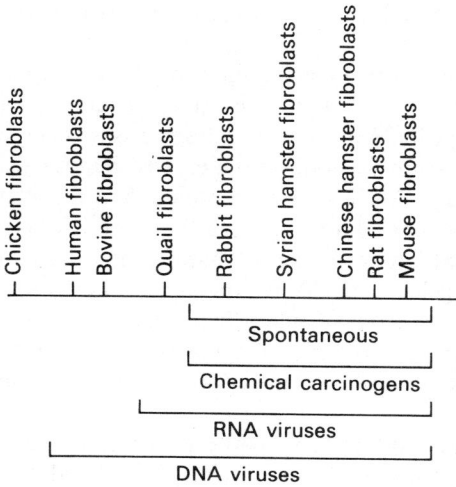

FIG. 1. Scale indicating the probability of obtaining a continuous cell line from fibroblast-like cells of different species. The phenomenon seems to be extremely rare with chicken fibroblasts even after treatment with different agents. Human fibroblasts from normal donors do not yield continuous cell lines but can do so after infection with certain DNA viruses. Bovine cells seem to be identical to human cells. Quail fibroblast produce continuous cell lines after infection with RSV. The rodent cells indicated on the scale become spontaneously established cell lines. In these cells the phenomenon is accelerated by chemical carcinogens and oncogenic viruses.

from adult donors have a lower division potential than those from embryos (Hayflick 1965). The relationship between a finite life span *in vitro* and aging was further established by comparison between embryonic and adult cells (Macieira-Coelho and Ponten 1969) and between cells originating from normal donors of different ages (Martin, Sprague, and Epstein 1970; Schneider, Mitsui, Tice, and Shiller 1975) and from patients with premature aging (Goldstein 1969; Goldstein, Littlefield, and Soeldner 1969).

Relationship between aging and cancer and the life span of cells *in vitro*

Some aspects of the relationship between the life span of cells *in vitro* and cancer already mentioned derive from the facility with which cell populations become immortal, either spontaneously or through the effect of carcinogens. But there are interesting features that have been discovered recently. Within the human species there seems to be a variability between skin fibroblasts originated from donors that have or are prone to neoplasia. Thus, it has been reported that skin fibroblasts from patients with lung or mediastinal neoplasmas become spontaneously permanent cell lines (Azzarone, Pedulla, and Romanzi 1976) and that skin fibroblasts from donors with the von Recklinghausen syndrome can be established by chemical carcinogens (Benedict, Jones, Lang, Igel, and Freeman 1975). This has never been reported for fibroblasts from normal donors. If cells that establish *in vitro* do not originate from micrometasteases disseminated through the body, these findings could mean that at least some neoplasmas are not localized diseases but rather are generalized pathological conditions expressed in other somatic cells. Hence individual variability seems to exist between human donors, and one could speculate that eventually this difference in the propensity to establish *in vitro* could be used as a test to check proneness to cancer. In that case it seems that one could build a separate scale within the human species (Fig. 2).

It seems obvious that knowledge of the mechanisms leading to growth decline will have important implications for aging and that, vice-versa, to know why the capacity to divide persists will contribute to understanding of how cancer develops. Decline of transfer of information was one of the earliest hypotheses used to explain aging, and investigators in this field have extended their theories to the phenomenon *in vitro*. Hypotheses varied according to the level at which failure occurred but most admitted that whatever the mechanism, it led to an accumulation of errors in proteins (Orgel 1963). The accumulation of errors in proteins has so far never been demonstrated and many investigators tend to believe that modifications described in the proteins of aging cells are due to post translational changes rather than to the incorporation of faulty amino acids (Gershon and Gershon 1976).

Even the problem of the rate of RNA and protein synthesis during aging *in vivo* and *in vitro* is still controversial. However, using a variety of procedures, we found a decline of RNA synthesis during aging *in vitro* of human and chicken fibroblasts (Macieira-Coelho, Ponten, and Philipson 1966; Macieira-Coelho and Lima 1973). Furthermore, among the different parameters that were measured the decline in the rate of protein synthesis was the earliest change detected during the life span of chicken embryonic fibroblasts (Figs. 3, 4, and 5).

On the other hand cortisone and hydrocortisone which prolong the life span of human embryonic fibroblasts (Macieira-Coelho 1966; Cristofalo 1970) also

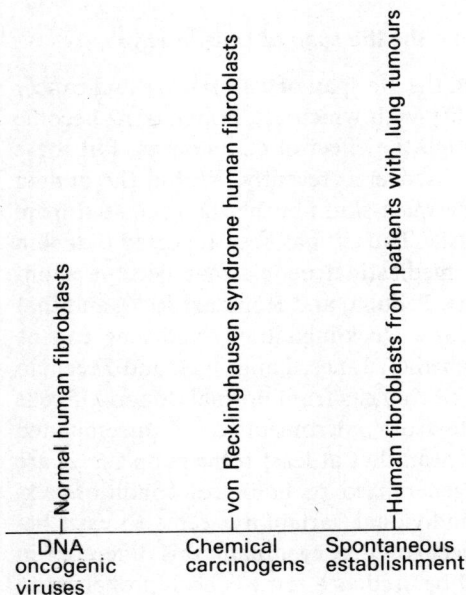

Normal human fibroblasts	von Recklinghausen syndrome human fibroblasts	Human fibroblasts from patients with lung tumours
DNA oncogenic viruses	Chemical carcinogens	Spontaneous establishment

FIG. 2. Tentative scale indicating the probability of obtaining a continuous cell line from human fibroblasts of different donors.

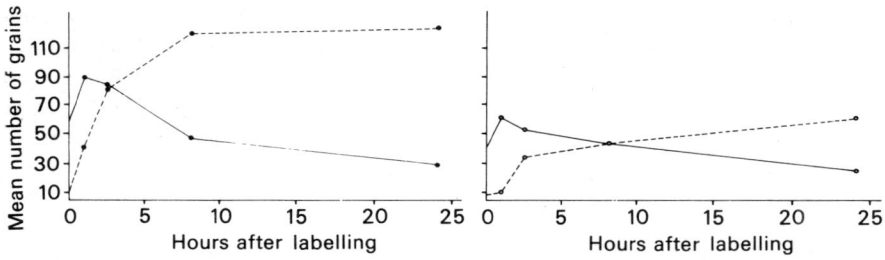

FIG. 3. RNA synthesis in the nucleus (●——●) and cytoplasm (○- - -○) of young (left side) and old (right side) human embryonic fibroblasts expressed as a function of the number of grains found after autoradiography of cells fixed at different times after a pulse labelling.

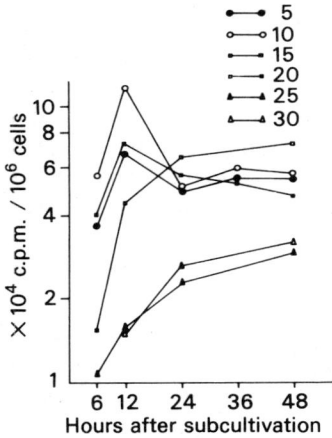

FIG. 4. Radioactivity found in the acid insoluble fraction after pulse labelling chicken embryonic fibroblasts with H³-uridine at different times after subcultivation. The numbers indicate the passage when the experiments were performed.

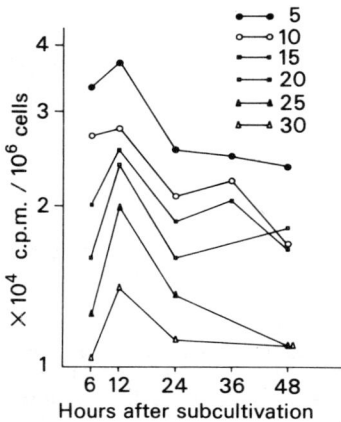

FIG. 5. Radioactivity found in the acid insoluble fraction after pulse labelling chicken embryonic fibroblasts with C¹⁴-amino acids at different times after subcultivation. The numbers indicate the passage when the experiments were performed.

stimulate RNA and protein synthesis in the same cells (Macieira-Coelho and Loria 1974). The withdrawal of hormone from cultures that had lived beyond the life span of the controls led to a rapid decline in the stimulation of RNA synthesis and to the death of the cells (Macieira-Coelho and Loria 1974). These findings suggest an association between the decrease of RNA and protein synthesis and the growth decline after a given number of doublings *in vitro*.

Effects of irradiation on fibroblasts of different species

As a matter of fact a decline in the rate of protein synthesis would be enough to explain the loss of division potential. The question is why is there a decline in RNA and protein synthesis and where does it originate? Why does it invariably happen in some cells and why is it that in other cells the protein-synthesizing machinery goes on forever? We have done some comparative work with cells represented at different points of the scale illustrated in Fig. 1, which suggest that the behaviours described above could be determined by a rearrangement of the cell genome.

Cells from the opposite ends of the scale illustrated in Fig. 1 (chicken and mouse fibroblasts) were irradiated with low-dose-rate radiation (100 rad each time at 0.27 rad min^{-1}). The irradiated chicken fibroblasts had survival curves parallel to those of the control cultures but the life span was shorter in the former cultures (Fig. 6). The total number of cells produced in each group decreased logarithmically with increasing doses of radiation (Fig. 11). The same experiment performed with mouse fibroblasts gave the opposite results, i.e., the control as well as the irradiated cultures acquired an infinite life span but the phenomenon occurred earlier in the latter (Figs. 7 and 8) so that the total number of cells produced in each group increased logarithmically with increasing doses of radiation (Fig. 11).

An acceleration of the immortalization of mouse fibroblasts can also be obtained by keeping the cultures under optimal nutritional conditions. The phenomenon is illustrated in Fig. 9. New-born mouse lung fibroblasts were

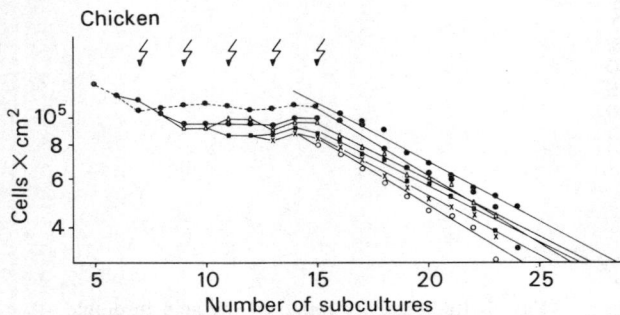

Fig. 6. Survival curves of chicken embryonic fibroblasts irradiated one (●——●), two (△——△), three (■——■), four (X——X), and five (○——○) times with 100 rads at a rate of 0.27 rad min^{-1}. Control cells (●‑‑‑●). Ordinate: cell density before each subculture; abcissa: passage number.

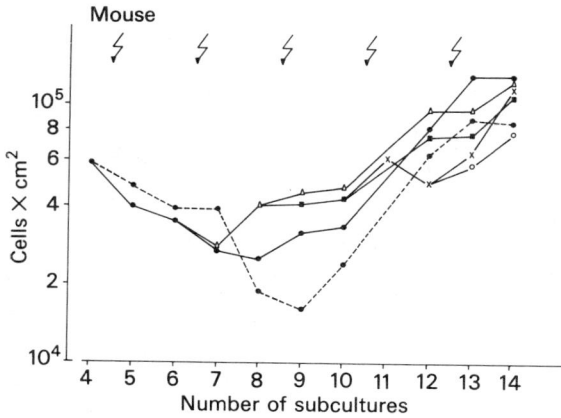

FIG. 7. Survival curves of mouse new-born fibroblasts irradiated one (●——●), two (△——△), three (■——■), four (X——X), and five (○——○) times with 100 rad at a rate of 0.27 rad min^{-1}. Control cells (●- - -●). Ordinate: cell density before each subculture, abcissa: passage number.

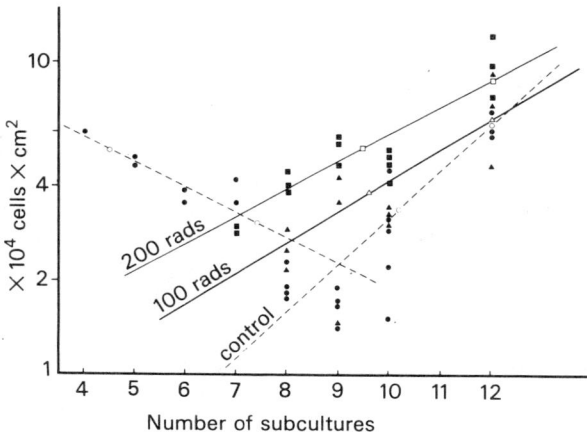

FIG. 8. Regression lines obtained with the cell counts illustrated in Fig. 7.

maintained in borosylicate milk dilution bottles. One group of cultures was carried in 30-ml nutrient medium and the other in 15-ml. The survival curve of the latter showed a growth decline with a long latency period where cell division almost stopped, followed by recovery and immortalization. The group carried in 30 ml of medium did not go through a growth decline and the cell population became a continuous line without any intermediate latent stage.

When the irradiation experiment was performed with human fibroblasts the results were intermediate to those obtained with the two other series: the life span of the irradiated cells was unchanged or slightly prolonged as compared with the controls (Fig. 10) and the total number of cells produced in each group

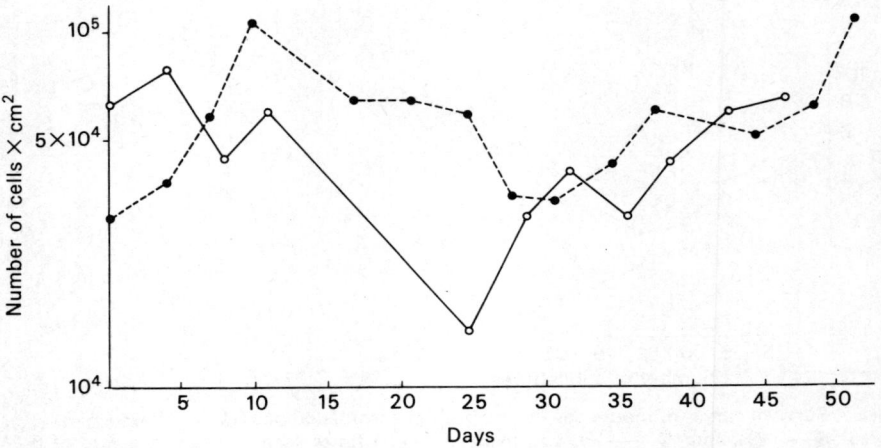

FIG. 9. Survival curves of mouse new-born fibroblasts kept in 30 ml (●---●) and 15 ml (○——○) of nutrient medium. Ordinate: cell density at each passage; abcissa : days in culture.

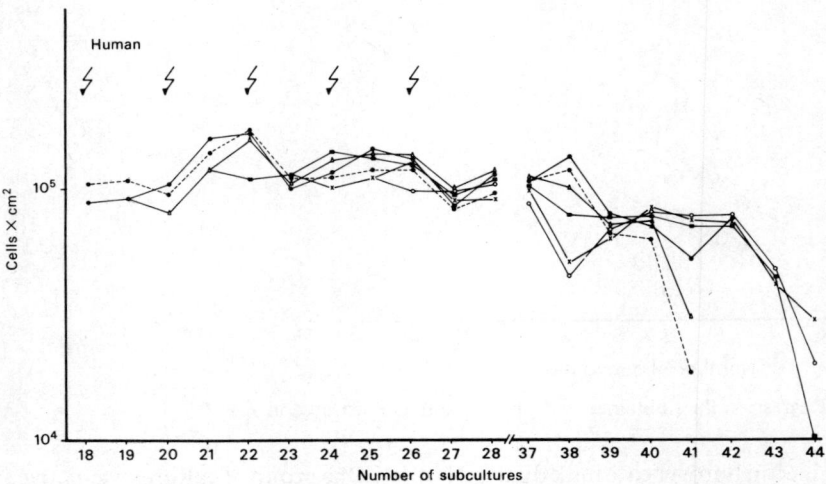

FIG. 10. Survival curves of human embryonic fibroblasts irradiated one (●——●), two (△——△), three (■——■), four (X——X), and five (○——○) times with 100 rad at a rate of 0.27 rad min⁻¹. Control cells (●---). Ordinate: cell density before each subculture; abcissa : passage number.

was unchanged (Fig. 11). So it seems that low dose rate ionization radiation accelerates growth decline in chick fibroblasts; in mouse fibroblasts, on the contrary, it accelerates the immortalization of the cells; and in human fibroblasts it does not lead either to an acceleration of aging or immortalization.

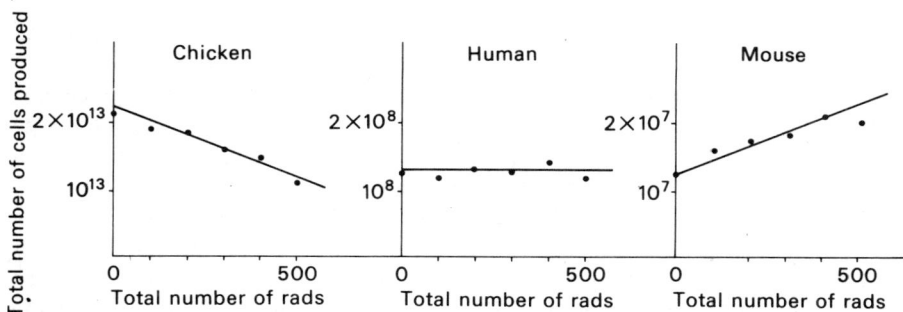

FIG. 11. Total number of cells produced in control and irradiated chicken, human, and mouse fibroblasts after different doses of ionizing radiation. The calculation for chicken and human cells was done up to the last passage. For mouse cells it was done up to the 20th passage when the cultures became well established.

Since the response to ionizing radiation of the fibroblasts from these three species corresponds to their relative positions in respect to stability of life span, it seems justified to think that the mechanisms involved in this stability are the same implicated in survival after ionizing radiation.

The role of DNA strand switching in cell aging and immortalization

Recent concepts developed from bacterial genetics (Kolata 1976) could form the basis for a model that would fit our data and could explain the phenomena of cell aging and immortalization in eukaryotes. It is well known that at each cell division there is DNA strand switching through sister chromatid exchanges. Transcription from these reorganized DNA strands will depend on the efficiency of repair and on the mutual influence between the chromatin regions that come together. Fibroblasts could differ both in capacity to repair and in fitness between distant chromatin regions.

The absence of some repair enzymes or the presence of a non-repairable substrate could cause gaps after DNA strand switching during cell division. At each cell cycle more and more breaks would remain unrepaired with the subsequent silencing of different genes due to loss of the normal regulation existing between neighbouring regions.

If repair takes place and new strands come together, new influences will be created which could depend on fitness between different chromatin regions. When there is a poor fit or the number of controlling elements with a good fit is small, most of the new regions that come together will not influence each other and the genes within them will not be transcribed, causing a decreased rate of RNA synthesis and protein synthesis. Although each protein would be correctly transcribed, the decreased rate of protein synthesis would lead to a protein pool containing a relative increase in degraded molecules due to postsynthetic changes. These are molecules that normally remain in the cell before being completely eliminated. The renewal of the protein pool will eventually become so small that it will be insufficient for such functions as cell division and cell attachment.

It is possible, though, that in cells where the number of controlling elements with a good fit is small the probability of immortalization can increase through the incorporation of external elements (e.g. transfection, transformation, cell hybridization) that would turn on the silenced regions.

On the other hand, in cells where repair mechanisms are efficient and there is a good fit between controlling elements and other chromatin segments the former would have a positive influence on the new adjacent regions. In cells such as these under conditions that increase DNA strand switching (cell division, ionizing radiation, chemical carcinogens) the probability of chromatin regions to meet controlling elements with a good fit will be high and thus DNA will still be transcribed. In fact, a stimulation of cell division by large volumes of medium/or ionizing radiation accelerates the acquisition of an infinite life span of mouse fibroblasts (Figs. 7 and 9). The hypothesis is schematically illustrated in Fig. 12.

In summary, DNA strand switching is the inevitable event that will determine the fate of the dividing cell. The probability of becoming immortal will be higher for some types of cells than for others, due to the presence either of efficient repair or of controlling elements with a good fit for other regions of the genome. The probability of immortalization will be increased through events that stimulate DNA strand switching or through the insertion of foreign DNA, that will lead to the creation of new regions which will develop into self-replicating units.

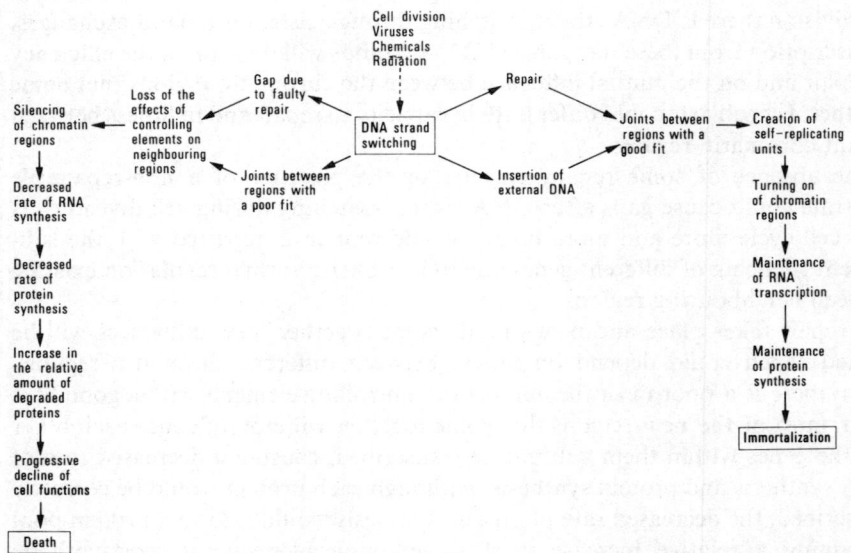

FIG. 12. Tentative model of the events leading to aging or immortalization of dividing cells. The same basic event (DNA strand switching) will have a different outcome depending on the genome organization of the cell.

References

AZZARONE, B., PEDULLA, D., and ROMANZI, C. A. (1976). *Nature, Lond.,* 262, 74.
BENEDICT, W. F., JONES, P. A., LANG, W. E., IGEL, H. J., and FREEMAN, A. E. (1975). *Nature, Lond.,* 256, 322.
CRISTOFALO, V. J. (1970. *Aging in cell and tissue culture,* p. 83. Plenum Press, New York.
EARLE, W. R. (1943). *J. Nat. Cancer Inst.,* 4, 165.
GEDER, L., LAUSCH, R., O'NEILL, F., and RAPP, F. (1976). *Science, N.Y.,* 192, 1134.
GERSHON, D. and GERSHON, H. (1976). *Gerontology,* 22, 212.
GIRARDI, A. J., JENSEN, F. C., and KOPROWSKI, H. (1965). *J. Cell comp. Physiol.,* 65, 69.
GOLDSTEIN, S. (1969). *Lancet,* i, 424.
——, LITTLEFIELD, J. W., and SOELDNER, J. S. (1969). *Proc. Nat. Acad. Sci. USA,* 64, 155.
HAYFLICK, L. (1965). *Exp. Cell Res.,* 37, 614.
—— and MOORHEAD, P. S. (1961). *Exp. Cell Res.,* 25, 585.
KOLATA, G. B. (1976). *Science,* 193, 392
MACIEIRA-COELHO, A. (1966). *Experientia,* 22, 390.
—— and PONTEN, J. (1969). *J. Cell Biol.,* 43, 374.
——, ——, and PHILIPSON, L. (1966). *Exp. Cell Res.,* 42, 673.
—— and LIMA, R. (1973). *Mech. Age. Dev.,* 2, 13.
—— and LORIA, E. (1974). *Nature (Lond.),* 251, 67.
MARTIN, G. M., SPRAGUE, C. A., and EPSTEIN, C. (1970). *J. Lab. Invest.,* 23, 86.
OGURA, H. and ERIIS, R. (1975). *J. Virology,* 16, 443.
ORGEL, L. E. (1963). *Proc. Nat. Acad. Sci. USA,* 49, 517.
PONTEN, J. (1971). *Virology Monogr.,* 8, 4.
SCHNEIDER, E. L. and MITSUI, Y. (1976). *Proc. Nat. Acad. Sci. USA,* 73, 3584–8.
TERZI, M and HAWKINS, T. S. C. (1975). *Nature, Lond.,*253, 361.

Eukaryotic cell differentiation: induction of differentiation of murine erythroleukaemia cells Paul A. Marks, Richard A. Rikfind, Arthur Bank, Masaaki Terada, Roberta Reuben, Eitan Fibach, Uri Nudel, Jane Salmon and Yair Gazitt

We have investigated the mechanism of eukaryotic cell differentiation employing an erythroid model system: induced erythropoietic differentiation of murine erythroleukaemia cells (MELC) transformed by Friend virus complex (Friend 1957; Friend, Scher, Holland, and Sato 1971; Marks, Rifkind, Bank, Terada, Maniatis, Reuben, and Fibach 1976). This chapter reviews studies elucidating events involved in the induction of MELC to differentiate to erythroid cells in culture with dimethylsulfoxide and other chemical inducers. MELC show a low level (< 1 per cent) of spontaneous erythroid differentiation in culture; but when cultured with various chemicals, a high proportion of the cells are induced to express a programme of erythroid differentiation. This programme of differentiation has many similarities to that observed in the erythropoietin-induced differentiation of foetal mouse liver erythropoiesis (Marks and Rifkind 1972), including morphological changes (Friend *et al.* 1971), accumulation of globin mRNAs (Ross, Ikawa, and Leder 1972; Ostertag, Melderis, Steinhoider, Kluge, and Dube 1972; Gilmour, Harrison, Windass, Affara, and Paul 1974; Singer 1975), alpha and beta globin synthesis (Boyer, Wuu, Noyes, Young, Scher, Friend, Priesler, and Bank 1972), increase in haeme synthesis (Ebert and Ikawa 1974), synthesis of proteins characteristic of erythrocytes, such as catalase and spectrin (Kabat, Sherton, Evans, Bigley, and Koler 1975; Arndt-Jovin, Ostertag, Eisen, and Jovin 1976), limited capacity for cell division (Friend *et al.* 1971; Gusella, Geller, Clarke, Weeks, and Housman 1976; Fibach, Reuben, Rifkind, and Marks 1977), and appearance of mature red cell specific antigens (Furasawa, Ikawa, and Sugano 1971).

MELC has a number of advantages for genetic and biochemical studies of mechanisms of induction of eukaryotic cells to differentiation. MELC can be maintained in continuous culture. A cell line has been developed in our laboratory which has a very low percentage (< 0.5 per cent) of spontaneous erythroid differentiation (Singer, Cooper, Maniatis, Marks, and Rifkind 1974); chemicals have been synthesized, such as hexamethylene bisacetamide (Reuben, Wife, Breslow, Rifkind, and Marks 1976), which can induce essentially 100 per cent of the cells in culture to differentiate to erythroid cells; and variatint cell lines have been developed, which are resistant to induction by one or another inducer (Ohta, Tanaka, Terada, Miller, Bank, Marks, and Rifkind 1976; Gusella and Housman 1976; Harrison, Gilmour, Affara, Conkie, and Paul 1974). MELC differ from normal mammalian erythropoiesis in not being dependent upon or sensitive to erythropoietin (Marks, Rifkind, Cantor, unpublished observations), and rarely proceed to a non-nucleated stage of differentiation which is characteristic of definitive mammalian erythropoiesis (Friend *et al.* 1971; Reuben *et al.* 1976).

MELC differentiation will be considered with respect to:

(1) accumulation of globin mRNA and globin synthesis during differentiation;
(2) structure of chemicals active as inducing agents;
(3) relation of the action of inducing agents and the cell division cycle;
(4) requirements for stable commitment to differentiation of MELC;
(5) differential effects of various inducers on the expression of globin genes in MELC.

Accumulation of mRNA for globin and globin synthesis

Studies of the effect of Me_2SO under conditions of clonal growth indicate that MELC are an essentially homogeneous population of transformed erythroid cells (Singer *et al.* 1974; Paul and Hickey 1974). There is evidence which suggests that the transformed cells correspond to proerythroblasts (Tambourin and Wendling 1971).

In MELC cultured with 280-mM Me_2SO, accumulation of mRNA for globin, assayed by cDNA:RNA hybridization, is first detectable at about 24 hours (Singer 1975). An increase in the rate of globin synthesis is also first detectable at approximately 24 hours (Singer 1975). These findings suggest that there is little lag in the accumulation of mRNA for globin and the onset of translation of globin mRNAs.

Chemical structure of compounds active as inducing agents

The induction by Me_2SO of the erythropoietic programme of differentiation in MELC prompted investigations on the chemical structural requirements for compounds active as inducing agents. It has been demonstrated (Tanaka, Levy, Terada, Breslow, Rifkind, and Marks 1975) that a series of planar-polar compounds, such as *N*-methyl acetamide, induce differentiation in MELC, as assayed by the proportion of cells becoming benzidine reactive, at concentrations significantly below that required for Me_2SO. Further, it was shown that dimerization of the inducing agent, *N*-methyl acetamide, by linkage at nitrogen through varying numbers of methylenes, resulted in a group of inducing agents, polymethylene bisacetamides, which were even more active than the simple monomer (Reuben *et al.* 1976). A variety of other chemicals have been shown to act as inducers including fatty acids, purine and purine derivatives, haeme, and inhibitors of DNA and RNA synthesis (Scher, Preisler, and Friend 1973; Dube, Gaedicke, Kluge, Weismann, Melderis, Steinheider, Crozier, Beckmann, and Ostertag 1973; Leder, Orkin, and Leder 1975; Gusella and Housman 1976; Ebert, Wars, and Buell 1976).

Among the compounds tested in this laboratory, the polar compound hexamethylene bisacetamide (HMBA) (Table 1) has been found to be most effective by the criteria:

(a) essentially the entire population of MELC is induced to differentiate;
(b) a greater proportion of the total protein synthesized is haemoglobin;
(c) a relatively low concentration is effective (Reuben *et al.* 1976).

For example, HMBA is an effective inducer at concentrations of 1 mM, and, at an optimal concentration of 5 mM, induces essentially all cells in culture to differentiate.

Table 1 Structure of compounds active as inducing agents

Dimethylsulphoxide	$CH_3\text{-}\overset{\overset{\textstyle O}{\|\|}}{S}\text{-}CH_3$
N-methylacetamide	$CH_3\text{-}\overset{\overset{\textstyle O}{\|\|}}{C}\text{-}NH\text{-}CH_3$
Dimethylacetamide	$CH_3\text{-}\overset{\overset{\textstyle O}{\|\|}}{C}\text{-}\underset{\underset{\textstyle CH_3}{\|}}{N}\text{-}CH_3$
Hexamethylene bisacetamide	$CH_3\text{-}\overset{\overset{\textstyle O}{\|\|}}{C}\text{-}NH\text{-}(CH_2)_6\text{-}NH\text{-}\overset{\overset{\textstyle O}{\|\|}}{C}\text{-}CH_3$

There is a direct relationship between the optimal concentration for induction and the concentration at which these compounds inhibit growth and cause cell death in culture. This is a consistent observation for the entire series of polar compounds effective as inducers (Tanaka *et al.* 1975; Reuben *et al.* 1976). These observations suggest that the mechanisms of induction may involve a change in the structure of a cellular component, which, if too extensive, is incompatible with cell survival. Alternatively, the inducers may have toxic effects on the cells which are independent of the action causing differentiation, but which is apparent at a concentration closely related to that which is optimal for induction. The data at present do not permit one to distinguish between these two possibilities.

The nature of the cellular site of the primary action of these polar compounds has not been established. Evidence will be summarized below which suggests that inducing agents cause a series of changes which may initially involve an effect at the level of the membrane and, subsequently, changes in chromatin and product of transcription of the chromatin associated with differentiation.

Induction of MELC and DNA synthesis (S-phase)

There is accumulating evidence that the transition to the synthesis of a differentiated protein requires DNA synthesis (Marks and Rifkind 1972; Holtzer, Weintraub, Mayne, and Mochan 1972; Rutter, Pictet, and Morris 1973; Dworkin, Higgins, Glenn, and Mandelstam 1972; McClintock and Papaconstantinou 1974; Levy, Terada, Rifkind, and Marks 1975; Marks *et al.* 1976). In MELC synchronized with respect to cell division cycle by exposure to high levels of thymidine (Levy *et al.* 1975), it was shown that the inducer must be present during DNA synthesis, and, possibly, shortly thereafter, for differentiation to erythroid cells to occur in culture. Thus, it was found that cells which were synchronized by culture for 44 h in 2-mM thymidine and 280-mM Me_2SO and released from cell division block by transfer to fresh medium without Me_2SO or thymidine, proliferated but did not differentiate. Cells which were removed from cell division block and transferred to fresh media with 280-mM Me_2SO and cultured for 4 h (a time sufficient for essentially all cells to enter S and, some cells, a portion of G_2), and then transferred to fresh media without inducer, proceed to differentiate over the ensuing five days. An additional condition in these studies for the induction of erythroid differentiation was that Me_2SO be present for at least 20 h prior to the release from cell division block. The preincubation period may, in part, be related to effects of the inducer which must occur prior to the critical S-phase (see below).

Transient inhibition of initiation of S-phase (prolongation of G_1) associated with induction of MELC

MELC cultured with Me_2SO develop a transient block in initiation of DNA synthesis, or a prolongation of G_1, which appears to be most marked at about

20 h in non-synchronous cultures. This was demonstrated by examining the rate of DNA synthesis, proportion of cells in S-phase and pattern of DNA accumulation in MELC grown in the presence and absence of Me_2SO and other inducing agents, such as butyric acid and dimethylacetamide (Terada, Fried, Nudel, Rifkind, and Marks 1977a).

These findings in these studies suggest that there is a transient inhibition of entry of MELC into the S-phase when cultured with Me_2SO. This conclusion was supported by analysis of the proportion of cells in S-phase (cells which become labelled during 20-min exposure to (^{3}H)thymidine) during culture with and without inducing agent, and by determining the relative DNA content per cell using the propidium iodide binding measure with flow microfluorometry (Terada *et al.* 1977a). There is a decrease in the proportion of cells in S-phase which occurs during the early period of culture with inducing agents, and is most marked, in comparison with uninduced cultures, at 20 h.

In addition, it has been found (Terada *et al.* 1977a) that there is a difference in the pattern of binding of the intercalating agent, propidium iodide, to chromatin in cells in G_1 phase of MELC cultured with or without Me_2SO. In control cells, cultured without inducer, there is an increase in the binding of propidium iodide as early as 10 h; this is not observed in cells cultured with Me_2SO. The Me_2SO-resistant cell line, DR-10, behaves like control DS-19 cells, even when cultured with Me_2SO.

These observations suggest that during prolongation of the G_1 phase of the cell cycle, there is an associated alteration in chromatin structure. These changes in G_1 may be related to the induction of MELC to erythroid differentiation.

Changes in DNA associated with induction of MELC

Further definition of the effects of inducing agents on MELC has been obtained from studies of DNA structure in cells cultured with and without inducers. Analysis of preparations of DNA on alkaline sucrose gradient shows a decrease in the rate of sedimentation of DNA prepared from MELC cultured with Me_2SO, as early as 27 h after onset of culture (Terada, Nudel, Rifkind, and Marks 1977b). This is approximately the time at which MELC begin to accumulate mRNA for globin (Singer 1975). No change in the rate of sedimentation of DNA is observed when analysed on neutral sucrose gradients. The decrease in rate of sedimentation of DNA in alkaline sucrose gradients is observed with DNA MELC cultured with other inducing agents, such as butyric acid and dimethylacetamide. On the other hand, Me_2SO does not induce a change in the sedimentation properties of DNA from Me_2SO-resistant DR-10 cells cultured with Me_2SO (Terada *et al.* 1977b). Analysis of the slowly sedimenting DNA recovered from the alkali sucrose gradient analysis of material from MELC cultured with inducer suggest it represents single strand DNA of relatively small size (corresponding to 120s to 150s). The alteration of DNA associated with induction of MELC may prove to be a critical event leading to the expression of the programme of differentiation. Alternatively, the changes in the properties of

DNA could be a feature or product of differentiation, subsequent to the events which are critical to the commitment of MELC to differentiate.

Commitment of MELC to differentiate

To evaluate the relationship of alterations in cell division cycle, changes in DNA and/or chromatin structure, and the action of the inducing agent during the S-phase of the cell cycle, to the commitment of MELC to differentiate, it is necessary to be able to study the kinetics of recruitment to differentiation at the single cell level and in a quantitative manner. A technique for the assay of commitment of individual cells to differentiate has been developed (Fibach *et al.* 1977). In this assay, following suspension culture with inducing agent, MELC are cloned in a semisolid medium in the absence of the inducer and clones scored for poliferative capacity (number of cells in a colony) and differentiation (number of colonies containing benzidine reactive cells). Employing this assay, it has been shown that the proportion of cells in the culture which are committed to differentiate is dependent both on the concentration of the inducing agent and the duration of exposure to the inducing agent in the pre-cloning suspension culture. For example, with HMBA, stabilized differentiation of MELC is essentially complete when the cells are cultured with 5-mM HMBA for 50 h. HMBA-induced erythroid differentiation is associated with a limitation in proliferative capacity, as is characteristic of normal erythropoiesis. By contrast, under conditions less than optimal for induction of differentiation, with respect to either the concentration of HMBA or the duration of pre-cloning culture with HMBA, induction to differentiation is not fully stabilized. This is indicated by the fact that a single cell can give rise to a colony containing both differentiated and undifferentiated cells (Table 2).

Employing this assay, committed cells are detected after 12 to 13 h of culture with HMBA. Colonies derived from cells which had been in suspension culture with HMBA are of three types as assayed by the benzidine reaction:

(a) uniformly benzidine negative cells;
(b) uniformly benzidine reactive cells;
(c) a mixture of benzidine reactive and non-reactive cells ('mixed colonies').

Pre-cloning culture with 5-mM HMBA for 53 h yielded colonies of which 96 per cent were uniformly benzidine reactive, 1 per cent were 'mixed colonies', and 3 per cent were benzidine non-reactive (Table 2). Exposure to 1-mM HMBA produced 7 per cent 'mixed colonies' and 28 per cent benzidine reactive. Thus, the contribution of 'mixed colonies' to the total population of differentiated (benzidine reactive) colonies is highest at suboptimal concentrations of HMBA or after short periods of exposure to HMBA. Careful inspection of the cultures immediately after inoculation indicated that 'mixed colonies' were very unlikely to be due to colony formation by more than one cell. This conclusion was confirmed by scoring 'mixed colonies' in plates inoculated with a range of concentrations from 5×10^2 to 5×10^3 per ml; under these conditions the proportion of

Table 2 Heterogeneity of colonies derived from MELC cultured with various concentrations of HMBA and for various times

1. *Studies with various concentrations of HMBA in pre-cloning culture for 53 h*

HMBA	Undifferentiated coloniest (per cent)	Differentiated colonies		
		A. Uniformly benzidine reactive (per cent)	B. 'Mixed colonies't (per cent)	C. Proportion of 'mixed colonies'§ (per cent)
mM				
0	100	0	0	—
0.5	95	2	3	60
1.0	65	28	7	20
2.0	19	76	5	6
3.0	8	90	2	2
4.0	5	94	1	1
5.0	3	96	1	1

2. *Studies with various times of pre-cloning culture with 5-mM HMBA*

Time (h)				
8	100	0	0	—
13	95	2	3	60
16	86	5	9	64
20	75	14	11	55
26	57	28	15	35
36	26	69	5	7
40	8	90	2	2
50	0	99	1	1

Cells were exposed in suspension culture to various concentrations of HMBA for 53 h (1) or to 5-mM HMBA for various periods before cloning (2) in semisolid medium in the absence of the inducer. Colonies were scored, 5 days from initiation of the experiments, by benzidine staining. See Fibach *et al.* (1977) for details.
†The criterion for an undifferentiated colony is the absence of any benzidine-reactive cells.
‡The criterion for a 'mixed colony' is the presence of benzidine-reactive and benzidine-unreactive cells in the same colony.
§$C = \dfrac{B}{A+B} \times 100.$

'mixed colonies' was independent of inoculant concentration. These observations suggest that under these conditions a committed cell may give rise to both differentiated and undifferentiated progeny.

As discussed above, inducer must be present during DNA synthesis and possibly during a portion of cell cycle thereafter, in order to induce differentiation of MELC. If exposure to inducer during S-phase of the cell cycle is sufficient to commit a cell to differentiate, then the rate at which cells enter S-phase will equal the rate of commitment to differentiation. Alternatively, if exposure to inducer during S-phase is required but not sufficient for commitment, then the rate of entry into S will exceed the rate of commitment. These alternatives were examined by scoring cells for DNA synthesis (by (^{3}H)thymidine uptake and radioautography) during HMBA induced differentiation. The rate of entry into S-phase as measured in this fashion was greater than the rate of commitment to differentiation, as measured by 'transfer out' from medium with HMBA to medium without inducer (Fibach *et al.* 1977). Taken together the present data suggest DNA synthesis (passage through S-phase of the cell cycle) is a necessary but not a sufficient condition leading to induced differentiation. The fact that the rate of entry of MELC into S-phase is greater than the rate of commitment suggests the possibility that additional steps or events with different kinetics are required to achieve stable commitment of MELC to differentiation. Gusella *et al.* (1976) reported on a quantitative analysis of the kinetics of induction of MELC to differentiation employing a similar technique for analysis of commitment, and suggested that commitment for each cell is made in a stochastic manner. Irreversible commitment to expression of differentiated functions occurs with a discrete probability per cell generation for many cell generations. In agreement with the observations in our laboratory (Fibach *et al.* 1977), these workers concluded that the value for this probability is a function of the concentration of inducer, which in their experiments was Me_2SO. In both the studies of Gusella *et al.* (1976) and Fibach *et al.* (1977), the temporal relationship between the kinetics of commitment and developmental of biochemical characteristics of differentiated erythroid cells, suggest that an irreversible commitment differentiation may precede or at least accompany the first detectable accumulation of globin mRNA and globin synthesis.

Differential effects of chemical inducers on the expression of beta globin genes

The proportion of MELC induced to differentiate and the average haemoglobin content achieved per cell vary with the strain of MELC and with the inducing agent used. For example, with MELC (DS-19), 5-mM HMBA induces essentially the entire population (over 99 per cent) of MELC, with marked haemoglobinization of all cells (Reuben *et al.* 1976). Butyric acid on the other hand induces a lower proportion of cells, approximately 60 per cent. It is not yet known whether the different agents induce the identical programme of erythroid differentiation or whether there are different patterns of differentiation characteristic of the various inducers. This question has been explored in experiments designed to examine one aspect of the problem, namely, the effects of different agents on the relative rates of synthesis of haemoglobin major (Hb^{maj}) and haemoglobin minor (Hb^{min}) (Nudel, Salmon, Terada, Bank, Rifkind, and Merks 1977). Hb^{maj} and Hb^{min} differ in amino acid sequence of the beta chain (Hutton, Bishop, Schweet, and Russell 1962; Popp and Bailiff 1973; Gilman, 1976a,b). On the basis of the available genetic and biochemical evidence (Popp and Bailiff 1973; Gilman 1976a,b), β^{maj} and β^{min} genes appear to be closely linked and β^{maj} and β^{min} globins appear to differ by a relatively few (6 to 9) amino acids in the primary structure.

The rate of synthesis of globin was measured with (^{35}S)-methionine as the radioactive amino acid precursor. Relative rates of synthesis of Hb^{maj} and Hb^{min} were calculated assuming 1 methionine in α and 2 methionines in each of the β chains. The planar-polar compounds tested, such as HMBA, Me_2SO, and methyl pyrolidinone, induced two to three times more Hb^{maj} than Hb^{min}

in both the Me_2SO-sensitive (DS-19) and Me_2SO-resistant cell lines (DR-10). Fatty acids, such as butyric acid and propionic acid, induce approximately equal amounts of both haemoglobins in DS-19 and induce relatively more Hb^{min} in DR-10. (Table 3). These differences in relative accumulation of Hb^{maj} and Hb^{min} are associated with similar differences in the rates of synthesis of β^{maj} and β^{min} globin and of accumulation of mRNA for β^{maj} and for β^{min} globins (Table 4) (Nudel *et al.* 1977). The ratio of the rates of synthesis of the two β globins in both DS-19 and DR-10 remain similar from day 2 through the duration of the period of culture (day 6) (Table 3). These findings suggest that the differences in the ratio of β^{maj} and β^{min} are not due to changing rates of of synthesis at different stages of erythroid differentiation.

The finding that the ratio of the relative rates of synthesis of β^{maj} to β^{min} globin reflects the relative content of poly(A)-containing mRNA in induced MELC (Nudel *et al.* 1977) suggests that the differences in the relative amounts of

Table 3 Ratio of synthesis of β^{maj} globin to β^{min} globin in MELC cell lines DS-19 and DR-10 cultured with different inducing agents

Cell line	Day	Inducing agent added			
		Me_2SO	HMBA	MPL	BA*
DS-19	2	2.1			1.1
	3	2.7	2.7		1.3
	4	2.1	2.5	2.4	1.1
	5	1.8	2.2		1.3
	6	1.9	2.4		1.2
DR-10	2			3.1	1.1
	3			2.5	1.0
	4		2.3	2.5	0.9
	5		2.1	2.2	0.8
	6		2.6	2.1	0.5

Cell extracts were prepared from cultures incubated with inducing agents for the indicated number of days. Incubation with [^{35}S]methionine separation and quantitation of globins were as described in Nudel *et al.* 1977. The ratio of synthesis of β^{maj} to β^{min} globin was determined by comparing the amount of radioactivity in each globin assuming that each β globin chain contains two methionine residues.

Table 4 Ratio of synthesis of β^{maj} globin to β^{min} globin in a wheat germ cell-free system with MELC poly(A)-containing RNA as template

Source of RNA	Inducing agent added				
	Me_2SO	HMBA	MPL	BA*	None
DS-19 cells	1.9	2.9		1.4	
DR-10 cells		3.1	2.4	0.9	
DBA/2 reticulocytes					3.7

MELC were cultured for 4 days with different inducing agents. Preparation and translation of RNA and quantification of β globins were as described in Nudel *et al.* 1977.
Ratio of rates of synthesis of β^{maj} globin to that of β^{min} in a wheat germ cell-free system to which was added poly(A)-containing RNA purified from the reticulocytes of DBA/2 adult mice.

the β globin observed with different types of inducing agents are not attributable to translational or post-translational regulatory mechanisms. The inducers ap- to act directly or indirectly to control the rates of synthesis of β^{maj} and β^{min} globins by affecting the transcription or processing of mRNA for these proteins.

Mechanism of action of inducing agents

On the basis of the observations summarized above, one can suggest a sequence of events which ensue in culture of MELC with inducing agents causing differ- entiation. It appears that the virus transformed cell is an erthroid precursor cell. We assume that the cell has developed to a point where it is 'set' to express a co-ordinated programme of protein synthesis characteristic of erythroid cells. Virus transformation causes a block in the responsiveness of these cells to erythropoietin or, alternatively, block the cells at a stage beyond which they are normally responsive to erythropoietin (Marks and Rifkind 1972).

When one considers the chemical nature of compounds which have been demonstrated to be active as inducers of differentiation in MELC, it is, at present, difficult to make a single generalizing statement as to the property which makes these compounds active. Several of the most active compounds are relatively highly polar and planar. It is assumed that the specificity of the effects of the inducing agent are due to the properties of the target cell.

One of the earliest detectable biochemical events characteristics of the expres- sion of the erythroid programme is the accumulation of mRNA for globin. This suggests that the inducers, either directly or indirectly, act to effect the transcrip- tion or processing of the product of the structural genes whose expression is characteristic of erythroid cells. (While this seems to be generally true for indu- cers with various lines of MELC, Harrison *et al.* (1974) have presented evidence which they interpret as suggesting that a Friend leukaemia line may be induced at a level involving translational control of expression of the mRNA for globin).

The evidence that the inducer must be present during a critical S-phase (DNA synthesis) for the transition to expression of the differentiated programme suggests DNA replication has a critical role in the onset of expression of globin and, other associated structural genes. Evidence has been provided that the stability of the protein–DNA complexes may be altered as the replication apparatus copies the DNA. There is evidence (Terada *et al.* 1977b) that changes in DNA protein complex occur in induced cells at a time just prior to or accom- panying the first detectable accumulation of mRNA for globin. The presence of an inducer during DNA synthesis is not sufficient for the stable expression of the differentiated programme in all progeny of a cell exposed to inducer (Fibach *et al.* 1977).

The finding that an early and transient increase in cAMP levels occurs during culture with the inducer suggests that an initial event in the induction may occur at the cell membrane and that effects on the regulation of transcription are secondary. That chemicals active as inducers of MELC do affect the cell membrane has been suggested by evidence that topical anaesthetics, which increase the fluidity of membranes *in vitro*, interfere with the effects of the inducers (Bernstein, Boyd, Crickley, and Lamb 1976) and that there is a correlation between the ability of inducers to cryoprotect erythocytes and the effectiveness as inducing agents (Preisler 1976).

One cannot exclude a direct effect of the inducing agents on the cell membrane as well as at the level of chromatin (Marks *et al.* 1976). In this regard, the findings of Nakanishi, Pastan, and co-workers (Nakanishi, Adhya, Gottesman, and Pastan 1974a,b), that Me_2SO and other DNA denaturing agents stimulate the synthesis of specific gal and lambda RNA transcripts from wild-type and promote defective templates of *E. coli in vivo* and *in vitro*, are of interest. Me_2SO can directly affect the stability of chromatin and of DNA (Lapeyre and Bekhor 1974).

As a working hypothesis, it is suggested that the induction to erythroid differentiation involves a series of events which include:

(a) an effect on the cell membrane which occurs early and leads to a transient increase in cAMP levels;
(b) a prolongation of G_1 which is associated with a structural alteration in chromatin, as evidenced by the restricted binding of intercalating dyes and the increased susceptibility to alkali degradation of the DNA of induced cells;
(c) 'reprogramming' of the chromatin for transctiption occurring during the subsequent S-phase of the cell cycle;
(d) additional stabilizing events occurring following this S, which are required to render differentiation irreversible.

Acknowledgements

Studies reported in this paper from the authors' laboratory were supported, in part, by grants from the NIGMS (GM-14552), NCI (CA-13696, CA-18314) and contract (NO1-CP-6-1008), and grant from the NSF (PCM 75-08696).

Masaaki Terada is a Hirschl Trust Scholar. Roberta Reuben and Eitan Fibach are Schultz Foundation Scholars.

Abbreviations

The following abbreviations are used in the text:
HMBA, hexamethylene bisacetamide; MPL, methyl pyrolidinone; BA, butyric acid.

References

ARNDT-JOVIN, D. J., OSTERTAG, W., EISEN, H., and JOVIN, T. M. (1976). Analysis by computer-controlled cell sorter of Friend virus-transformed cells in different stages of differentiation. In *Modern trends in human leukemia II* (eds. R. Neth, R. C. Gallo, K. Mannweiler, and W. C. Moloney). J. F. Lehmanns Verlag, Munich. [Series: Hamatologie and Blattransfusion, *Band* 19.]

BERNSTEIN, A., BOYD, A. S., CRICKLEY, V., and LAMB, V. (1976). Induction and inhibition of Friend leukemic cell differentiation: the role of membrane-active compounds. In *Biogenesis and turnover of membrane macromolecules* (ed. J. S. Cook), pp. 93–103. Raven Press, New York.

BOYER, S. H., WUU, K. D. NOYES, A. N., YOUNG, R., SCHER, W., FRIEND, C., PRIESLER, H. D., and BANK, A. (1972). Hemoglobin biosynthesis in murine virus-induced leukemic cells in vitro: Structure and amounts of globin chains produced. *Blood*, **40**, 823–835.

DUBE, S. K., GAEDICKE, G., KLUGE, N., WEISMANN, B. J., MELDERIS, H., STEINHEIDER, G., CROZIER, T., BECKMANN, H., and OSTERTAG, (1973). Hemoglobin synthesizing mouse and human erythroleukemic cell lines as model systems for the study of differentiation and control of gene expression. *Proceedings of the 4th International Symposium of the Princess Takamatsu Cancer Research Fund*, pp. 99–132. University Park Press, Tokyo.

DWORKIN, M., HIGGINS, J., GLENN, A., and MANDELSTAM, J. (1972). Synchronization of the growth of bacillus subtilis and its effect on sporulation. *Spores*, **5**: 233–7.

EBERT, P. S. and IKAWA, Y. (1974). Induction of δ-aminolevulinic acid synthetase during erythroid differentiation of cultured leukemia cells. *Proc. Soc. exp. Biol. Med.* **146**, 601–4.

——, WARS, I., and BUELL, D. N. (1976). Erythroid differentiation in cultured Friend leukemia cells treated with metabolic inhibitors. *Cancer Res.*, **36**, 1809–13.

FIBACH, E., REUBEN, R., RIFKIND, R. A., and MARKS, P. A. (1977). Effect of hexamethylene bisacetamide on the commitment to differentiation of murine erythroleukemia cells. *Cancer Res.*, **37**, 440–4.

FRIEND, C. (1957). Cell-free transmission in adult Swiss mice of a disease having the character of a leukemia. *J. exp. Med.*, **105**, 307–18.

——, SCHER, W., HOLLAND, J. G., and SATO, T. (1971). Hemoglobin synthesis in murine virus induced leukemic cells *in vitro*: Stimulation of erythroid differentiation by dimethyl sulfoxide. *Proc. Nat. Acad. Sci. (USA)*, **68**, 378–82.

FURUSAWA, M., IKAWA, Y., and SUGANO, H. (1971). Development of Erythrocyte membrane-specific antigen(s) in clonal cultured cells of Friend virus-induced tumor. *Proc. Japan Acad.*, **47**, 220–24.

GILMAN, J. (1976a). Mouse haemoglobin beta chains: Sequence data on embryonic *y*-chain and genetic linkage of the y-chain locus to the adult β-chains locus Hbb. *Biochem. J.*, **155**, 231–41.

—— (1976b). Mouse haemoglobin beta chains: Comparative sequence data on adult major and minor beta chains from two species, *mus musculus* and *mus cervicolor*. *Biochem. J.*, **159**, 43–53.

GILMOUR, R. S., HARRISON, P. R., WINDASS, J. W., AFFARA, M., and PAUL, J. (1974). Globin mRNA synthesis and processing during haemoglobin induction in Friend cells. I. Evidence for transcriptional control in clone M2. *Cell Differentiation*, **3**, 9–22.

GUSELLA, J. and HOUSMAN, D. (1976). Differentiation *in vitro* by purine and purine analogs. *Cell*, **8**, 263–9.

——, GELLER, R., CLARKE, B., WEEKS, V., and HOUSMAN, D. (1976). Commitment to erythroid differentiation by Friend erythroide leukemia cells: a stochastic analysis. *Cell*, **9**, 221–9.

HARRISON, P. R., GILMOUR, R. S., AFFARA, N. A., CONKIE, D., and PAUL, J. (1974). Globin messenger RNA synthesis and processing during haemoglobin induction in Friend cells. II. Evidence for post-transcriptional control in clone 707. *Cell Differentiation*, 3, 23–30.

HOLTZER, H., WEINTRAUB, H., MAYNE, R., and MOCHAN, B. (1972). The cell cycle, cell lineages and cell differentiation. *Curr. Topics Dev. Biol.*, (eds. A. A. Moscana and A. Monroy), Vol. 7, pp. 229–56.

HUTTON, J. J., BISHOP, J., SCHWEET, R., and RUSSELL, E. S. (1962). Hemoglobin inheritance in inbred mouse strains. I. Structural differences. *Proc. Nat. Acad. Sci.*, 48, 1505–13.

KABAT, D., SHERTON, C. C., EVANS L. H., BIGLEY, R., and KOLER, R. D. (1975). Synthesis of erythrocyte-specific proteins in cultured Friend leukemia cells. *Cell*, 5, 331–8.

LAPEYRE, J. and BEKHOR, I. (1974). Effects of 5-bromo-2'deoxyuridine and dimethylsulfoxide on properties and structure of chromatin. *J. mol. Biol.*, 89, 137–62.

LEDER, A., ORKIN, S., and LEDER, P. (1975). Differentiation of erythroleukemic cells in the presence of inhibitors of DNA synthesis. *Science, N.Y.*, 190, 893–4.

LEVY, J., TERADA, M., RIFKIND, R. A., and MARKS, P. A., (1975). Induction of erythroid differentiation by dimethylsulfoxide in cells infected with Friend virus: relationship to the cell cycle. *Proc. Nat. Acad. Sci.*, 72, 28–32.

MARKS, P. A. and RIFKIND, R. A. (1972). Protein synthesis: Its control in erythropoiesis. *Science, N.Y.*, 175, 955–61.

——, ——, BANK, A., TERADA, M., MANIATIS, G. M., REUBEN, R. C., and FIBACH, E. (1976). Erythroid differentiation and the cell cycle. In *Growth kinetics and biochemical regulation of normal and malignant cells* (eds. D. Drewinko and R. M. Humphrey) pp. 329–45. Williams and Wilkins, Baltimore.

MCLINTOCK, P. R., and PAPACONSTANTINOU, J. (1974). Regulation of hemoglobin synthesis in a murine erythroblastic leukemic cell: the requirement for replication to induce hemoglobin synthesis. *Proc. Nat. Acad, Sci.*, 71, 4551–5.

NAKANISHI, S., ADHYA, S., GOTTESMAN, M., and PASTAN, I. (1974a). Activation of transcription at specific promoters by glycerol. *J. Biol. Chem.*, 249, 4050–6.

——, ——, ——, and —— (1974b). Effects of dimethylsulfoxide on the E. coli *gal* operon and on bacteriophage lambda *in vitro*. *Cell*, 3, 39–46.

NUDEL, U., SALMON, J. E., TERADA, M., BANK, A., RIFKIND, R. A., and MARKS, P. A. (1977). Differential effects of chemical inducers on expression of β globin genes in murine erythroleukemia cells. *Proc. Nat. Acad. Sci.*, 74, 1100–4..

OHTA, Y., TANAKA, M., TERADA, M., MILLER, O. J., BANK, A., MARKS, P. A., and RIFKIND, R. A. (1976). Erythroid cell differentiation: murine erythroleukemia cell variant with unique pattern of induction by polar compounds. *Proc. Nat. Acad. Sci.*, 73, 1232–326.

OSTERTAG, W., MELDERIS, H., STEINHEIDER, G., KLUGE, N., and DUBE, S. (1972). Synthesis of mouse hemoglobin and globin mRNA in leukemic cell cultures. *Nature New Biol.*, 239, 231–4.

PAUL, J. and HICKEY, I. (1974). Haemoglobin synthesis in inducible, uninducible and hybrid Friend cell clones. *Exp. Cell Res.*, 87, 20–30.

POPP, R. A. and BAILIFF, E. G. (1973). Sequence of amino acids in the major and minor beta chains of the diffuse hemoglobin from Balb/c mice. *Biochem. Biophys. Acta*, 303, 61–7.

PREISLER, H. D. (1976). *In vitro* and preliminary *in vivo* studies of compounds which induce the differentiation of Friend leukemia cells. In *Modern trends in human leukemia II* (ed. R. Neth, R. C. Gallo, K. Mannweiler, and W. C. Moloney) J. F. Lehmanns Verlag, Munich. (Series: Hamatologie and Bluttransfusion, *Band* 19).

REUBEN, R. C., WIFE, R. L., BRESLOW, R., RIFKIND, R. A., and MARKS, P. A. (1976). A new group of potent inducers of differentiation in murine erythroleukemia cells. *Proc. Nat. Acad. Sci.*, **73**, 862–6.

ROSS, J. (1976). A precursor of globin mRNA. *J. mol. Biol.*, **106**, 403–20.

——, IKAWA, Y., and LEDER, P. (1972). Globin mRNA induction during erythroid differentiation of cultured leukemia cells. *Proc. Nat. Acad. Sci.*, **69**, 3620–3.

RUTTER, W. J., PICTET, R. L., and MORRIS, P. W. (1973). Toward molecular mechanisms of developmental processes. *Ann. Rev. Biochem.*, **42**, 601–46.

SCHER, W., PREISLER, H., FRIEND, C. (1973). Haemoglobin synthesis in murine virus-induced leukemic cells *in vitro. J. cell. phys.*, **81**, 63–70.

SINGER, D. (1975). Ph.D. Dissertation. Columbia University, New York.

——, COOPER, M., MANIATIS, G. M., MARKS, P. A., and RIFKIND, R. A. (1974). Erythropoietic differentiation in colonies of Friend virus transformed cells. *Proc. Nat. Acad. Sci.*, **71**, 2668–70.

TAMBOURIN, P., and WENDLING, F. (1971). Malignant transformation and erythroid differentiation by polycythaemia-inducing Friend virus. *Nature, New Biol.*, **234**, 230–3.

TANAKA, M., LEVY, J., TERADA, M., BRESLOW, R., RIFKIND, R. A., and MARKS, P. A. (1975). Induction of erythroid differentiation in murine virus infected erythroleukemia cells by highly polar compounds. *Proc. Nat. Acad. Sci.*, **72**, 1003–6.

TERADA, M., FRIED, J., NUDEL, U., RIFKIND, R. A., and MARKS, P. A. (1977). Transient inhibition of initiation of S-phase associated with dimethylsulfoxide induction of murine erythroleukemia cells to erythroid differentiation. *Proc. Nat. Acad. Sci.*, **74**, 248–52.

——, NUDEL, U., RIFKIND, R. A., and MARKS, P. A. (1978). Changes in DNA associated with induction of erythroid differentiation by dimethylsulfoxide in murine erythroleukemia cells. *Cancer Res.*, **38**, 835–40.

Session 11

Biological prospects for life extension

Introduction George A. Sacher

People who debate the social and ethical implications of life prolongation—proponents and opponents alike—seem to agree that it is a single, undifferentiated problem, about which they can have a single viewpoint, favourable or unfavourable as the case may be. This is understandable, for the biological gerontologists, from whom their guidance presumably comes, also tend to treat the problem in rather simple terms. I prefer to avoid direct quotation, but I believe a fair paraphrase of the common view is that biological research seeks ways to slow down the rate of aging, and that success in this quest will make it possible to defer the onset of senescent debility and disease, and thereby confer individual and social benefit.

It must be pointed out that this is an inadequate presentation of the biological situation, and that reliance on it can lead to erroneous assessments of the socio-economic consequences of life extension. There are, in fact, two fundamentally different approaches to life extension, and they would have very different consequences for the productivity, the dependency ratios, and the *per capita* health care costs for the populations employing them. Analysis of the demographic consequences of life table modification leads to the realization that a life extension regime can defer the onset of senescence, and increase the maximum span of life, but nevertheless be disadvantageous in terms of socio-economic criteria such as those listed above. Let us briefly consider the reasons for this paradoxical situation.

The shape of the survivorship curve for an adult population of mice or men is determined by two basic parameters. The meaning of these parameters is best shown by consideration of the age-specific mortality rate, shown in Fig. 1, which gives a schematic representation of the age-specific mortality rates in relation to age. Since these rates increase approximately exponentially with age, a plot of death rates on a logarithmic scale against age on a linear scale yields a straight line. Two numbers are needed to characterize a straight-line: the *slope coefficient*, which measures the inclination of the line, and the *intercept coefficient*, which specifies the vertical, y, axis value of the line for a reference value of the horizontal, x, axis. In the present case the slope measures the *rate of actuarial aging*, and we will denote it as α (alpha). The intercept value is found by extending the straight line back to birth, so it is an estimate of the *initial vulnerability to age-related disease*. If the reference age is zero (i.e., birth), then the vulnerability parameter is called q_0. Vulnerability is fundamentally different from aging.

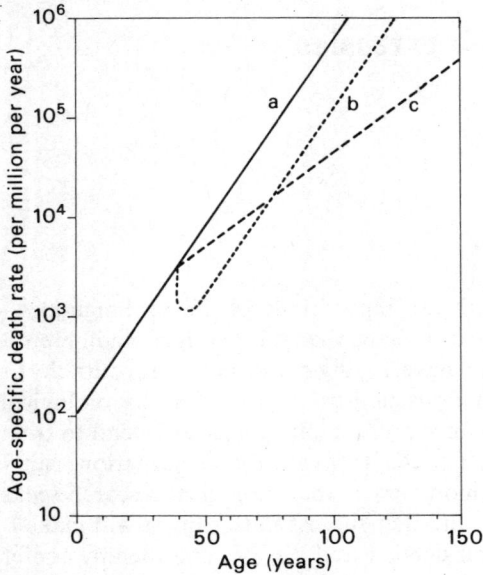

FIG. 1. Diagrammatic representation of the effects of the two basic life-extension regimes on the age-specific mortality rate for a model human population. The unmodified population is represented by line a. Treatment begins at age 40. The two cases are: (1) decrease of the rate of aging (slope) by a factor of two (curve c); or (2) decrease of the vulnerability by a constant factor of 5 (curve b).

Figure 1 shows the two ways in which mortality rate trends can be modified, starting at age 40 years. The line labelled c models the situation in which the rate of aging, alpha, is reduced while q_{40}, the vulnerability at age 40, is left unchanged. Line b represents the case in which the vulnerability coefficient is decreased by a factor of 5, beginning at age 40, while leaving alpha unaltered.

The consequences of these two alternations for the subsequent survivorship curve are shown in Fig. 2. Reduction of alpha (curve c) has little effect initially, but has a cumulative effect overall, so that survival is much increased at advanced ages. Reduction of q_{40} (curve b) leads to a pronounced reduction of mortality in the first few years, giving an advantage over the reduced alpha regime, but this advantage is lost at more advanced ages. In this example, the increase of life expectation was set equal for the two regimes.

How shall we assess the relative desirability of these two regimes? In regard to maximum attainable life span, the reduced alpha regime is clearly preferable. However, if we consider the question of dependency ratios, the ranking is reversed. The decrease of slope due to reducing the aging rate (alpha) means that the population so altered dwells for a longer time in the phase of increased morbidity, and therefore should be expected to show a higher prevalence of disability and chronic disease. This can be illustrated by comparing the hatched areas, which give the number of person-years lived by the last 10 per cent of the

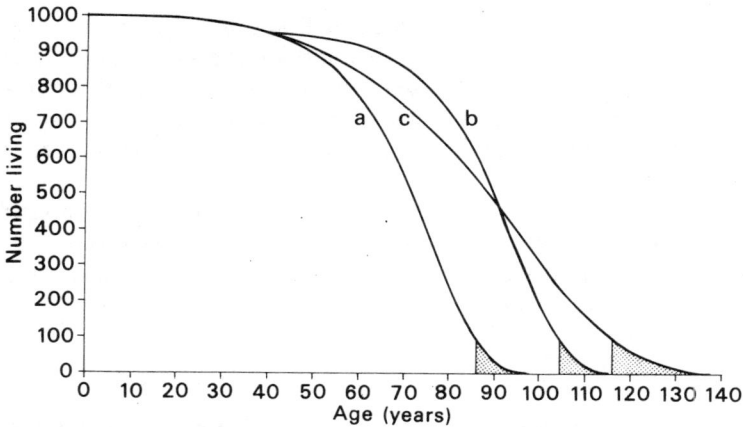

FIG. 2. Effects of the two life-extension regimes on the survival of the treated populations. Note that decrease of aging rate (curve c) has progressively greater effect with increasing age, while decreasing vulnerability (curve b) effectively shifts the curve to the right. The hatched areas are the number of person-years at risk for the last 10 per cent of each population. For curve b this number is equal to curve a, while for curve c the number of person-years in this risk group is doubled. [From Havighurst, R. J. and Sacher, G. A. (1977). Prospects of lengthening life and vigor. in *Extending the human life span: social policy and social ethics* (ed. B. L. Neugarten and R. J. Havighurst), pp. 13–18. National Science Foundation, NSF/RA 770123.]

reduced-alpha and the reduced-vulnerability populations. These populations can be expected to be equally debilitated, and comparable to the last 10 per cent of the untreated population. That area is twice as great for the reduced-alpha population as for the reduced-vulnerability or control populations, and in consequence the *dependency ratio*, defined by the ratio of the person-years in the last 10 per cent of survivors to the person-years in productive ages, is also about twice as great for that population, as compared to the population with reduced vulnerability coefficient.

There is a simple numerical index of the actuarial consequences of a modification of the life table parameters, given by the ratio q_x/α. This is a dimensionless number, which we can call the *actuarial risk index*, for it is low in youth and increases with age, and it is lower for a healthy population at a specified age than for a malnourished or otherwise weakened population at the same age. Decrease of alpha alone *increases* the actuarial risk index, and decrease of vulnerability coefficient, q_x, alone *decreases* the index, as compared to the unmodified population. Therefore, despite its reduced aging rate and deferred mortality the reduced-alpha population will, by all demographic indices, resemble an older population.

Hence, the widely expressed desire to reduce the rate of aging would, if carried out literally, precipitate a demographic catastrophe by producing a more aged population in terms of actuarial risk. Decrease of vulnerability alone would, on the other hand, decrease the dependency ratio, and decrease the actuarial risk index, so that the population would be biologically better off. Whether it would also be benefited in socio-economic terms would depend on whether the added potential for productive work was utilized effectively.

The possibility that an 'anti-alpha' treatment will appear in the near future would seem to be remote, for none of the putative anti-aging drugs that have been tested on animals have produced a decrease of the mortality rate slope (alpha), although a few have effected significant decreases of the vulnerability parameter. However, this was not the theoretically expected outcome, so the mechanism of these effects is still in question.

We should forgo our arguments about the desirability of life extension until we have done the kind of biologically-based actuarial and socio-economic modelling that would give us at least a rough idea about the actual consequences of various patterns of life table alteration.

Acknowledgement

This work was supported by the U.S. Department of Energy under contract No. W-31-109 ENG-38.

Prospects for human life extension by genetic manipulation
Leonard Hayflick

Introduction

Since this chapter is to be confined to 'genetic possibilities' for life extension, it is important at the outset to determine first whether genetic factors even play a role in aging before considering how those factors might be manipulated. Perhaps of even greater importance is a consideration of the apparent assumption by those who requested this contribution that increasing the human life span is desirable. But let us consider first whether genetics does play a role in aging.

Most gerontologists believe that a cell's genetic apparatus is the major arena in which occur the primary events that lead to the decrements associated with biological aging. The principal evidence that aging is, at least in part, genetically determined is based upon the following kinds of observations:

1. *Species-specific life spans*. It is generally agreed that all animal species age and that each species has a characteristic life span. This suggests that regardless of the kind and degree of trauma suffered by individual animals during their lifetime, there are genetically determined factors which operate independently of the environment.

Differences in life spans of members of various animal groupings argue strongly in favour of a species-specific genetic basis for longevity. The eagle owl (*Bubo bubo*) has a maximum recorded longevity of 68 years whereas the crowned pigeon (*Goura cristata*) lives a maximum of 16 years (Comfort 1964). Marions tortoise (*Testudo sumeiri*) has survived at least 152 years while the loggerhead turtle (*Caretta caretta*) lives only 33 years (Comfort 1964). In mammals, the longest-lived species is man (about 115 years) and the shortest-lived species are small rodents; the golden hamster (*Cricetus auratus*), for example, lives between 2 and 3 years (Comfort 1964).

2. *Hybrid vigour*. The effect of genetic constitution on longevity is perhaps best exemplified by those experiments in which 'hybrid vigour' or heterosis has been demonstrated. In 1923, Pearl, Parker, and Gonzalez found that the F_1 hybrid of two *Drosophila melanogaster* strains had a greater longevity than either parental strain. Clarke and Maynard-Smith (Clarke and Maynard-Smith 1955; Maynard-Smith 1959) obtained even more striking results when they crossed two geographically isolated strains of *Drosophila subobscura* and found that the hybrid lived longer and had a less variable life span than its inbred parents. Most explanations of heterosis suggest that recessive, harmful, but non-lethal, mutations are produced by inbreeding; hence hybrid vigour results from the reciprocal dominance between wild-type alleles of one strain and the recessive, sub-optimal genes of the other parental strain. Nevertheless, it is worth considering that the increased longevity seen in heterosis has not been shown to exceed the life span of wild strains. Heterosis may simply be the restoration of the life span characteristic of wild strains that has been lost by inbreeding.

3. *Sex and longevity*. Sex differences in longevity are well-established facts. In the human population, the penalty for maleness is that almost every disease has a higher incidence in males than in females. This difference in vulnerability is also expressed in life span, where a white female born in the United States today can expect to outlive her male counterpart by 7.6 years (Siegel 1976). If genes carried on the sex chromosomes dictate life span, then factors on the X-chromosome may decrease vulnerability to degenerative diseases. Contrariwise, genes on the Y chromosome may exert life-shortening effects that are incidental to their main function. In spite of the fact that the male sex is the shorter-lived in most animal species, some mouse and rat strains show quite the opposite state of affairs (Oliff 1953; Wooley 1946) as do pigeons (Levi 1957). Regardless of which sex might be favoured, the fact that one is, strongly suggests that there is a fundamental genetic basis for the difference.

4. *Influence of parental age*. Actuarial data for man leads to the conclusion that genetic factors play a principal role in determining individual longevity. Figure 1 graphically shows that life expectation for persons, both of whose parents attained the age of 75 or greater, live longer than persons whose parents died under the age of 60. Figure 2 shows that fathers of long-lived sons live longer than fathers of short-lived sons. Conversely, sons of long-lived fathers live longer than sons of short-lived fathers. Pearl and Pearl (1934a,b) found that the summed ages at death of the six immediate ancestors of centenarians and nonagenarians were significantly greater than in a control series. Long-lived persons (older than 70) had at least one long-lived parent. In nonagenarians, 48.5 per cent had two such parents and 53.4 per cent of centenarians had two long-lived parents. All of these figures are significantly higher than those found in control groups. Kallman and Sander (1948, 1949) found that in 1062 pairs of twins, the mean difference in longevity between dizygotic twin individuals was twice that found in mono-zygotics.

American and Canadian life insurance
cos issues 1869–99

Metropolitan Life Insurance Co.
ordinary issues 1899–1902

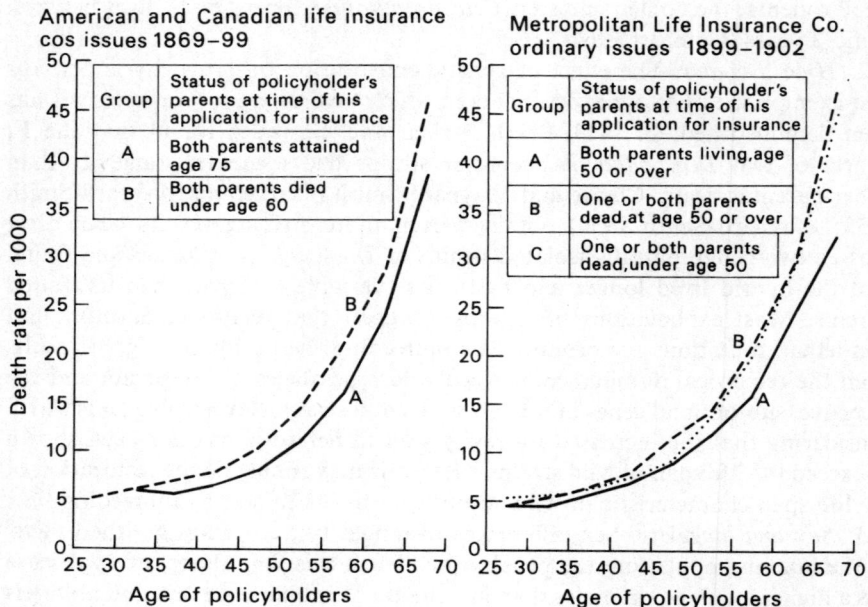

FIG. 1. Inheritance of longevity. Death rates at successive ages among white male policy-holders classified according to longevity of parents. (From Dublin, Lotka, and Spiegelman (1949).)

These principal lines of evidence, although by no means complete, constitute a reasonable basis for the notion that genetic factors play an important role in those events that lead to the aging and death of individual members of a species. It should be stressed, nevertheless, that non-genetic factors must also play a role in those decrements that lead to manifestations of aging. Changes that occur in molecular structures and biochemical reactions over time are certainly not all governed by genetic events. The cross-linking of collagen may be one good example of the kind of change that occurs over time and that is probably not directly influenced by a genetic programme, yet might contribute to senescent changes. Thus at the level of macromolecules, a 'programme' could be the stability of the macromolecule itself, which does not require any genetic basis. The accumulation of lipofuscin and the denaturation of organelles and enzyme molecules having regular turnover rates may represent other examples of molecular changes occurring over time that do not necessarily require instructions from information-containing molecules. Other extrinsic aging mechanisms are endocrine and neural factors which apparently regulate age changes in target cells (Finch 1976). However, a clear demonstration that these factors are not under the control of gene expression has not been made.

If genetic mechanisms do play a role in longevity, the next question to be answered is: What is the mechanism? Current thought on this question has led to speculation within four general categories.

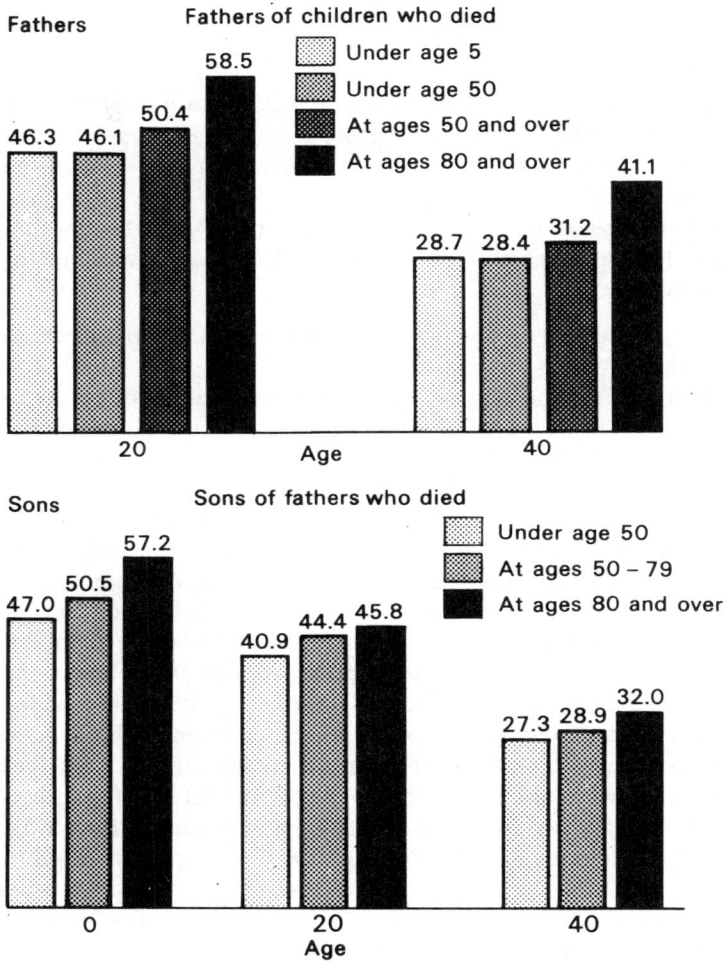

FIG. 2. Expectation of life of (a) fathers according to longevity of their children, (b) sons according to longevity of their fathers. (From Pearl (1931) and Pearl and Pearl (1934a) as reproduced in Dublin *et al.* (1949).)

A. *Unprogrammed senescence.*

1. Instability of the genome. This is unprogrammed senescence resulting from the acquisition of genetic damage.

2. Slow accumulation of non-genetic damage which has a minor influence on an individual's survival before reproductive maturity. These events would not cause evolutionary selection of compensating genetic properties.

B. *Programmed senescence.*

1. The presence of 'aging genes', that is, genes that slow down or shut down vital processes. This would be an active process where genes are selected through evolution because they confer a direct advantage to survival of the species but at the expense of individual death.

2. Programmed senescence where the degenerative processes of aging are accidentally incurred as a passive by-product of the genetic selection of advantageous properties.

A detailed description of several theories applicable to some of the above mechanisms has been outlined previously (Hayflick 1975).

In any consideration of the role of genetics or any other possible root cause of aging, one must come to terms with at least two important biological principles. The first principle is that death from old age is almost certainly confined to man and those animals that he chooses to protect, that is his domestic or zoo animals. Animals in the wild are generally killed by predators or struck down by disease or accidents well before they exhibit physiological decrements analogous to those expressed in very old humans. The prolongation of the life span beyond reproductive maturation therefore has no survival value for the species. In cold biological terms, people over the age of, say, 40 do not contribute to the biological survival of the species. Says Bidder (1925): 'If primitive man begat a son, the species had no more need of him by 37, when his son could hunt for the food for the grandchildren.' Aging, as we recognize its most profound expressions in man, simply does not occur in wild animals. One must cope with the thought that man's success in dealing with his environment to the extent that his life expectation is now well beyond the period of reproductive maturity and child-rearing, has simply revealed a Pandora's Box of vicissitudes that were never intended to be seen by him.

The second principle that impacts on any consideration of the role of genetics or any other root cause of aging is to account for those biological systems that have seemingly escaped from its inevitability (Hayflick 1976). These are the continuity of the germ cells (precursors of egg and sperm cells) and continuously reproducing cancer-cell populations. It may be possible to explain the immortality of cancer-cell populations by the suggestion that genetic information is exchanged between somatic cells or viruses and somatic cells in the same way that the genetic cards are reshuffled when egg and sperm fuse. Thus, exchange of genetic information may serve to reprogramme or reset the biologic clock. By this mechanism, species survival is guaranteed, but the individual members are ultimately programmed to failure.

Having established that genetic factors do play a role in human longevity and that speculation is rife as to possible mechanisms, the remaining considerations are, first: How can we tamper with the machinery? and second: Is it desirable to do so? Before considering the answers to these questions, it is important to discuss the recent epidemiological trends in aging as they have occurred over the

past several decades. It is only against this background that an intelligent consideration of the desirability and practicability of increasing human longevity
can be made.

Epidemiology of human aging

If the future can be judged by the past, then the impact of biomedical research
on human longevity in the next twenty-five years in this country should be to
extend life expectancy considerably beyond the present 70 years. Yet the likelihood of a net increase occurring by the year 2000 of the magnitude seen since
1900 is very doubtful. Life expectancy at birth in 1900 was about 49 years and
in 1950 it was about 68 years—a net gain of 19 years. From 1950 to 1974 however, the gain has been only 3.8 years, and it has continued to level off (Siegel
1976) (Fig. 3). Why has there been such a profound increase in life expectation
in the first half of this century and, in the beginning of the second half, an equally
profound levelling off? That this has occurred is even more impressive if one
accepts the common notion that the extent of advances made in biomedical
research in the past 25 years has been greater than those made in all previous
years. The answer to this apparent dilemma derives from a consideration of the
important distinction to be made between life expectancy and life span.

It is generally believed that the human life span, of about 100 years, has not
changed since recorded history, but what has changed is the larger number of

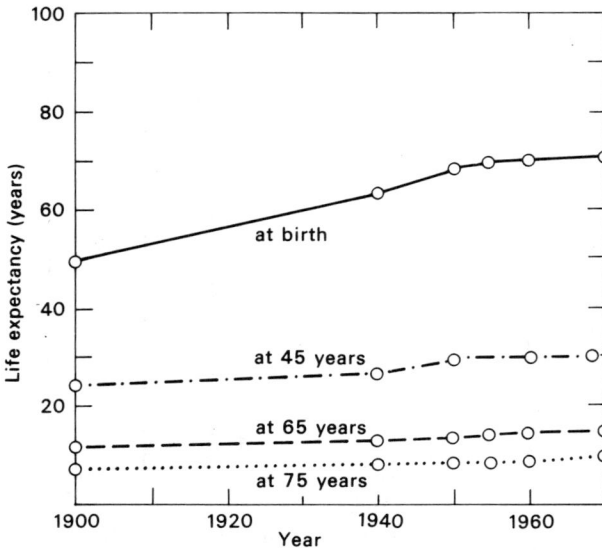

FIG. 3. Life expectation at birth and at ages 45, 67, and 75 since 1900.

people surviving to this apparent limit (Fig. 4). Medical achievements have simply resulted in the fact that more people are reaching the limit of what appears to be a fixed life span. Deaths in the early years are becoming increasingly less frequent, resulting in life tables that are simply becoming more rectangular as indicated by the direction of the arrow in Fig. 5. In many privileged countries, you can now reasonably expect to become old, which is a very new phenomenon, indeed.

In a world where the two leading current causes of death would be resolved, the elimination of all vascular diseases and cancer will yield a net increase of about nineteen years in life expectation at birth and only slightly less at age 65 (Table 1). This figure is almost identical to the net increase in life expectation achieved at birth in this country from 1900 to 1950 (Fig. 3). The increase in life expectation at birth during the first half of this century resulted from the resolution of deaths which occurred before the age of 65. The gain in life expectation at ages 65 and 75 from 1900 to 1950 was, respectively, only 1.9 and 1.3 years and from 1950 to 1974, 1.8 and 1.4 years.

If there is reason to believe that deaths from vascular diseases and cancer will be resolved in the next 25 years, then life expectancy will show an increase in the second half of this century as profound as that which occurred in the first half. After that spectacular accomplishment, the leading cause of death will be accidents, which because of their statistical nature are not likely to yield to total elimination. Thus the social, psychological, political, and economic impacts of

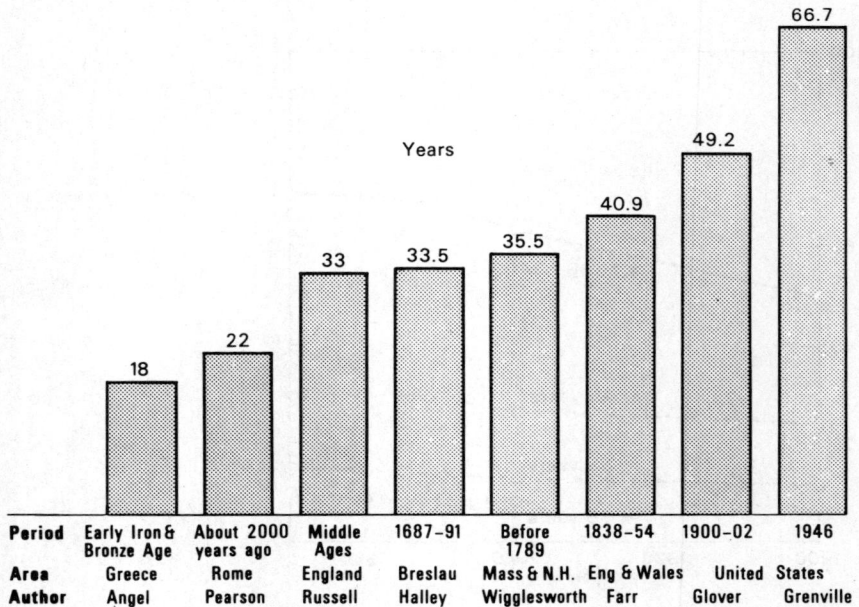

Period	Early Iron & Bronze Age	About 2000 years ago	Middle Ages	1687–91	Before 1789	1838–54	1900–02	1946
Area	Greece	Rome	England	Breslau	Mass & N.H.	Eng & Wales	United States	Grenville
Author	Angel	Pearson	Russell	Halley	Wigglesworth	Farr	Glover	

FIG. 4. Average length of life from ancient to modern times. (From Dublin *et al.* (1949).)

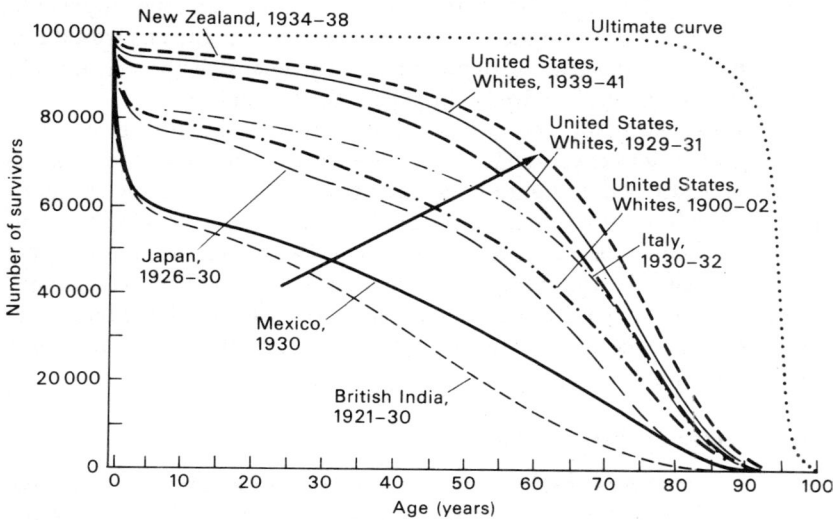

FIG. 5. Life expectancy curves for various countries at different periods of this century. (Adapted from Comfort (1964).)

Table 1 Gain in expectation of life at birth and at age 65 due to elimination of various causes of death

Cause of death	Gain in years in expectation of life if cause was eliminated	
	At birth	At age 65
Major cardiovascular–renal diseases	11.8	11.4
Heart diseases	5.9	5.1
Cerebrovascular diseases	1.2	1.2
Malignant neoplasms	2.5	1.4
Motor vehicle accidents	0.7	0.1
Accidents excluding those caused by motor vehicles	0.6	0.1
Influenza and pneumonia	0.5	0.2
Diabetes mellitus	0.2	0.2
Infectious and parasitic diseases (excluding tuberculosis)	0.2	0.1
Tuberculosis	Less than 0.05	Less than 0.05

Source: Hayflick (1976).

resolving the two leading causes of death on life expectation in the next half-century can be assessed reasonably by studying like changes that have occurred in the first half of this century when a similar increase in life expectation occurred.

Let us also consider a world in which all causes of death resulting from disease and accidents are totally eliminated (Table 1). What would be the effect on human longevity and the human life span? The effect on human longevity would be to realize the ultimate rectangular curve (Fig. 5) in which citizens would live out their lives, free of the fear of premature death, but with the certain fate that on the eve of their one-hundredth birthday, they would die.

This situation is occurring and will continue to evolve because biomedical research has trained its heavy artillery almost exclusively on the disease-associated causes of death. Scant attention has been paid to the underlying causes of biological aging that are not disease-associated but which, in clock-like fashion, dictate for each species a specific maximum life span. To be sure, the physiological decrements that occur in advancing years increase vulnerability to disease but unless more attention is paid to the fundamental non-disease-related biological causes of aging, then the fate of all inevitably will be death on or about our one-hundredth birthday.

Prospects for increasing human longevity

As a consequence of these considerations there are two approaches by which the efforts of biomedical research can be expected to extend human longevity in the next 25 years. The first is to reduce or eliminate the major causes of death, in particular, vascular diseases and cancer. The results of ameliorating minor diseases will be minimal. For example, if tuberculosis were completely eliminated, there would be a mere 18-day gain in life expectancy at birth or at age 65 (Table 1). Thus it could be argued that if an increase in life expectation becomes the main goal of biomedical research, all such research should be directed toward the elimination of the two major causes of death. This position, although less than humane, and not likely to attract many adherents, is none the less the most logical conclusion to be derived from life-table studies and the projections dealt with in Table 1.

The second way in which biomedical research can deal with human longevity is to address itself specifically to the underlying non-disease-related fundamental biological causes of age changes. These are not diseases but are the basic biological changes that produce the physiological decrements characteristic of aging and upon which are often superimposed an increasing vulnerability to disease. Such an approach then does not directly concern itself with efforts to increase human life expectancy but rather to extend what appears to be a genetically determined fixed life span.

If one can measure the current effort put forth toward these two approaches by the expenditure of funds for each, then funds spent on vascular disease and cancer research are one hundred times greater than those funds spent in gerontology. It is also probable that the number of researchers, and consequently the amount of effort, in both these areas also differs by a hundredfold. Consequently, the likelihood that any significant increase in human longevity will occur in the next 25 years depends upon (1) significantly better cure rates for vascular diseases and/or cancer, and/or (2) significant advances in our understanding and ability to manipulate the biological clock(s) that sets a mean maximum life span for man.

If potential success in either of these endeavours can be measured by the current attitudes and priorities of the biomedical research establishment, then it is clear that the search for vascular disease and cancer cures are much more likely to effect human longevity than would be efforts made by gerontologists to develop some kind of 'genetic fix'. Notwithstanding this, there is the further conclusion that by curing these two diseases a maximum of 14 years of additional life expectancy could be attained but with successful efforts to increase the life span itself by genetic or other means, no fixed end-point is ruled out. Furthermore the conquest of the two leading killers will in no way reverse or halt the decline in physiological decrements characteristic of age changes whereas efforts to increase the life span could lead to such a reversal. Clearly research in vascular diseases and cancer should not be stopped but, if our goal is to maximize opportunities to effectively increase human longevity, then our current priorities are seriously out of balance. If this imbalance continues unchanged then the likelihood that the research accomplishments of a handful of underfunded biogerontologists will affect the human life span is very small indeed.

I am very pessimistic that ways will be found in the next 25 years to manipulate our genetic machinery in such a way as to affect human longevity. Having said that, I suppose I have properly discharged my responsibility to discuss the genetic possibilities for life prolongation. Nevertheless I would prefer to consider the question in its global sense, that is, are there any practicable ways, genetic or otherwise, by which the human life span might be extended, in the next 25 to 50 years? I risk doing this because this broader question is not covered at this conference and I believe it to be a pivotal point in achieving the conference's stated goals. Before considering possible means for lengthening human life span, let us consider why the likelihood of achieving this by manipulation of our gene pools is unrealistic. The best approach is to deal with the principal lines of evidence that support the notion that aging is influenced by gene expression and then consider ways in which manipulation of each might be accomplished. The principal lines of evidence, considered earlier, are:

1. *Species-specific life spans.* All animal species have characteristic life spans that are presumably under genetic control. We know so little about this presumptive association that to argue that an understanding of the mechanism will occur such that it could be manipulated in the foreseeable future is unrealistic.

2. *Heterosis.* The progeny of animals from two inbred strains have life spans longer than either of the parental strains. There is clearly no hope that this fact could benefit man. Inbred human strains do not exist and even if they did, the political, social, and economic consequences of human 'hybrid vigour' are too painful to contemplate.

3. *Longer female life expectation.* In humans, female life expectation at birth in the United States in 1974 was 7.6 years more than for males. This well recognized fact has no immediate hope of being exploited to increase human longevity, unless a means were to be found by which only females would be produced. Although this might satisfy our most militant feminists, it is the surest means of leading *Homo sapiens* to extinction.

4. *Long-lived parents*. Parents who die at ages beyond the average life expectation have children who are more likely to live longer as well. The only way to exploit this finding is to adhere to the old saw 'Choose your parents wisely'.

Some immediate possibilities

In spite of these pessimistic views there is, in the judgment of many gerontologists, at least one comparatively innocuous way in which the human life span undoubtedly can be extended significantly. However it does not seem to have a direct genetic basis. The method derives from classic studies made by McCay in the 1930s and since confirmed in many laboratories for a number of animal species including rats in which it was first described (McCay, Maynard, Sperling, and Barnes 1939; McCay, Pope, and Lunsford 1956). The method is simply to reduce the caloric intake to such a level that undernutrition, but not malnutrition, occurs. This is done by providing an animal with a diet sufficient in all necessary nutrients but very low in calories. Longevity can then be increased by as much as 50 per cent. The effects are most pronounced if caloric restriction diets are initiated when animals are very young. This results in a stretching-out of the developmental stages such that infancy, puberty, maturity, adulthood, and aging simply occur at later than usual points in time so that the total life span is increased.

On the assumption that undernutrition in man would yield similar results, it is of interest to observe that in the forty years since this has been known, no human has consciously chosen to do it: not even the biologists who know the data best. Considering the number of nostrums and treatments that have been foisted on a gullible public as anti-aging regimens, the lack of interest in underfeeding is remarkable. On the supposition that the method is widely known, that it works, and that it is not dangerous, the main conclusion that can be drawn from the notable lack of interest in it is that for most people the quality of life is more important than its quantity.

If this is so, then an important lesson can be learned. Any method that might increase human longevity is unacceptable even if it minimally affects the enjoyment of life. It might be amusing to consider the reciprocal question: Will many people opt for a treatment that would accelerate aging and presumably give twice the pleasure (and twice the grief) in half the time?

Another aspect of this question bears on whether any method shown to increase human longevity will, in fact, be used. The notion that any method guaranteed to reduce illness or extend life would not be used may at first seem to be naïve, but we are, none the less, surrounded by that reality. Consider poliomyelitis and its tragic consequence. Even with the availability of a highly effective prophylaxis in what surely must be considered to be the most painless form of administration (one drop of a sweet-tasting solution on the tongue), nearly half of all pre-school age children in the United States are not immunized. When the vaccine first became available, long lines of people waited for treatment. The current apathy is due largely to the fact that, unlike the older generation, young adults have never seen a polio victim. Consequently, a strong motivation to voluntarily immunize their children is lacking, and were it not for the legal requirement that immunization is necessary for school admission, the likelihood is that immunization against polio would fade to zero in a few years. In order to maintain a proper level of motivation to immunize, the best method probably would be to allow a sufficient number of crippled polio victims to hobble around the streets as constant reminders of the threat. Perhaps it would be more humane to secretly employ paid actors for this purpose.

It would be my guess that like the one example cited of the many that could be given, any regimen designed to increase longevity, even one as simple as a drop of sweet-tasting fluid on the tip of the tongue, would fail one generation after its initial use. Quite obviously if no one ever saw an aged individual the likelihood is nil that he could be persuaded that for lack of treatment he might age.

To sleep, per chance to dream . . .

There remains yet another method for increasing life expectancy that bears consideration. Although it will not result in an extension of life on an absolute time scale it is interesting to consider a form of increased longevity based on the self-evident supposition that life can be lived only when individuals are at least mentally active. Since, for most individuals, sleep consumes nearly one-third of our lives, any method that reduces the time spent sleeping should result in an increase in productive occupation and the enjoyment of life—that is if sleep itself is not considered to be either productive or enjoyable. Sleep researchers tell us that no detectable effect on health has been observed in those individuals who have learned how to make a modest reduction in the length of time usually spent asleep. The impact of this change would be profound, for if we were to reduce by one hour the time we now spend sleeping, the net effect on 'life-extension' would be an increase of more than 2 years. This 'increase in life expectancy' would be equivalent to living in a society where cancer deaths are totally eliminated.

Other alteratives

The patchwork method of resolving individual diseases and other public health prophylactic measures is of predictably limited value if our goal is to increase human longevity by greater than twenty years. Such results, although certainly desirable, will not further increase the length of vigorous life since most vascular diseases and cancers are associated with advancing years. To resolve diseases occurring late in life would mean that those who were saved would merely continue to suffer those physiological decrements to which the aged are prone. Taken together, the characteristics of these decrements, their predictable occurrence at specific periods of time in the life of each individual, and the uniform life span for all animal species strongly suggests the presence of a clock-like mechanism that dictates the occurrence of age changes.

There is the distinct possibility that a complete understanding of the fundamental mechanism of aging is unnecessary in order to permit us to alter the process even at the present level of our ignorance. Analogous to this reasoning is the view that many human illnesses are currently dealt with adequately without a full understanding of the mechanism and, in several cases, even without proof of aetiology. Based on this argument it may not be premature even today to initiate studies on the age-decelerating effects of a variety of potentially useful treatments. It has been suggested that one reason for not testing such presumably innocuous means for extending human life span as calorie restriction is that the human life span affects not only the investigated but also the investigator (and the granting agency). Consequently, it is argued, gerontologists are unwilling to undertake experiments whose outcome may only become known to their children or the children of grant administrators.

Nevertheless, it is believed by Comfort (1969, 1972) that a battery of short-term tests for rate-of-age-changes that could be measured over a decade or less might adequately substitute for measurements made over a lifetime. Models for this approach have, in fact, been developed to assess the possible age accelerating effects of irradiation on Hiroshima survivors. One could simply assess the rate of change in a number of unrelated physiological decrements over a five- or ten-year period in treated and untreated human subjects with the expectation that if all or most of these variables were affected that this could be extrapolated to effect longevity (Comfort 1969, 1972). Studies of similar design and magnitude to this proposal are now underway to test, for example, the effects of diet on heart disease. An approach such as this has a great deal of appeal, not the least of which is the fact that it is currently feasible to do and we know of several possible age-decelerating treatments that would probably be morally and ethically acceptable if a sufficient number of volunteers could be found. In particular caloric restriction and the effect of anti-oxidants could be studied immediately. Caloric restriction is inherently safe since it is both voluntarily and involuntarily practised by many people and anti-oxidants, existing as they do as food preservatives, have already gained acceptance by the Food and Drug Administration for human ingestion.

Thus the arguments in favour of this kind of approach, rather than the control of specific diseases or an understanding of the role of gene action in aging, can be summarized as follows:

1. Disease elimination will not retard the processes of aging, but approaches designed specifically to affect the rate of age changes will.
2. The approach is currently feasible from the standpoint of several practical considerations including cost, ethics, logistics, and time.
3. It is easier to affect a biological rate than it would be to prevent its occurrence. It should be easier, for example, to postpone the occurrence of cancer or atheroma than to cure these conditions (Comfort 1972).

Tampering with our biological clocks

If the control of aging were possible by genetic manipulation or otherwise, one profoundly important question arises: How desirable is it to be able to manipulate our biological clocks? The answer to this question is not simple. The fact that it must be asked is further evidence of the distinction that must be made between disease-oriented biomedical research and biogerontological research. Who would ask: What are the goals of cancer research or what are the goals of cardiovascular or stroke research? The answers are so obvious as to preclude asking the question. But the goals of gerontological research are quite a different matter because we are not certain whether the 'resolution' of the physiological decrements of old age will indeed benefit the individual or society as a whole. Many different biological resolutions of age changes are possible and each has an important potential side effect. Take, for example, the possibility that research into the biology of aging might result in the total elimination of all age-related physiological decrements. If this were achieved and no control were had on the biological clock itself, the result would be a society whose members would live full, physically vigorous, youthful lives until death claimed them at the stroke of midnight on their one-hundredth birthday. If, on the other hand, we were to learn how to tamper with our biological clocks, with what goal in mind would one choose to reset his clock? Surely one wouldn't choose to spend an additional ten years suffering from the infirmities of old age—yet that might, initially, be the only way to intervene. Is society prepared to cope with individuals whose only choice might be between naturally occurring death and ten or more years spent with the vicissitudes of old age? We can hardly deal with a mean maximum life span of say 80 years to say nothing of the further social, economic, and political dislocations that might occur if we add a decade to this figure. Aside from this possibility, it is also worth considering the prospect of clock tampering in which the choice would be to spend more years at a particular stage of our lives than we now do. The clock might be stalled for ten years at, for example, a chronological age of 20. Is this desirable? Each of us, after pondering this provocative question would likely agree that the time at which we would like our biological clocks arrested should correspond to those years in which maximum life satisfaction and productivity occurred. Yet if we were forced to make such a decision, it would probably have to be made prospectively, which means that we would have to know at what time maximum life satisfaction would occur before having experienced it. Even more complex is the question of when in the human life span individuals are most productive. An interesting and exhaustive study of this question was made by Lehman in 1953 and the conclusion reached from these data was that, depending upon the particular area of human endeavour, the time of maximum productivity can occur almost anywhere throughout the human life span. Thus clock tampering becomes a game that very few of us are capable of playing.

Although simple to state and conceptually easy to understand, I have purposely avoided the notion of biological immortality. I have done this for one principal reason—that to attain it is so far beyond any practical realization that any discussion of it would be more science fiction than likely science fact.

Furthermore, one of the most serious effects of even a modest success by biogerontologists in increasing human life expectancy are the societal consequences. Most gerontological sociologists are persuaded that even as little as a 5-year increase in life expectancy at say age 75 would be so profound as to rupture our present economic, medical, and welfare institutions.

In spite of the apparent dilemma in stating goals for gerontological research there is, I believe, one goal that appears to be wholly desirable and even attainable as a short-range objective. That would simply be to reduce the physiological decrements associated with biological aging so that vigorous, productive, non-dependent lives would be led up until the mean maximum life span of, say, 80 years. Implicit in this notion is that the quality of life is more important than its quantity.

The goal of gerontological research in the future should be to understand the biological basis of aging in order to extend the number of vigorous and productive years and to reduce the time spent in senility and the infirmities of old age.

Of what value is immortality, if by achieving it one extends the infirmities? Two modern versions of this theme exist in Aldous Huxley's *After many a summer dies the swan* and Oscar Wilde's *The picture of Dorian Gray*. In fact the American Gerontological Society itself has as its motto: 'To add life to years not years to life'. I would therefore challenge the view that the goal of research in aging is simply to increase longevity.

If longevity is to be increased merely by extending the years of our infirmities, then the goal is not worth seeking. This indeed is the modern dilemma faced by many physicians who are torn between using every means for prolonging the terminal stages of disease in the name of prolonging life but at the expense of continuing the agony of certain death. The goal that appears to be not only more desirable but indeed more attainable is not the extension of longevity *per se*, but the extension of our most vigorous and productive years. If tampering with our biological clocks ever becomes a reality, I believe that it would be tragic in the extreme if such clock-tampering would result only in the extension of those years spent in declining physical and mental health.

Prognostications

In any attempt at 'futurology' it is wisest to base predictions on similar events that may have happened in the past. To the question, what will be the impact of achieving in the future a 5-, 10-, or even 20-year increase in human life expectancy, we have only to look back at the same question being asked in 1900. For it is only during the period 1900–50 that increases in human longevity of these magnitudes did, indeed, occur. It is therefore safest to conclude that any further increase in human life expectancy is likely to incur the same sets of problems that occurred in the model system that embraces the first half of this century. The question then is: To prepare for a potential increase in human longevity, what should we now do that is different from what was or was not done in 1900? The chief medical problem during the first half of the twentieth century was infectious diseases and the chief biomedical accomplishment during that time was their virtual elimination. As a result society now finds itself burdened with unprecedented numbers of disabled and indigent old people who have survived infectious diseases but who will not survive old age. We do not wish to prolong old age by keeping people alive well beyond their years of vigour; medical science has essentially achieved this dubious goal. What we want to do is what the science of gerontology is all about.

As to making predictions about the future likelihood of increasing human longevity some consideration should be given to recent efforts in which such prognostications have been made. These studies were conducted by eliciting the opinions of scientists as to their expectations (Bender, Strack, Ebright, and von Haunalter 1969; Gordon and Helmer 1964; Gordon, Gerjuoy, and Anderson 1976). Polls are a poor way to conduct scientific research, but for what it might be worth the results from two of these studies were as follows. In the Rand Study (Gordon and Helmer 1964) scientific prognosticators concluded that an increase in longevity of 50 years will occur by the year 2020. In the Smith, Kline, and French study (Bender *et al.* 1969) a median estimate of a 50-year increase in longevity is considered attainable by the early-1990s. I find these predictions wildly optimistic.

Yet since life expectancy has increased so dramatically in the last half-century anyone could foresee the possibility of some small degree of further extension. All that needs to be done to produce this is to improve upon the hygienic, health care, and nutritional deficiencies of that substantial proportion of the world's population now denied these basic human needs. Thus there is no requirement for a new intellectual basis of understanding the biology of aging to materially increase the longevity of a substantial portion of our society. All that it takes is motivation and money. This achievement would increase life expectation but, of course, would not affect the life span or the rate of aging. Nevertheless, it is something that could be done now without requiring any new scientific innovations. For significant increases in longevity to take place, spectacular scientific achievements will be necessary. To increase life expectancy at birth by 11.8 years, resolution of all vascular diseases would have to occur (Table 1). To increase longevity by 2.5 years at birth, cancer would have to be eliminated (Table 1). Both accomplishments would yield a net gain of about 14 years but beyond that, significant extension would occur only by understanding the basic mechanisms of age changes and having the ability to slow the rate or otherwise manipulate the clock.

Summary

The consensus of scientific opinion is that the fundamental underlying causes of age changes, like developmental changes, are somehow programmed within the genetic apparatus but that their expression can be influenced by extrinsic factors. It is in the genetic apparatus that the clock is undoubtedly located. A fruit fly is old in 30 days, a mouse in 3 years, and a man in 90 years. The genetic control of these widespread differences is more or less self-evident. The rate of aging (or degree of vulnerability) per gram of mouse tissue is 30 times faster than it is per gram of human tissue. Further clues that genetic processes control age changes can be seen from the sex differences in human and animal life expectation. Perhaps the best examples are actuarial data which clearly show that the children of long-lived parents are themselves long-lived. Demographic data leads to the provocative conclusion that the best possible circumstances necessary to achieve maximum longevity are to be a white, highly educated, wealthy, Swedish female with centenarian parents and grandparents (Siegel 1976). One wonders what she would have to say to her poor old, black, sick counterpart living in an American ghetto.

The conclusion to be reached is that if, in the next 25 years, biomedical research were to triumph to the extent that deaths caused by vascular disease and cancer would be preventable, a net increase in life expectancy of about 21 years would occur. Advances made in preventing deaths caused by other diseases would not have much impact on human longevity. However, the greatest potential impact on human longevity would be research directed toward reducing the rate of the fundamental non-disease-related biological causes of age changes which are undoubtedly genetically determined.

If our social, political, and economic institutions are likely to be severely dislocated by these achievements, what right do we have to encourage this kind of research?

Acknowledgement

This work was supported in part by the Glenn Foundation for medical resarch, Rauharset New York, and by Grant 1 R01AG 00850 from the National Advisory Council on Aging, MIH, Bethesda, M.d., U.S.A.

References

BENDER, A. D., STRACK, A. E., EBRIGHT, G. W., and VON HAUNALTER, G. (1969). *Futures*, **1**, 289.

BIDDER, G. P. (1925). *Nature, Lond.*, **115**, 495.

CLARKE, J. M. and MAYNARD-SMITH, J. (1955). *J. Genet.*, **53**, 172.

COMFORT, A. (1964). *Ageing: the biology of senescence.* Holt, Rinehart & Winston, Inc. New York.

—— (1969). *Lancet*, **ii**, 1411.

—— (1972). *Mech. Ageing Dev.*, **1**, 101.

DUBLIN, I., LOTKA, A. J., and SPIEGELMAN, M. (1949). *Length of life.* The Ronald Press Co., New York.

FINCH, C. E. (1976). *Quart. Rev. Biol.*, **51**, 49.

GORDON, T. J. and HELMER, D. (1964). Report on a long-range forecasting Study. Report No. P-2982, Rand Corp., Santa Monica, California.

GORDON, T. J., GERJUOY, H., and ANDERSON, M. (1976). A study of life-extending technologies. Report 272–46–18/01. The Futures Group, 124 Hebron Ave., Glastonbury, Connecticutt.

HAYFLICK, L. (1975). *Fed. Proc.*, **34**, 9.
—— (1976). *New Engl. J. Med.*, **295**, 1302.
KALLMAN, F. J. and SANDER, G. (1948). *J. Hered.*, **39**, 349.
—— and —— (1949). *Amer. J. Psychiat.*, **106**, 29.
LEHMAN, H. C. (1953). *Age and achievement*. Princeton University Press, Princeton, New Jersey.
LEVI, W. M. (1957). *The pigeon*. Sumter, South Carolina.
MAYNARD-SMITH, J. (1959). In *Ciba Foundation colloquia on aging* (eds. G. E. W. Wolstenholme and M. O'Connor), Vol. 5, p. 269. Little, Brown, Boston.
McCAY, C. M., MAYNARD, L. A., SPERLING, G., and BARNES, L. L. (1939). *J. Nutrition*, **18**, 1.
——, POPE, F., and LUNSFORD, W. (1956). *Bull. N. Y. Acad. Med.*, **32**, 91.
OLIFF, W. D. (1953). *J. Anim. Ecol.*, **22**, 217.
PEARL, R. (1931). *Hum. Biol.*, **3**, 245.
——, PARKER, S. L., and GONZALEZ, B. M. (1923). *Amer. Naturalist*, **57**, 153.
—— and PEARL, R. DE W. (1934a). *The ancestry of the long-lived*. Oxford University Press, London.
—— and —— (1934b). *Hum. Biol.*, **6**, 98.
SIEGEL, J. S. (1976). *Demographic aspects of aging and the older population in the United States*. Current Population Reports, Series P–23, No. 59. U.S. Government Printing Office, Washington, D.C.
WOOLEY, G. (1946). In Hamilton, J. B. (1946). *Rec. Prog. Hormone Res.*, **3**, 257. ·

Possibilities and hazards of genetic engineering
Maxine F. Singer

Introduction

The techniques commonly referred to as 'recombinant DNA experiments' have caused unprecedented discussions in both scientific and public communities around the world. The explanation for this extraordinary situation can be found in the nature of the experiments. They permit the construction, in the laboratory, of organisms with unique properties—organisms that are not known to develop by natural processes. The DNA of animals and plants can be inserted into bacteria and replicated therein; the DNA of bacteria can be inserted into the genomes of animal viruses and then be replicated along with the viral DNA. These new capabilities allow us to approach previously intractable problems in biology and medicine. Opportunities have opened in many areas—including the biology of aging. But in addition to the optimistic predictions concerning the enormous scientific rewards to be gained from these techniques, involved scientists recognized, from the start, that the techniques had a potential for harmful effects when applied to certain situations (Singer and Söll 1973; Berg, Baltimore, Boyer, Cohen, Davis, Hogness, Nathans, Roblin III, Watson, Weissman, and Zinder 1974; Berg, Baltimore, Brenner, Roblin III, and Singer 1975). This combination of great promise for research, and the possibility of creation of hazards, has captured the interests of individuals, national governments, and international organizations. It has forced scientists and scholars to participate in the establishment of public policy, and it has forced policy-makers to become acquainted with some esoteric aspects of biology.

Yet the issues raised by recombinant DNA experiments are simple compared to the issues that will arise if recombinant DNA technology, or other developments, lead to what is more generally understood as 'genetic engineering'. The presently feasible experiments involve the insertion of foreign genes into bacteria, or into cells of higher organisms growing in tissue culture. Should the deliberate modification of the genetic constitution of complex organisms, including humans, become feasible in the future, either for the correction of individual genetic defects or for the alteration of heritable characteristics, much more complex and difficult problems will arise. Broad discussion of the philosophical, moral, and ethical questions of concern to individuals and society will be necessary to inform both private and public decision-making.

Some experiments using recombinant DNA methodology

To understand the opportunities that recombinant DNA methodology offers in the field of research on aging it is helpful to look at some of the experiments that have already been carried out (for a more detailed review see Sinsheimer 1977). The experiments can be defined as involving molecules that consist of different segments of DNA which have been joined together in cell-free systems, and which have the capacity to infect and replicate in some host cell, either autonomously, or as an integrated part of the host's genome. Figure 1 depicts a generalized recombinant DNA experiment and defines certain terms as they are commonly used.

At the upper left is a cell containing chromosomal DNA and several small independent genetic elements. These small independent DNA molecules are isolated from the cell and will serve as one portion of the recombined DNA, the segment termed the vector. Such elements may be circular DNA molecules such as plasmids, or viral DNAs, and they can be cleaved by endonucleases, as shown, to yield linear duplex DNA segments which either have sticky ends, or have ends that can be made sticky by appropriate modification. The term 'sticky' means that the ends can come together, under appropriate conditions in solution. In general 'stickiness' is attained by the formation of hydrogen-bonded base pairing between single-stranded regions at the ends of the DNA segments.

At the upper right of Fig. 1 another cell is shown as a rectangle. This cell will serve as the source of DNA to be joined to the vector. This DNA is termed the foreign DNA. The rectangular cell can represent a cell of the same species as the first cell or one from any other species. As shown here, the foreign DNA might contain chromosomal DNA or independent DNA elements, or both. It too can be cleaved to yield fragments of various lengths with sticky ends, or ends that can be made sticky. The foreign DNA fragments are then mixed with the vector and

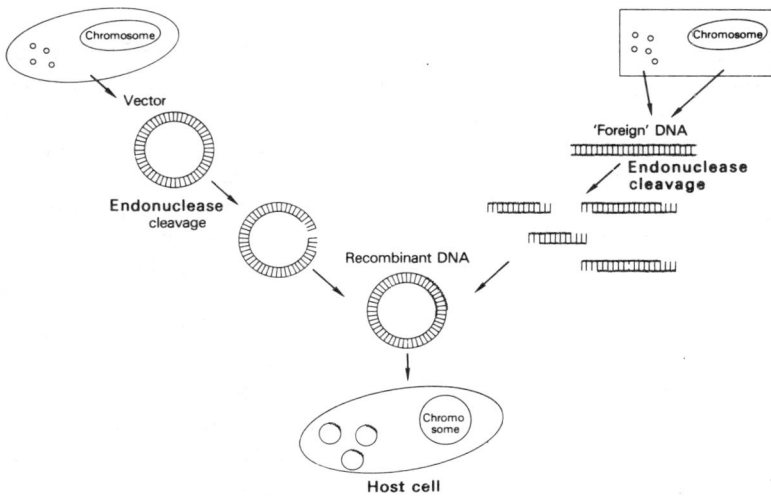

FIG. 1. A typical recombinant DNA experiment.

joined to the vector DNA by duplex formation at the sticky ends, followed by enzymatic closure of the internucleotide bonds. The recombinant DNA is inserted into a recipient cell, which is called the host. The host cell will most likely be of the same species as that used for the isolation of the vector. It is the genetic information encoded in the DNA of the vector which ultimately will be responsible for the continued existence and replication of the recombined DNA in the recipient cell. The cells are then placed under conditions where either they or the recombined DNA can replicate.

At present, and probably in the near future, only a limited number of cell-types will serve as host cells. In order to be useful as a host, the species must be associated with well-characterized, independently replicating DNA elements that can be used as vectors. The vector molecules must be obtainable in a pure state and must be capable of being reinserted into cells of the host species after being combined with foreign DNA. The DNA of certain bacteriophage and plasmids that infect *E. coli* meet these requirements and are being used as vectors in many laboratories. After a brief time at an elevated temperature in the presence of Ca^{2+}, plasmid DNA can be taken up by *Escherichia coli* cells (Cohen, Chang, and Hsu 1972). Similarly, naked bacteriophage DNA can be inserted into *E. coli*. The DNA genomes of certain animal viruses are also useful vectors for recombinant DNA experiments. In this instance, the host cells are appropriate animal cells in tissue culture. For example, the genome of simian virus 40, has been used as a vector for foreign DNA from the bacteriophage lambda in conjunction with monkey kidney cells as host (Ganem, Nussbaum, Davoli, and Fareed 1976; Goff and Berg 1976).

Selection and cloning of desired DNA recombinant

The experiment shown in Fig. 1 describes the use of a mixture of DNA fragments containing all of the sequences present in the genome of origin. This type of experiment is called a 'shotgun' experiment in current jargon. Clearly, however, only one segment, corresponding to a particular gene, a linked group of genes, or a regulatory sequence, will be the object of a given experiment. If the shotgun approach is used then it will be necessary to clone, from a population of host cells, that cell containing the sequence of interest. Alternatively, a desired DNA fragment can be purified first, and the purified fragment used for insertion into the vector. In both cases some means for selecting the clone or clones of interest is required. Even with the purified fragment it is necessary to remove host cells that did not receive the foreign DNA, or those which might contain a fragment derived from a minor impurity in the original fragment.

One approach to selection of the desired recombinant involves identification of the DNA sequence of interest in a mixture of recombinants, by hybridization with a characterized radioactive nucleic acid containing that sequence. This approach is useful when the sequence in question is available independent of the recombination experiment. Examples of such sequences are tRNA molecules, or purified messenger RNAs, or DNA segments that occur in multiple copies in normal genomes—the latter include, for example, the genes for ribosomal RNA, or histones, or segments of viral genomes.

DNA segments containing the genes for sea urchin histones were cloned in this manner (Kedes 1976), using an *E. coli* plasmid as a vector. The initial experiment was a 'shotgun'. Populations of *E. coli* containing the random recombinants were examined, after repeated multiple dilutions, for the presence of cells containing sequences homologous to highly purified histone messenger RNA. Several of the desired recombinants were cloned in this way. Investigation of the resulting purified recombined plasmids has already revealed information on:

(1) the organization of the five genes for the common histones in relation to one another and in relation to unread spacer sequences between them;
(2) the transcription of the genes into messenger RNA.

The determination of the nucleotide sequence of the genes and the regulatory spacer units is in progress.

Elegant techniques for selection and cloning of the desired recombinants by nucleic acid hybridization have been developed (Grunstein and Hogness 1975). A large number of colonies of recipient host cells are formed on nitrocellulose filters with a reference set prepared by replica plating. The DNA of the colonies is then fixed on the filter and hybridized with the radioactive nucleic acid probe of interest. Colonies containing the desired fragment can then be identified by autoradiography. In addition to the great convenience afforded by the method, its use significantly decreases the escape of potentially hazardous organisms from the laboratory because it avoids large-scale liquid culture of uncharacterized recombinant organisms.

These methods have been used to obtain a variety of DNA fragments from the Drosophila genome. *In situ* hybridization of pure fragments to Drosophila polytene chromosomes indicated that they were derived from specific chromomeres, or from the chromocentre (Wensink, Finnegan, Danelson, and Hogness 1974). Thus, the problem of chromosome organization as well as of DNA organization can be elucidated as a result of recombinant DNA technology.

Another approach to selection is to look for complementation of a non-reverting bacterial mutant—complementation that is dependent on the inserted 'foreign' DNA. If the mutation is in the gene for a protein, this assay assumes that the foreign DNA is both translated and transcribed in its new host, and that a functional gene product is produced. The procedure has been used (Struhl, Cameron, and Davis 1976) to isolate *E. coli* cells relieved of a growth requirement for histidine by virtue of insertion of recombinant DNA composed of a bacteriophage vector and fragments of yeast DNA. It was demonstrated that the complementation of the missing enzyme, imidazol glycerol phosphate dehydratase, depended on the presence of the yeast DNA. However, direct demonstration of the synthesis of the enzyme has not been reported, as yet. Indeed, the production of a complete and functional eukaryote gene product in prokaryote host cells, remains to be proven.

Another approach to isolation of specific genes is illustrated by several recent investigations concerning globin genes (Maniatis, Kee, Efstratiadis, and Kafatos 1976; Rabbits 1976; Rougeon, Kourilsky, and Mach 1975). Highly purified messenger RNA for globin is isolated from reticulocytes and double-stranded DNA copies of the messenger RNA are prepared with the aid of DNA polymerases. These DNA preparations can then be inserted into vectors and the DNA amplified. If the DNA copies are true and full length, this type of approach may yield regulatory sequences which are not translated into protein at either end of the message. However, regulatory sequences for transcription, that may flank the messenger sequences in the original gene, will not be isolated by such procedures. The availability of pure DNA in good quantity may allow the selection of the corresponding DNA complete with transcription regulators from a 'shotgun'-type experiment.

This brief description of some of the work that is presently going on, gives an idea of the varied number of questions that can be attacked when recombinant DNA technology is coupled with the other methods of molecular biology. Restriction endonucleases, in addition to generating sticky ends, are powerful tools for the generation of specific fragments of DNA (Nathans and Smith 1975). Recent advances in methods for sequencing DNA make it feasible to obtain readily the nucleotide sequence of DNA fragments over a hundred residues long (Maxam and Gilbert 1977). Well-defined experiments concerning regulation and gene structure in normal and abnormal conditions are forthcoming.

These developments are truly revolutionary—biology can proceed in new directions. By classical procedures the isolation of specific bits of DNA, corresponding to particular genes, is a formidable if not impossible task when one starts with a complex organism whose DNA contains thousands of genes. With recombinant DNA technology, relatively large quantities of individual genes can be obtained after recombination into simple bacteria or viruses. Equally important, this DNA will be purer than anything one could possibly isolate from the original source. In addition to the use of this method for elucidating problems in biology such as those already described, there are potential practical applications of recombinant DNA technology. For example, if eukaryote genes can be efficiently transcribed and translated in bacterial cells, then such cells can be used for the manufacture of a variety of eukaryote proteins and enzymes that are important clinically and industrially.

New approaches to unresolved questions about aging organisms are readily imagined—genes from aging tissues, or cells, can be prepared in the requisite amounts by cloning techniques, and their structures can be compared in detail with those of the same genes from young, or germ line, cells. A direct resolution of whether faulty transcription or faulty translation occur in given instances is feasible. General studies on control signals and regulatory sequences will allow comparison of these processes in young and aging organisms. The isolation of sequences involved in hormonal responses will permit study of such sequences and their specific binding proteins in aging organisms.

Possible hazards of recombinant DNA technology

The exciting prospects posed by recombinant DNA technology reflect the novelty of the method—an ability to combine, at will, genetic information from unrelated species and to perpetuate the recombined genes in easily grown living cells. In nature, recombination is known to occur with some frequency during mating, but that involves the genes of members of the same species. Interspecies recombination is also known to occur in nature between certain micro-organisms. We do not know whether interspecies recombination takes place across species barriers at some low but significant frequency among higher organisms, or between prokaryotes and eukaryotes. We also know very little about how genes foreign to any particular cell will behave inside it. For these reasons, biologists, and others have been concerned that cells containing DNA recombined in the laboratory might acquire new, unpredictable, and possibly hazardous properties. For example, under the direction of a new gene a cell could produce a protein not normally found in the host cell, and with undesirable effects either on the host itself, or after release of the protein from the host into a human or other ecologically important environment. Or, a host bacterium might serve as a vehicle for carrying the foreign DNA fragment into a human, animal, or plant cell in contact with the host bacterium or virus vector. If the DNA combined, secondarily, with the DNA of the new species, the foreign DNA fragment might interfere with normal cell function. Or, the DNA fragment might alter the properties of the recipient host cell itself and change benign cells into pathogenic ones. Current knowledge is insufficient to analyse these possibilities with any accuracy:

indeed, the imagined dangers may not exist. To date, no known hazardous agent has been produced in recombinant DNA experiments. Nevertheless, the chance that research might inadvertently cause harm demands responsible action. The development and promulgation of guidelines for assessment of possible risk, and for appropriate precautions, promises a substantial reduction of the risk of an unacceptable result. Such guidelines have been published by government agencies in the United States and the United Kingdom (Singer 1977; Tooze 1976). In many other countries committees to oversee the safe conduct of recombinant DNA experiments have been or are being formed. Several international organizations, including the European Molecular Biology Organization, the World Health Organization, the European Science Foundation, and the International Council of Scientific Unions, have active working committees and are excellent sources of information. Several of these organizations, as well as national groups are planning training courses both in the technology itself, and in safety procedures.

The search for new knowledge always carries certain risks. Since the answers being sought are not known in advance, the extent of the hazards attendant upon discovery cannot be defined. Consequently, the assessment of risks and the adequacy of the precautions designed to eliminate or minimize such risks, are matters of judgement based on objective, intuitive, and value considerations. Undeniably, more information is needed to assess fully the risks in this research. That information can be gained with minimal risk by expecting and insisting that scientists engaged in this work, wherever they are, adhere diligently to both the intent and letter of the guidelines operative in their own institutions and countries. As those concerned with the problem of aging begin to apply this technology they will need to join in the discussion of risks. The information gathered must be added to ongoing re-evaluations of risks and of guidelines. Each experiment will have to be considered not only for its scientific merit, but for its potential for harm. And the evaluations may need to be defended to concerned laymen or public officials as well as scientific colleagues. The experience may be painful and discouraging. But it can also be rewarding: it is an opportunity to share the excitement of discovery—and to instruct others in matters that are, after all, as important to them as they are to the scientific community.

Addendum

The field of recombinant DNA research has moved rapidly during the past two years. Highly significant scientific achievements have been published, important information relevant to speculations concerning possible hazards resulting from the experiments has accumulated, and public policy regarding the experiments has taken new directions. This attempt to summarize briefly the events since 1977 must be fragmentary and thus unsatisfactory. Even a listing of all important references would take many pages and therefore only a small number of examples can be given here.

Scientifically, investigators in various fields have been quick to perceive the many opportunities provided by recombinant DNA techniques. The pages of any of the leading journals in biochemistry or molecular biology will lead the interested reader to the details of experiments dealing with the genomes of a variety of organisms. Among the highlights are reports concerning the cloning and expression in *E. coli* of DNA copies of messenger RNA for insulin (Ullrich, Shine, Chirgwin, Pictet, Tischer, Rutter, and Goodman 1977; Villa-Komaroff, Efstratiadis, Broome, Lomedico, Tizard, Naber, Chick, and Gilbert 1978), the cloning and expression of a synthetic gene for somatotropin (Itakura, Hirose, Crea, Riggs, Heyneker, Bolivar, and Boyer 1977), the cloning and determination of the structure of genes and messenger RNAs for globin (Efstratiadis, Kafatos, and Maniatis 1977; Tilghman, Tiemeier, Seidman, Peterlin, Sullivan, Maizel, and Leder 1978), ovalbumin (Mandel, Breathnach, Gerlinger, LeMeur, Gannon, and Chambon 1978; Dugaiczyk, Woo, Lai, Mace, McReynolds, and O'Malley 1978), and immunoglobin (Bernard, Hozumi, and Tonegawa 1978; Seidman, Leder, Edgell, Polsky, Tilghman, Tiemeier, and Leder 1978). These and other experiments yielded the surprising fact that a single eukaryote gene need not be contained in a single contiguous linear stretch of DNA, but rather, that genes may be interrupted by non-coding (intervening) sequences that are lacking in the corresponding messenger RNAs. Furthermore, present data indicate that in the case of immunolgobulin genes, DNA sequences themselves are rearranged during somatic differentiation in order to bring constant and variable regions together (Bernard, Hozumi, and Tonegawa 1978).

There has been a continuous refinement of vectors and host cells for recombinant DNA experiments with *E. coli*: some of these developments have centred in the construction of systems with extremely limited capacity to grow and multiply except under special laboratory conditions (Curtiss III, Pereira, Hsu, Hull, Clark, Maturin, Goldschmidt, Moody, Inoue, and Alexander 1977). Increasingly, host–vector systems other than *E. coli* are being used to great advantage. Current work includes the use of yeast (Hinnen, Hicks, and Fink 1978) and animal viruses such as simian virus 40: globin genes have been inserted into the simian virus 40 genome and the recombinants are being used to study regulation of eukaryote gene expression (Mulligan, Howard, and Berg 1979).

The speculation that recombinant DNA experiments might lead to the formation of micro-organisms with unpredictable and possibly hazardous properties has received considerable attention. Discussion has been informed by experts in pathogenicity and epidemiology, by accumulating experience with organisms containing recombinant DNA, and by experiments designed for the express purpose of assessing possible risks (Israel, Chan, Rowe, and Martin 1979; Chan, Israel, Garon, Rowe, and Martin 1979). There has been extensive analysis of the available data as, for example, in the reports of the Falmouth Conference (Gorbach 1978) and of the joint US–EMBO workshop on eukaryote viruses (Federal Register 1978a). To date, the available information and analyses indicate that many of the speculative hazards are highly unlikely or impossible.

The dramatic scientific successes of recombinant DNA techniques as well as the reassuring results of risk assessment have brought about changing attitudes concerning containment requirements. In the United States extensive modifications of the guidelines promulgated by the National Institutes of Health (Federal Register 1978b) have been made. Many experiments widely believed to present no possibility for hazard are now exempt from any required containment conditions and the containment mandated for many other types of experiments has been significantly lowered.

References

BERG, P., BALTIMORE, D., BOYER, H. W., COHEN, S. N., DAVIS, R. W., HOGNESS, D. S., NATHANS, D., ROBLIN III, R. O., WATSON, J. D., WEISSMAN, S. M., and ZINDER, N. D. (1974). *Science, N.Y.* **185**, 303.

——, ——, BRENNER, S., ROBLIN III, R. O., and SINGER, M. F. (1975b). *Proc. Nat. Acad. Sci. USA*, **72**, 1981.

BERNARD, O., HOZUMI, N., and TONEGAWA, S. (1978). *Cell*, **15**, 1133.

CHAN, H. W., ISRAEL, M. A., GARON, C. F., ROWE, W. P., and MARTIN, M. A. (1979). *Science, N.Y.* **203**, 887.

COHEN, S. N., CHANG, A. C. Y., and HSU, L. (1972). *Proc. Nat. Acad. Sci. USA*, **69**, 2110.

CURTISS III, R., PEREIRA, D. A., HSU, J. C., HULL, S. C., CLARK, J. E., MATURIN, L. J., GOLDSCHMIDT, R., MOODY, R., INOUE, M., and ALEXANDER, L. (1977). In *Recombinant molecules: impact on science and society* (eds. R. F. Beers, Jr. and E. G. Bassett), p. 45. Raven Press, New York.

DUGAICZYK, A., WOO, S. L. C., LAI, E. C., MACE, M. L., MCREYNOLDS, L. A., and O'MALLEY, B. W. (1978). *Nature, (Lond.)* **274**, 328.

EFSTRATIADIS, A., KAFATOS, F. C., and MANIATIS, T. (1977). *Cell*, **10**, 571.

FEDERAL REGISTER (USA) (1978a). *Federal Register*, 31 March 1978, Part III, p. 13 748–55.

—— (1978b). *Federal Register*, 22 December 1978, Parts VI and VII, p. 60 080–131.

GANEM, D., NUSSBAUM, A. L., DAVOLI, D., and FAREED, G. C. (1976). *Cell*, **7**, 349.

GOFF, S. and BERG, P. (1976). *Cell*, **9**, 695–705.

GORBACH, S. L. (ed.) (1978). *J. infect. Dis.*, **137**, 613.

GRUNSTEIN, M. and HOGNESS, D. S. (1975). *Proc. Nat. Acad. Sci. USA*, **72**, 3961.

HINNEN, A., HICKS, J. B., and FINK, G. R. (1978). *Proc. Nat. Acad. Sci. USA*, **75**, 1929.

ISRAEL, M. A., CHAN, H. W., ROWE, W. P., and MARTIN, M. A. (1979). *Science, N.Y.* **203**, 883.

ITAKURA, K., HIROSE, T., CREA, R., RIGGS, A. D., HEYNEKER, H. L., BOLIVAR, F., and BOYER, H. W. (1977). *Science, N.Y.* **198**, 1056.

KEDES, L. (1976). *Cell*, **8**, 321.

MANDEL, J. L., BREATHNACH, R., GERLINGER, P., LEMEUR, M., GANNON, F., and CHAMBON, P. (1978). *Cell*, **14**, 641.

MANIATIS, T., KEE, S. G., EFSTRATIADIS, A., and KAFATOS, F. C. (1976). *Cell*, **8**, 163.

MAXAM, A. and GILBERT, W. (1977). *Proc. Nat. Acad. Sci. USA*, **74**, 560–4.

MULLIGAN, R. C., HOWARD, B. H., and BERG, P. (1979). *Nature, (Lond.)* **277**, 198.

NATHANS, D. and SMITH, H. O. (1975). *Ann. Rev. Biochem.*, **44**, 273.

RABBITS, T. H. (1976). *Nature, (Lond.)* **260**, 221.

ROUGEON, F., KOURILSKY, P., and MACH, B. (1975). *Nucleic Acids Res.*, **2**, 2365.

SEIDMAN, J. G., LEDER, A., EDGELL, M. H., POLSKY, F., TILGHMAN, S. M., TIEMEIER, D. C., and LEDER, P. (1978). *Proc. Nat. Acad. Sci. USA*, **75**, 3881.

SINGER, M. F. (1977). *Gene*, **1**, 123–39.

—— and SÖLL, D. (1973). *Science, N.Y.* **181**, 1114.

SINSHEIMER, R. L. (1977). *Ann. Rev. Biochem.*, **46**, 415–38.

STRUHL, K., CAMERON, J. R., and DAVIS, R. W. (1976). *Proc. Nat. Acad. Sci. USA*, **73**, 1471.

TILGHMAN, S. M., TIEMEIER, D. C., SEIDMAN, J. G., PETERLIN, B. M., SULLIVAN, M., MAIZEL, J. V., and LEDER P. (1978). *Proc. Nat. Acad. Sci. USA*, **75**, 725.

TOOZE, J. (1976). *Trends biochem. Sci.*, **1**, N246.

ULLRICH, A., SHINE, J., CHIRGWIN, J., PICTET, R., TISCHER, E., RUTTER, W. J., and GOODMAN, H. M. (1977). *Science, N.Y.* **196**, 1313.

VILLA-KOMAROFF, L., EFSTRATIADIS, A., BROOME, S., LOMEDICO, P., TIZARD, R., NABER, S. P., CHICK, W. L., and GILBERT, W. (1978). *Proc. Nat. Acad. Sci. USA*, **75**, 3727.

WENSINK, P. C., FINNEGAN, D. J., DONELSON, J. E., and HOGNESS, D. S. (1974). *Cell*, **3**, 315.

Effects of environmental factors and life patterns on life span

Role of exercise in aging J. L. Hodgson and E. R. Buskirk

Introduction

Several reviews on physiological aging are available with particular attention paid to the possible role of physical exercise (Shock 1967; Simonson 1957, 1971; Skinner 1970; Taylor and Montoye 1972). The deterioration of the capacity of the respiratory and circulatory systems to deliver oxygen to the working muscles is well documented between the ages of 25 and 65 in these and other studies (Astrand 1960; Dehn and Bruce 1972; Robinson 1938; Shephard 1966). Detailed information beyond about 60 to 65 years or the age of retirement is limited (Strandell 1964). Simonson (1957) has summarized the changes in several components of physical work capacity related to age. The largest deterioration, as stated above, was related to the cardiovascular and respiratory function. Muscular strength at age 40 was reported to be 90 per cent of peak but was about the same at age 50. Maximum isometric grip strength did not change from age 20 to 60 years (Petrofsky and Lind 1975; Shephard 1969). In the absence of neuromuscular disease, speed of repetitive movements in small muscles, and motor co-ordination in both small and large muscles is maintained with age (Simonson, Enzer, and Benton 1943). Simple reaction time and discrimination reaction time have been shown to increase with age (Spirduso 1975).

Rate of aging

There have been several reports of the decrement in $\dot{V}_{O_2}$max with age (Astrand 1960; Binkhorst, Pool, von Leeuwen, and Bouhuys 1966; Robinson 1938; Skranc 1968; and others) but few reports (Dehn and Bruce 1972) are available that describe the rate of decrease of aerobic capacity or the ability to deliver oxygen to working muscle as affected by regular participation in exercise.

The concept of aerobic capacity as the maximal oxygen intake ($\dot{V}_{O_2}$max) as an objective measure of cardio-respiratory performance has been discussed in detail by Taylor, Buskirk, and Henschel (1955).

The rate of decline in $\dot{V}_{O_2}$max with age as observed from literature reviews of cross-sectional studies is fairly consistent and uniform. Shephard (1966) reported a decline of 0.45 ml kg^{-1} min^{-1} y^{-1} which agreed with the value of 0.41 obtained by Hodgson (1971) in a review of sedentary men. Twenty-three studies with a total of 1800 observations of men age 18 to 60 were included in these pooled data. Dehn and Bruce (1972) calculated the rate from 17 studies with 700 observations and reported it to be 0.398 ml kg^{-1} min^{-1} y^{-1}. A similar review (Hodgson 1971) of 9 studies with approximately 350 physically active men yielded a regression coefficient of 0.44 ml kg^{-1} min^{-1} y^{-1}. Five cross-sectional studies with a total of 116 athletes who had maintained their active status provided a regression coefficient of 0.48 ml kg^{-1} min^{-1} y^{-1}.

A much lower rate of decline in $\dot{V}_{O_2}$max was observed among control groups of men aged 40 through 60 and free of coronary heart disease in Minneapolis and at Pennsylvania State University (Taylor, Buskirk, and Remington 1973). Both groups were at moderately high risk of coronary heart disease (CHD) and were subjects in a study of the feasibility of physical activity trials for CHD prevention. In Minnesota, 115 men were recruited from 1546 men in the age group (40–60 years) from a Minneapolis suburb and from a cluster of central city census tracts. At Penn State 189 men were recruited from 1623 employees of the University. Both groups were recruited using a stepwise process to allow evaluation of bias created by the recruitment process. Evidence was obtained that the subjects volunteering in Minnesota were similar to the population sampled with respect to body weight, blood-pressure, and serum cholesterol concentration. Men who smoked cigarettes tended to volunteer less frequently and men regularly pursuing physically active recreation tended to volunteer more frequently.

The regression of $\dot{V}_{O_2}$max in the pooled control groups from age 40 to 60 yielded a decrease of only 0.20 ml kg^{-1} min^{-1} y^{-1}. Nevertheless, the average $\dot{V}_{O_2}$max of 30.4 ml kg^{-1} min^{-1} at age 60 agreed well with the literature review for 60-year-old sedentary men, 29.5 ml kg^{-1} min^{-1}. The difference in slope of the regression line of $\dot{V}_{O_2}$max on age between the above study and the cross-sectional studies suggests that pooling data from a number of heterogeneous studies may be somewhat misleading and that the use of a linear regression equation to describe the entire age range conveys an oversimplified view.

In addition, the conclusion from the reviews of cross-sectional studies, that the rate of decline in $\dot{V}_{O_2}$max is uniform regardless of physical activity, does not agree with the report of Dehn and Bruce (1972). Their longitudinal data reported on 40 inactive men over a period of 2.5 years indicated a decline in $\dot{V}_{O_2}$max which was more than double that observed from the cross-sectional studies, i.e. 0.94 vs. 0.398 ml kg^{-1} min^{-1} y^{-1}. The greater rate was the same as that found in the longitudinal investigations of Dill, Robinson, and Ross (1967), who studied 13 former champion runners over a 24-year period, and Hollman (1972) who studied 56 sedentary men over a 12–15-year interval (1.04 and 0.93 ml kg^{-1} min^{-1} y^{-1}, respectively). It is likely, as Dehn and Bruce have stated, that cross-sectional studies have samples which are not representative of the population and produce biased results that include more fit individuals willing to be tested to maximum effort. They conclude that valid changes with aging can only be established by paired observations in the same persons and indicate that the lesser factors contributing to the decline in $\dot{V}_{O_2}$max with age may be the changes in body weight and composition. Further exploration of the differences in rate of aging between longitudinal studies and cross-sectional studies is necessary to clarify the issues involved.

The decline in cardiovascular function with age involving perhaps a lesser ability to partition and regulate regional blood-flow may be related to poorer temperature regulation with age during work in the heat. Work in our laboratory at Pennsylvania State University has provided evidence that after acclimation older men (McCormick and Buskirk 1974) and pre-adolescent boys (Haymes, McCormick, and Buskirk 1975) tolerated work in the heat less well than young men. Wagner, Robinson, Tzankoff, and Marino (1972) at Indiana University reported that after acclimation thermoregulation during work in the heat was significantly improved in all age groups. However, young men and older boys were superior to the pre-adolescent boys and older men with respect to time of toleration of a standard work–heat stress and maintained lower heart rates, and rectal and skin temperatures, and greater evaporative rates in relation to mean rectal and skin temperatures. During work in the heat the older men and pre-adolescent boys were more limited in the sensitivity and secretory capacity of the sweating mechanism than the young men and the older boys. The older men had lower coefficients of heat conductance and finger blood-flow in the heat than the young men.

Strength. Static muscle strength and endurance time in submaximal static work have been reported to change little with age in men (Petrofsky and Lind 1975; Shephard 1969). The work of Miles (1950) with 604 men and 553 women using a simultaneous grip test with two hand dynamometers indicated a fairly linear decrease with age in both men and women from age 30 to 70 (approximately 0.20 kg yr^{-1}). Also Burke, Tuttle, Thompson, Janney, and Weber (1953) have shown that grip strength endurance as well as grip strength decreased with age in 147 subjects from 20 to 79. In both studies grip strength in men was reduced at a greater rate between 60 and 80 than between 30 and 60.

Petrofsky, Burse, and Lind (1975) have reported a significant and linear decrease in isometric grip strength with age in 83 healthy women, aged 19 to 65 years. The rate of decrease of strength was 0.23 kg yr^{-1}. However, along with the grip strength decrease, there was an increase with age in duration of a 40 per cent of maximum isometric contraction. In both men and women heart rate responses to the static endurance work tended to decrease with age. About half of the difference (17 beats/min) between young women and older women during 40 per cent of maximum contraction could be attributed to the decrease in resting heart rate with age (8 beats/min). The systolic blood-pressure response to the static endurance work increased with age in both men and women. The diastolic blood-pressure response did not change with age.

The effect of physical conditioning

From age 20 up to the age of 65 there is little doubt about the effect of endurance-type exercise on the improvement of endurance for dynamic work and maximum work capacity (Saltin, Hartley, Kilbom, and Astrand 1969). In the examination of the literature of cross-sectional studies (Hodgson 1971) sedentary men after a conditioning programme were examined as a separate group. Seventeen age categories from 11 studies with a total of 203 observations were included in the data. At age 30 the increase in $\dot{V}_{O_2}$max with conditioning was 16.7 per cent and at age 60 the increase was 11.5 per cent. This increase in $\dot{V}_{O_2}$max placed each group at about the same level as the moderately active groups of the same age with a similar rate of decline in $\dot{V}_{O_2}$max with age (0.53 ml kg^{-1} min^{-1} y^{-1}).

The preceding constitutes a simplified summary of the effect of conditioning because of the lack of uniformity regarding the frequency, intensity, and duration of the exercise programme. It is also important to note that the effects of short-term conditioning programmes (usually 10 to 20 weeks) after years of inactivity may be different than regular exercise conducted over a lifetime. In addition, the conclusion of Dehn and Bruce, from the examination of longitudinal studies, was that sedentary men had a significantly greater annual decrement in $\dot{V}_{O_2}$max than habitually active individuals. Astrand, Astrand, Hallbäck, and Kilbom (1973) reported data on 44 women and 42 men studied both in 1949 and 1970. Most of the subjects were physical education teachers and were, with few exceptions, physically active. In the 21-year period, from age 26 to 47, the average rate of decline in $\dot{V}_{O_2}$max for the men was 0.64 ml kg^{-1} min^{-1} y^{-1} and for the women from age 22 to 43 only 0.44 kg^{-1} min^{-1} y^{-1}. For the men this represented a 23 per cent decrease from 58.7 ml kg^{-1} min^{-1} and for the women a 19 per cent decrease from 47.6. For the men this rate of decline is greater than that reported for active men from cross-sectional studies but is still less than the rate of decline reported by Dehn and Bruce for sedentary men. The change in $\dot{V}_{O_2}$max with exercise over a 10-year period was studied by Kasch and Wallace (1976). Sixteen men, initially 32 to 56 years, were trained with running or swimming at an intensity above 60 per cent of $\dot{V}_{O_2}$max. The average weekly running distance was 25 km. Mean $\dot{V}_{O_2}$max was unchanged over ten years at 44 ml kg^{-1} min^{-1}. No significant changes were seen in body weight, resting heart rate, or resting blood-pressure. How long $\dot{V}_{O_2}$max will remain unchanged is an important question. Based on the review of cross-sectional studies a 'normal' decrease in $\dot{V}_{O_2}$max with age should occur in these subjects over the ensuing 10-year period. Hopefully, the group will be followed further.

The circulatory effects of endurance conditioning on sedentary middle-age and older men (38 to 55 years) was examined in detail by Hartley, Saltin, Grimby, and others (Hartley, Grimby, Kilbom, Nilsson, Astrand, Bjure, Ekblom, and Saltin 1969; Saltin, Hartley, Kilbom, and Astrand 1969). Fifteen men participated in an endurance training programme which consisted of running for 3 one-half hour periods per week for 8 to 10 weeks. $\dot{V}_{O_2}$max increased an average of 14 per cent. This increase was achieved with a 13 per cent increase in maximal cardiac output. Heart rate was 8 to 17 beats/min lower during submaximal exercise. The maximal heart rate decreased by 6 beats/min. Stroke volume increased 16 per cent at maximal exercise. After training mean arterial blood-pressure was on the average 5 mm Hg lower at a given submaximum oxygen uptake and no change was observed at maximal exercise. Heart volume determined from radiographs did not change.

In many of the reported studies the improvement in $\dot{V}_{O_2}$ max with conditioning was related inversely to the initial $\dot{V}_{O_2}$ max. Those with an initial $\dot{V}_{O_2}$ max of 30 ml kg^{-1} min^{-1} had approximately a 20 per cent increase in $\dot{V}_{O_2}$ max and those with an initial $\dot{V}_{O_2}$ max of 50 ml kg^{-1} min^{-1} had approximately a 10 per cent increase. The improvement shown by the older subjects tended to be less than younger subjects if their initial aerobic capacity was the same at the onset of conditioning. Whether this trend continues into the 70s and 80s is not known. One study by Benestad (1965) provided some evidence that the effect of conditioning on $\dot{V}_{O_2}$ max may be minimal at these advanced ages. During a 5–6-week conditioning period, 13 men, aged 70 to 81, showed no change in $\dot{V}_{O_2}$ max. The primary effect of the conditioning was to decrease heart rate at a set submaximal work load.

After 6 weeks of an exercise conditioning programme with 68 men, aged 52 to 88, deVries (1970) reported a significant increase in the integrated work output (watts/min) up to a heart rate of 145 (approximately 90 per cent of maximum). Resting systolic and diastolic blood-pressure decreased significantly. Other significant increases occurred in strength (elbow flexion), vital capacity, minute volume (BTPS), and ventilation equivalent at an exercise heart rate of 145. At the end of 42 weeks with 8 subjects the integrated work, up to heart rate 145, remained increased but not significantly. Resting systolic blood-pressure was the same as before conditioning. Resting systolic blood-pressure was 5 mm Hg less but this decrease was not statistically significant. Strength, muscle girth, vital capacity, oxygen pulse at heart rate, 145, and minute ventilation at heart rate 145 were significantly greater. The exercise programme above consisted of a 15–20-minute warm-up period of calisthenics, a progressive run–walk programme of 15 to 20 min and a 15–20-min static stretching period or aquatics period. During the run–walk period the pulse rate was kept below 145 beats/min. A modified exercise programme was administered to seven subjects because of asymptomatic myocardial ischaemias or arrythmias. The participants were limited to a heart rate of 120 instead of 145 for normal subjects. This was done by eliminating the run–walk phase and substituting a progressive walking programme. The changes observed after six weeks with the walking programme were similar to those reported in the 'normal' programme except that resting blood-pressure, vital capacity, and strength were not significantly changed.

The conclusion that the trainability of older men with respect to physical work capacity is probably greater than had been suspected was supported in a survey of Soviet literature on physical activity and aging (Gore 1972a, b, c). One ten-year longitudinal study of the effect of exercise by Deshin (1972), with 6 men and 16 women, aged 51 to 74, reported no deterioration in physical condition. Improvement, most marked at the end of 3 to 5 years, was reported for some variables. Resting ECG, pulmonary function, and blood tests were made. Orthostatic tests, balance time with eyes shut, and several physical and motor performance tests were also conducted. The improvement in performance on these tests was noteworthy. Several tests involving strength (sit-ups, push-ups, throwing a 2-kg medicine ball, sustaining a 70 to 90° angle with outstretched legs), balance, and jumping in place, demonstrated quantitative improvement. The number of longitudinal studies in the Soviet literature dealing with physical activity and aging is impressive. It is unfortunate that the central haemodynamic and $\dot{V}_{O_2}$ max data are not available for comparison with the cross-sectional studies of Europe and North America.

Reaction and movement time. Few studies of reaction time and movement time have included elderly athletic or other active groups. Most samples for study of aging and neuromuscular parameters have been comprised of institutionalized rather than non-institutionalized subjects. Spirduso (1975) reported results of reaction and movement time on 60 male volunteers from the University of Texas at Austin. Four groups of 15 each were formed: older active sportsmen (OA = 57.2 years); older non-active men (ONA = 56.3 years); young non-active men (YNA = 25.4 years) young active (YA = 23.6 years). The effects of age and activity level were significant for simple reaction time (SRT), discrimination reaction time (DRT), and movement time (MT). The active groups, when averaged over age reacted and moved faster than the non-active. The ONA group was significantly slower from the other three groups in all of the above variables. The OA group had slower MT than the YA group but faster MT than the YNA group. SRT and DRT in the OA group was about the same as for the YNA group. The results indicated that physical activity may play a more dominant role than age in determining reaction time and movement time. The average decrement in these parameters that might be attributed to age was 8 per cent in the active group and non-significant, whereas the ONA men were on the average 22.5 per cent slower than the NA men.

Chapman, deVries, and Swezey (1972) reported the effects of exercise on joint stiffness in young and old men. Two groups of 20 men were formed; older men age 63 to 88 and young high school boys age 15 to 19. Baseline values in strength and stiffness of both right and left index fingers were obtained with one side as a control for half the subjects and the opposite side for the remainder. Joint stiffness was measured by the torque and energy requirements necessary to oscillate the index finger passively about its metacarpophalangeal joint. There was a significantly greater joint stiffness in the old men than in the young. There was no significant difference between the two groups in measured strength. After a 6-week training programme (weight training with the index finger according to the method of Delorme and Watkins (1951), significant increases in strength and decreases in joint stiffness were seen in both the young and older groups. The authors concluded that joint stiffness in both young and old men in the absence of arthritis or other joint disease is a reversible phenomenon and suggested a need to re-examine our ideas concerning the trainability of older individuals.

Extension of longevity

The effects of exercise on longevity were first evaluated by comparing the age at death of men who participated in athletics during their youth with those who did not. Many of these studies included former high school and college athletes. This area of investigation has been reviewed extensively by Montoye (1974) and a summary revealed that there was little difference in life expectancy for former college athletic award winners compared to their college classmates. Montoye suggested that regular engagement in physical activity and control of body weight to prevent over-fatness throughout life may be more important in the meso-morphic (athletic) body type, as compared to other body types, in order to maintain a healthy cardiovascular system. The study of risk factors in development of heart disease, in particular the Framingham study (Gordon and Kannel 1973) support the concepts that weight control and regular physical activity for middle-aged men will minimize their chances of developing coronary heart disease. Perhaps the relationship of physical activity and longevity should be approached in a manner similar to the studies of nutrition and aging. Stuchlíková, Juricová-Horaková, and Deyl (1975), using male Wistar rats, golden hamsters, and mice gave restricted diets of exactly one-half the amount of food cosumed by controls. They found that food restriction put upon animals at any stage of individual life, if chronic, produced a distinct increase in life span.

These findings have also been obtained with such species as the Rotifer, *Tokophyra infusorum*, and Daphnia (Shock 1970) and confirm the findings of McCay, Maynard, Sperling, and Barnes (1939). Studies of longevity of rodents where the factors of exercise and caloric restriction are controlled may provide more understanding of the effects on man. However, as Shank (1972) has pointed out, there are no data from man that would support the thesis that chronic underconsumption of food (and we would add, chronic exercise) will increase life expectancy.

References

ASTRAND, I. (1960). *Acta Physiol. Scand.*, **49**, 169.

ASTRAND, P. O., HALLBACK, I., and KILBOM, A. (1973). *J. appl. Physiol.*, **35**(5), 649.

BENESTAD, A. M. (1965). *Acta. Med. Scand.*, **178**(3), 321.

BINKHORST, R. A., POOL, J., VON LEEUWEN, P., and BOUHUYS, A. (1966). *Arbeitsphysiol.*, **22**, 10.

BURKE, W. E., TUTTLE, W. W., THOMPSON, C. W., JANNEY, C. D., and WEBER, R. J. (1953). *J. appl. Physiol.*, **5**, 628.

CHAPMAN, E. A., DEVRIES, H. A., and SWEZEY, R. (1972). *J. Gerontol.*, **27**(2), 218.

DEHN, M. M. and BRUCE, R. A. (1972). *J. appl. Physiol.*, **33**(6), 805.

DELORME, T. H. and WATKINS, A. L. (1951). *Progressive resistance exercise*. New York, Appleton-Century-Crofts.

DESHIN, D. F. (1972). *Gerontol. Clin.*, **14**, 78.

DEVRIES, H. A. (1970). *J. Gerontol.*, **25**(4), 325.

DILL, D. B., ROBINSON, S., and ROSS, J. C. (1967). *J. Sports Med.*, **7**, 4.

GORDON, T. and KANNEL, W. B. (1973). *Geriat.*, **28**, 80.

GORE, I. Y. (1972a). *Gerontol. Clin.*, **14**, 65.

—— (1972b). *Gerontol. Clin.*, **14**, 70.

—— (1972c). *Gerontol. Clin.*, **14**, 78.

HARTLEY, L. H., GRIMBY, G., KILBOM, A., NILSSON, N. J., ASTRAND, I., BJURE, J., EKBLOM, B., and SALTIN, B. (1969). *Scand. J. clin. Lab. Invest.*, **24**, 335.

HAYMES, E. M., McCORMICK, R. J., and BUSKIRK, E. R. (1975). *J. appl. Physiol.*, **39**(3), 457.

HODGSON, J. L. (1971). Ph.D. Dissertation, University of Minnesota.

HOLLMANN, W. (1972). *J. appl. Physiol.*, **33**(6), 805.

KASCH, F. W. and WALLACE, J. P. (1976). *Med. and Sci. in Sports*, **8**(1), 5.

McCAY, C. M., MAYNARD, L. A. SPERLING, G., and BARNES, L. L. (1939). *J. Nutr.*, **18**,

McCORMICK, R. J. and BUSKIRK, E. R. (1974). *Federation Proc.*, **33**, 441.

MILES, W. R. (1950). *Methods in medical research 3*. Year Book Publishers, Chicago.

MONTOYE, H. J. (1974). *Science and medicine of exercise and sport*, (2nd edn.) (eds. W. R. Johnson and E. R. Buskirk). Harper and Row, New York.

PETROFSKY, J. S. and LIND, A. R. (1975). *J. appl. Physiol.*, **38**(1), 91.

——, BURSE, R. L., and LIND, A. R. (1975). *J. appl. Physiol.*, **38**(5), 863.

ROBINSON, S. (1938). *Arbeitsphysiol.*, **10**, 251.

SALTIN, B., HARTLEY, H., KILBOM, A., and ASTRAND, I. (1969). *Scand. J. clin. Lab. Invest.*, **24**, 323.

SHANK, R. E. (1972). *DHEW Publication* (NIH), 75.

SHEPHARD, R. J. (1966). *Arch. Environ. Health*, **13**, 664.

—— (1969). *Arch. Environ. Health*, **18**, 982.

SHOCK, N. W. (1967). *Canad. Med. Assoc. J.*, **96**, 836.

—— (1970). *J. Amer. Dietetic Assoc.*, **56**(6), 491.

SIMONSON, E. (1957). *Geriat.* **12**(1), 28.

—— (1971). *Physiology of work capacity and fatigue*. Charles C. Thomas, Springfield.

——, ENZER, N., and BENTON, R. W. (1943). *J. Lab. clin. Med.*, **28**, 1555.

SKINNER, J. S. (1970. *Phys. Activity and Aging: Med. and Sport*, **4**, 100.

SKRANC, O. (1968). *Teor. Praxe tel. Vych.*, **16**(6), 15.

SPIRDUSO, W. W. (1975). *J. Gerontol.*, **30**(4), 435.

STRANDELL, T. (1964). *Acta Med. Scand.*, **175**, 414.

STUCHLIKOVA, E., JURICOVA-HORAKOVA, J., and DEYL, Z. (1975). *Exp. Gerontol.*, **10**, 141.

TAYLOR, H. L., BUSKIRK, E. R., and HENSCHEL, A. (1955). *J. appl. Physiol.*, **8**, 73.

——, ——, and REMINGTON, R. D. (1973). *Fed. Proc.*, **32**, 1623.

—— and MONTOYE, H. J. (1972). *DHEW Publication* (NIH) 75.

WAGNER, J. A., ROBINSON, S., TZANKOFF, J. P., and MARINO, R. P. (1972). *J. appl. Physiol.*, **33**(5), 616.

Influence of obesity on longevity in the aged   Reubin Andres

Introduction

Obesity has been shown to be associated with a large number of major life-shortening illnesses, such as coronary heart disease, hypertension, and diabetes (Bray 1975, 1976). Furthermore, a very large insurance study (Society of Actuaries 1959) emphasized that there is a continuous direct relationship between obesity and mortality extending over the entire distribution of relative body weight except, perhaps, for those extremely underweight (Keys, Aravanis, Blackburn, Van Buchem, Buzina, Djordjevic, Fidanza, Karvonen, Menotti, Puddu, and Taylor 1972).

It was, therefore, surprising that the present review of publications dealing with the effect of obesity on longevity in the aged has led to conclusions which are strongly at variance with these commonly held perceptions. There are difficulties in comparing data from the diverse populations studied, yet none of the studies in recent years supports such statements as: 'In affluent societies . . . survival is more likely in those as lean as possible' (Kannel and Gordon 1974). Indeed, the results of this literature search show that the 'ideal' or 'desirable' body weight for middle-aged and elderly adults is considerably higher than that presented in the most commonly used height–weight tables (*Statistical Bulletin* 1959).

The scope of this chapter will be sharply limited to the relation between obesity and mortality. Obesity may exert its effects on mortality in a variety of ways:

(1) It may influence known risk factors for disease. Thus, obesity has been shown to be associated with elevated serum lipids, glucose, and uric acid.
(2) It may influence the development of specific illnesses directly, that is, via mechanisms which have not been elucidated.
(3) It may influence mortality by more general mechanisms (not via specific diseases) which in some manner influence the ability to survive.

These associations are made even more complex by the influences of biological aging. Thus aging leads to changes in body composition with loss of lean body mass and with either relative or absolute increase in adipose tissue mass. Aging processes also influence the risk factors noted above; there are changes with age in the serum levels of the lipids and of glucose, for example. Other aging processes undoubtedly influence the rate of development of such diseases as atherosclerosis. These complex interactions are noted here in order to emphasize the goal of this paper which is to examine the impact of obesity at different ages on overall mortality, since mortality does represent, in effect, the integrated total of all the other 'intermediary' processes.

Early surveys of the relation between obesity and mortality

Underlying this analysis is the assumption that obesity has been accurately assessed. The techniques available for quantification of obesity range from measurement only of height and weight to complex procedures suitable only for the study of small numbers of individuals under laboratory conditions (Grande 1975). The large-scale community surveys which provide the bulk of the evidence reviewed in this chapter rely on height and weight measurements only. It is still necessary to convert these two measures into a single number which expresses the degree of overweight of each individual. This is generally accomplished by computing the 'relative body weight' or the Obesity Index, that is, the subject's weight is divided by a reference weight. The reference weight commonly used (Statistical Bulletin 1959) is provided from tables of heights and frame sizes for men and women derived from data of the large insurance study (The Society of Actuaries 1959). In these tables, an upper and lower range of desirable body weight is given for each height interval and for each of three frame sizes. Since there are no criteria for classifying an individual's frame size, the common practice is to take the mean of the range of values for the medium frame size and to assign that value as the desirable weight for a given height.

The Society of Actuaries report (1959) is an extensive compilation of data on persons insured from 1935 to 1953 and traced to 1954. Figure 1 presents an extract of those data for men and women aged 40 to 69 years.† It shows a linear relation between overweight and excess mortality. As noted above, this study has had a profound effect on physicians and, through them, on the public. The study has, however, been subjected to a number of criticisms, some dealing with the certainty of various biases in the insured population and with poorly standard- ized measurements of height and weight, etc., (Blackburn and Parlin 1966) and some with the assumption that a linear model gives the best fit of the data (Seltzer 1966). Those papers should be consulted for details of criticisms. If we turn now to more recent epidemiological studies, the results are quite different.

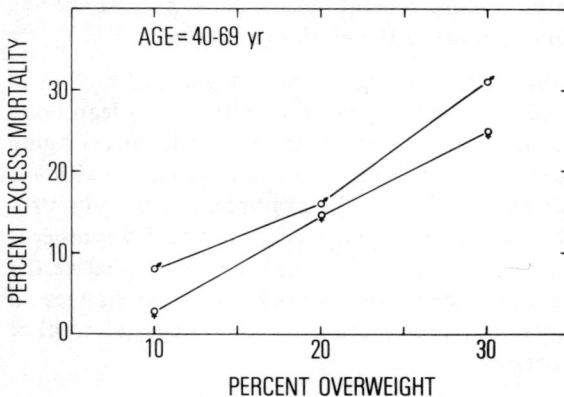

FIG. 1. Effect of overweight on excess mortality. The data are from the Society of Actuaries Building and Blood Pressure Study, 1959. The figure is drawn from data for 'Cases without known minor impairments' and includes subjects who 'were insured either as standard risks, or were rated as substandard risks only because of weight, having no other impairment that would bar them from obtaining standard insurance' (*Stat. Bull.*, Feb., 1960, p. 8, and Mar., 1960, p. 2).

† The men and women included in this figure 'were insured either as standard risks, or were rated as substandard risks only because of weight, having no other impairment that would bar them from obtaining life insurance' (*Stat. Bull.* 1959, **41** (Feb); 6–10 and 1959, **41** (Mar), 1–4). 'Overweight' in this figure represents percentage over average weight of the insured population. Since the average weight is considerably higher than the desirable weight (as defined above), the overweight values of 10, 20, and 30 per cent in Fig. 1 are equivalent to obesity indices of 1.25, 1.36, and 1.49 for men and of 1.31, 1.43, and 1.54 for women.

Recent epidemiological studies of the relation between obesity and mortality rate

1. *The Framingham Study.* This study of a 5209-person sample of the community of Framingham, Massachusetts was initiated in 1948. Participants were followed at 2-year intervals and a 16-year follow-up has been reported (Kannel and Gordon 1974; Shurtleff 1970). Figure 2 groups men and women over the broad age range of 45 to 74 years. Note that minimal mortality occurred in the men at an obesity index level of 1.25 to 1.39. The minimal level for women is broader, perhaps 1.05 to 1.24.

The data have also been presented for each decade of life studied (Fig. 3). Note especially the 45–54-year age group, labelled 5: there is a strongly negative relationship between obesity and mortality rate. The other age groups do not show as strong a tendency but regressions are negative for them as well.

2. Another community study on 6928 adult men and women was carried out in *Alameda County*, a typical California urban community (Belloc 1973). A five and one-half year follow-up of mortality rate as related to obesity has been reported. Note that for each of the four decades studied, the men (Fig. 4) showed a minimal mortality distinctly above the so-called 'ideal' obesity index of 1.0. Note further the upswing in mortality in the groups with indices greater than 1.3; these groups include that small fraction of extreme ('morbid') obesity present

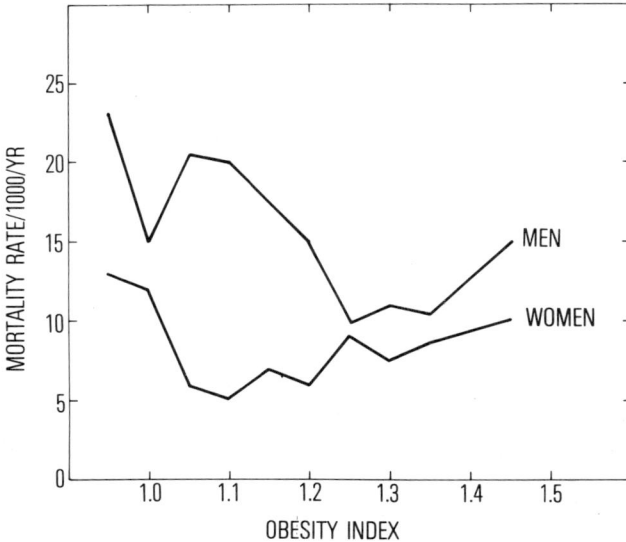

FIG. 2. Relation of obesity to mortality—The Framingham Study. The mortality rate is reported as the annual incidence per 1000 population at risk at examination (Kannel and Gordon 1974). Data for men and women are grouped for ages 45–74 y. The data plotted at obesity index 1.0, 1.1, etc., represent the subjects who ranged from 1.00 to 1.04, 1.10 to 1.14, etc.

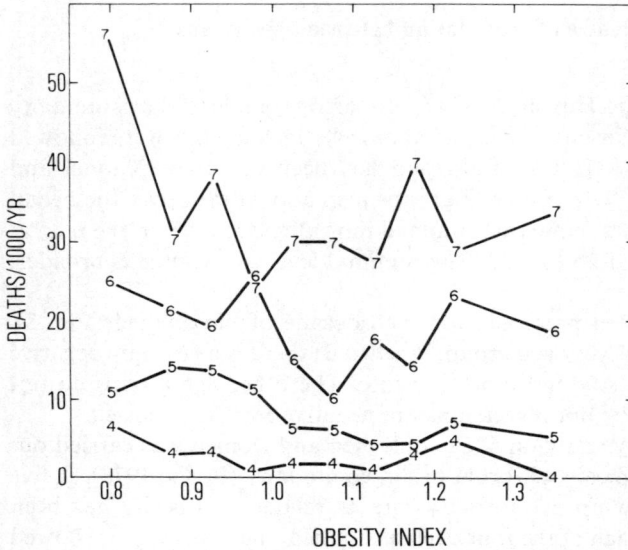

FIG. 3. Relation of obesity to mortality in men—The Framingham Study. Deaths are reported as the annual incidence per 1000 population at risk at examination. Data were derived from Table 12-8-B (Shurtleff 1970). Subjects aged 35–44 years at exam are labelled 4 and so forth up to subjects 65–74 years who are labelled 7.

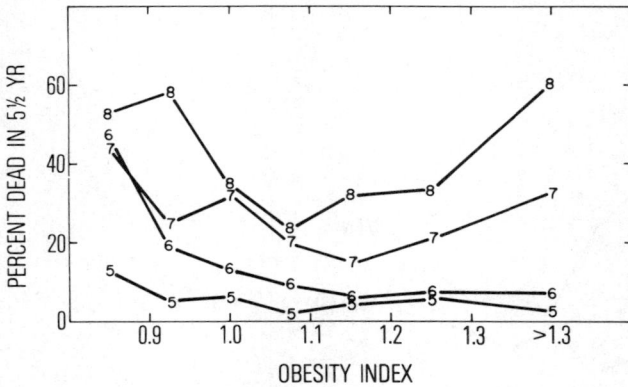

FIG. 4. Relation of obesity to mortality in men—the Alameda County study (Belloc 1973). Death rates are reported in per cent in a 5½ year period. The symbols are the same as in Fig. 3.

in all populations. Obesity has generally less impact on mortality in the women (Fig. 5).

3. The *Chicago Peoples Gas Company Study* (Dyer, Stamler, Berkson, and Lindberg 1975) involved 1233 male employees aged 40 to 59 years at first examination. They have been followed for 14 years (Fig. 6). Note that the minimal mortality for the 50–59-year age group occurred at an obesity index of

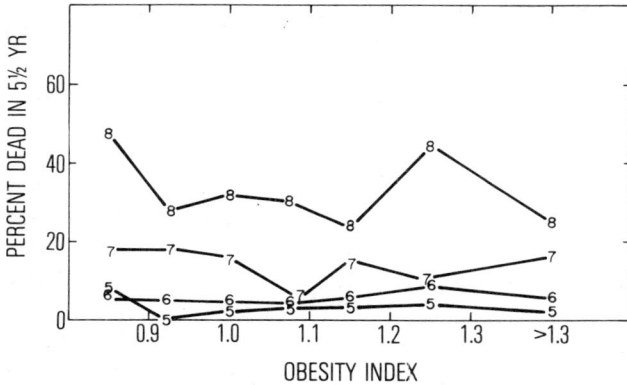

FIG. 5. Relation of obesity to mortality in women—the Alameda County Study (Belloc 1973). See legend to Fig. 4.

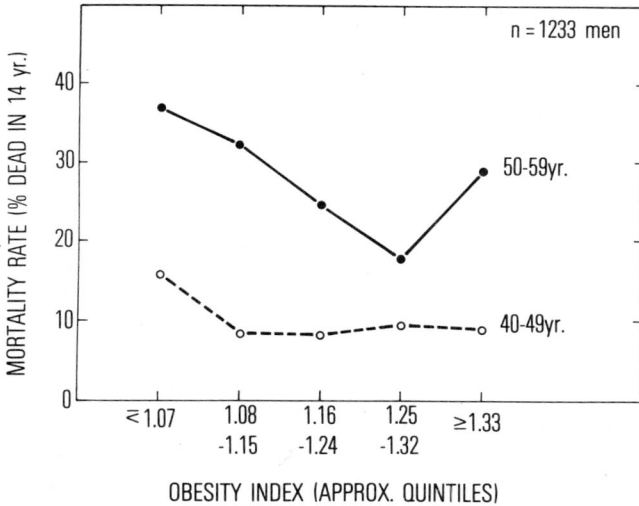

FIG. 6. Effect of obesity on mortality—the Chicago Peoples Gas Company Study (Dyer *et al.* 1975). Mortality rates are reported as the per cent dead in the 14-year follow-up period. Subjects were divided into approximate quintiles on the basis of their obesity indices at the initial examination.

1.25 to 1.32. The 40–49-years age groups showed little effect of obesity except that the leanest quintile had the highest mortality.

4. A 9–10-year follow-up study of 387 men aged 55 to 64 years in *Staveley*, Derbyshire, Great Britain, has been reported (Cole 1974). The measure of obesity used in this study was computed as log (wt) − 2 log (ht). The subjects were divided into approximate thirds on the basis of this index, the cut-points being 2.95 and 3.20. The exact interpretation of these values is difficult, but the effect of obesity on mortality rate is clear enough. The lightest third had the highest

annual mortality rate, 7.7 per cent, as the male subjects progressed from age 55–64 to age 65–74 years. Mortality rates for the middle and most obese thirds were 2.2 and 3.5 per cent, respectively.

5. A study of only 44 men, the *Human Aging Study*, is of interest because of the age of the participants, 65 to 91 years at first examination (Libow 1974). They were followed-up at 5 and 11 years after the initial examination. The date relevant to obesity were presented only in terms of the mean weights of three groups of subjects at initial examination: those who survived 11 years, those who died between five and 11 years, and those who failed to survive five years. The mean weights of these three groups were 71.0, 66.0, and 60.4 kg, respectively. These results were statistically significant at the $p < 0.05$ level.

6. The *Baltimore Longitudinal Study of Aging* was initiated in 1958 and has followed over 1100 men who range mainly from 25 to 90 years of age. Obesity has been assessed by a variety of techniques including the computation of percent fat in the body from detailed anthropometric measurements. The participants who have died have been compared to those who have survived. For each of the four decades, 50 to 89 years, the survivors are slightly but not statistically significantly less obese than the group that has not survived, the difference in per cent fat being about 1 per cent for each age group. But, again, no striking effect of obesity on mortality was present.

Conclusions

The implications of this literature review are complex. The hypothesis that obesity is a graded variable in its impact on mortality and that even minor degrees of obesity are detrimental cannot be supported by data from many recent studies. It is, however, important to stress that minor degrees of obesity may very well be harmful for specific subsets of the general population. It was not the purpose of this review to examine the evils of obesity in the hypertensive, the coronary patient, the diabetic, the osteoarthritic, etc. Nor have we examined the effect of obesity on the serum lipids, uric acid, or glucose levels. Those tasks are beyond the scope of this communication. There is a vast literature on these topics (Bray 1976) but each aspect of the impact of obesity and of the efficacy and practicality of weight-losing regimens deserves critical review.

The fact remains, however, that the general public, at the urging of physicians and of health information agencies, has been repeatedly instructed that minor deviations in weight from the sacrosanct 'desirable weight' tables will doom one to an early grave. We are quite accustomed to hearing that in affluent societies obesity is the number one health problem. In view of a great deal of evidence that the therapy of obesity is dismal indeed, it behoves the responsible physicians and health authorities to be very certain in the recommendations made to the general public. The impact of this health advice on the anxiety levels of that large fraction of the public that exceeds their 'desirable weight' is difficult to measure, and the impact of this anxiety on the development of other diseases and on a general sense of well-being is also unknown. It is an important postulate of programmes for the screening of disease and risk factors that the perils of the factor be clearly demonstrated, that the screening technique be accurate (false positives and false negatives should both be minimal), and that something can be done about the risk factor when it is correctly identified. The interesting feature about obesity as a risk factor is that the screening procedure is as available as the nearest bathroom scale. It behoves us to provide more realistic standards for judging obesity than those so readily available to the public and to physicians.

Another implication of this analysis of the literature is that a great deal of research remains to be done. The undoubted relation of obesity to specific important diseases which should, but do not, increase overall impact of obesity on mortality suggests that there are counterbalancing benefits to the obese state which have not received the attention of epidemiologists or of clinical investigators or of laboratory scientists. The literature is replete with articles and book chapters on the risks and hazards of obesity. There must be another side to the coin. With increased research, it should be possible to dissect out the mechanisms of both the hazards and the benefits in such a way as to minimize the one and to promote the other.

References

BELLOC, N. B. (1973). *Prevent. Med.*, **2**, 67.

BLACKBURN, H. and PARLIN, R. W. (1966). *Ann. NY Acad. Med.*, **134**, 965,

BRAY, G. A. (Ed.) (1975). *Obesity in perspective*, p. 527. DHEW Publication No. (NIH) 75–708.

——— (1976). *The obese patient*. W. B. Saunders Co., Philadelphia.

COLE, T. J. (1974). *Bull. Physio-pathol. Resp.*, **10**, 657.

DYER, A. R., STAMLER, J., BERKSON, D.M., and LINDBERG, H. A., (1975). *J. chron. Dis.*, **28**, 109.

GRANDE, F. (1975). In *Obesity in perspective* (ed. G. A. Bray), p. 189. DHEW Publication No. (NIH) 75–708.

KANNEL, W. B., and GORDON, T. (1974). In *Obesity symposium* (ed. W. L. Burland, P. O. Samuel, and J. Yudkin), p. 24. Churchill Livingstone, Edinburgh.

KEYS, A., ARAVANIS, C., BLACKBURN, H., VAN BUCHEM, F. S. P., BUZINA, R., DJORDJEVIC, B. S., FIDANZA, F., KARVONEN, M. J., MENOTTI, A., PUDDU, V., and TAYLOR, H. L. (1972). *Ann. intern. Med.*, **77**, 15.

LIBOW, L. S. (1974). Geriatrics, **29**(11), 75.

SELTZER, C. C. (1966). *New Engl. J. Med.*, **274**, 254.

SHURTLEFF, D. (1970). In *an epidemiological investigation of cardiovascular disease* (ed. W. B. Kannel and T. Gordon), Section 26, Table 18–8–B. U.S. Government Printing Office, Washington, D.C.

SOCIETY OF ACTUARIES (1959). *Build and blood pressure study*, p. 268. The Society of Actuaries, Chicago.

STASTICAL BULLETIN (1959). *Statist. Bull.*, **40**, 2.

Smoking as a risk factor in longevity Leonard M. Schuman

Gains in longevity

Man's subconscious quest for a measure of immortality continues unabated; yet, paradoxically he jeopardizes his small share in the immortality of his species by his actions. Man strives for an improvement in his longevity, yet contradicts this striving with certain of his habit patterns and environmental exposures. The gains in life expectancy at birth among so-called Western cultures in the 75 years since 1900 are only slightly, if at all, transmitted to the older age groups in our population. These gains are not added to man's longevity at the upper end of his life span. The major contributions to this large increase in life expectancy in the youngest age groups included the decline in infant mortality from 100 deaths per 1000 live births in 1915 to 16.1 in 1975 and the control of communicable diseases in childhood, chiefly respiratory and enteric diseases, by means of immunization and sanitation respectively (US Department of Health, Education, and Welfare 1979a; Section 2, Part A, pp. 2–3). In Table 1(a) and (b) the dramatic gains in

Table 1 Average remaining lifetime in years at specified ages: (a) for whites by sex: 1900–2 and 1975, USA; (b) for non-whites by sex: 1900–2 and 1975, USA

(a) Age	White male			White female		
	1900–2†	1975	Gain	1900–2	1975	Gain
0	48.2	69.4	21.2	51.1	77.2	26.1
1	54.6	69.6	15.0	56.4	77.1	20.7
10	50.6	60.9	10.3	52.2	68.4	16.2
20	42.2	51.4	9.2	43.8	58.6	14.8
30	34.9	42.2	7.3	36.4	49.0	12.6
40	27.7	33.0	5.3	29.2	39.4	10.2
50	20.8	24.3	3.5	21.9	30.3	8.4
60	14.4	16.8	2.4	15.2	21.9	6.7
70	9.0	10.9	1.9	9.6	14.4	4.8
80	5.1	6.7	1.6	5.5	8.6	3.1

(b) Age	Non-white male			Non-white female		
	1900–2†	1975	Gain	1900–2	1975	Gain
0	32.5	63.6	31.1	35.0	72.3	37.3
1	42.5	64.4	21.9	43.5	73.0	29.5
10	41.9	55.8	13.9	43.0	64.4	21.4
20	35.1	46.3	11.2	36.9	54.7	17.8
30	29.3	38.0	8.7	30.7	45.3	14.6
40	23.1	29.8	6.7	24.4	36.2	11.8
50	17.3	22.4	5.1	18.7	27.9	9.2
60	12.6	16.3	3.7	13.6	20.7	7.1
70	8.3	11.3	3.0	9.6	14.4	4.8
80	5.1	8.5	3.4	6.5	11.0	4.5

†10 states and D.C. in 1900–2; entire U.S. in 1975.
Source: U.S. Department of Health, Education, and Welfare (1979b), Sec. 5, Life Tables.

early life are readily discernible for both white and non-white segments of the US population and for both sexes. Equally interesting are the relatively insignificant gains in life expectancy at ages over 40 or 50 (US Department of Health, Education, and Welfare 1979b; Section 5, Part A, pp. 5–13).

Impediments to longevity—smoking

It is my thesis that a significant retardant to improvement in life expectancy at the middle and later years of life is the entire category of environmental hazards in which I include certain personal habit patterns, particularly smoking, which hazards initiate or promote chronic processes exhibiting themselves in the middle and later years of life. This thesis is supported by a number of observations and findings in analyses of mortality data in relation to smoking.

In Table 2 it will be noted that the diseases related to tobacco use contributed 52.0 per cent of the total US mortality in 1975 (US Department of Health, Education, and Welfare 1979c; Section 1, Part A, pp. 1–100). Even if we consider only those entities for which a causal relationship is considered to be firm or highly probable, their contribution is still 41.0 per cent of total mortality.

In the Report of the Advisory Committee on Smoking and Health to the Surgeon General of the US Public Health Service, data derived from the Dorn (1958) study of US veterans could be utilized to compare the death rates by age among cigarette smokers and non-smokers. The results are presented in Fig. 1 (US Department of Health, Education, and Welfare 1964; p. 88). Throughout the age-scale cigarette smokers show a distinctly greater mortality than non-smokers and the ratios of smoker to non-smoker mortality are greater for the middle years of life. These data, however, do not take into account the varying

Table 2 Mortality from selected chronic diseases related to tobacco use: United States, 1975

Diseases	Number of deaths
Causally related:	
Cancer of lung, bronchus, trachea (162)†	82 040
Chronic bronchitis and emphysema (490–2)	23 507
Cancer of larynx (161)	3237
Cancer of lip (140)	158
Probably causally related:	
Coronary heart disease (410–13)	642 719
Cancer of bladder (188)	9369
Cancer of buccal cavity and pharynx (141–9)	7851
Cancer of esophagus (150)	6997
Possibly causally related:	
Cerebrovascular disease (430–8)	194 038
Aortic aneurysm (non-syphlitic) (441)	13 634
Total	983 550
Total mortality, all causes	1 892 879

†I.C.D. No.—International List of Causes of Death, Eighth Revision.
Source: US Department of Health, Education, and Welfare (1979c), Mortality Part A, Sec. 1.

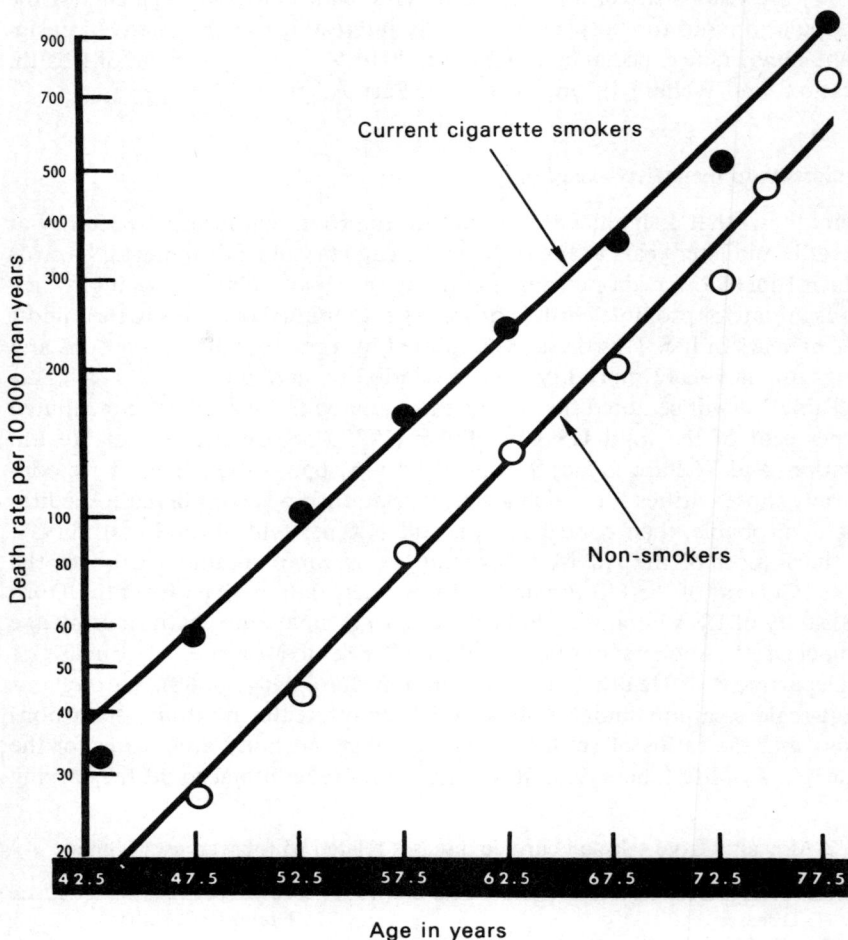

FIG. 1. Death rate (logarithmic scale) plotted against age—prospective study. of mortality in US veterans (US Department of Health, Education, and Welfare 1964).

contributions which smoking makes to disease-specific mortality, nor the percentage of smokers in the population. In some of these diseases the death rate differential (relative risk or mortality ratio) between smokers and non-smokers is far greater (e.g. lung cancer) than in others (e.g. coronary heart disease). Furthermore, even with a large death rate differential between smokers and non-smokers, a population with very few smokers would have very few excess deaths and a specific entity with a low overall death rate would likewise contribute very little excess mortality from the smokers affected by it. Thus, a combination of information is required to calculate the public health significance of smoking as a contributor to mortality in a given population. An indicator of the magnitude of the smoking problem would be the total excess deaths accounted for by smoking. These excess or additional deaths are those occurring per year among smokers above those deaths which would have occurred if smokers had had the same death rates as those who did not smoke. These additional deaths are expressed as a percentage of *all* deaths occurring in that age and sex group.

Horn (1967) utilizing the data derived from the Dorn study (Kahn 1966) and the 25-state study by Hammond (1966) calculated that for men between the ages of 35 and 60, approximately *one-third* of all their deaths would not have occurred if cigarette smokers had had the same death rates as non-smokers. With the size of the smoking population in this age group, the impact of prevention of mortality on longevity by not smoking is obvious.

Cause-specific mortality

Table 3 presents the contributions which the several specific causes of mortality make to the excess deaths calculated as due to smoking in the seven large-scale prospective studies (US Department of Health, Education, and Welfare 1964; p. 108). It will be noted that although the relative risk for coronary artery disease among smokers is far lower than for lung cancer, the former contributes the largest number of deaths to the smoking excess. Lung cancer contributes the second largest amount followed by chronic bronchitis, emphysema, and other heart disease.

Early mortality

Early mortality of necessity reduces life expectancy for later years. Despite the popular misconception that smoking-related diseases produce mortality only at

Table 3 Percentage of total number of excess deaths of cigarette smokers due to different causes[†]

Underlying cause	British doctors	Men in 9 States	U.S. veterans	California occupa-tional	California Legion	Canadian veterans	Men in 25 States
Coronary artery disease	32.9	51.9	38.6	43.5	43.5	44.2	51.7
Other heart disease	9.8	3.1	6.8	1.4	4.5	5.9	5.5
Cerebral vascular lesions	6.1	4.5	4.9	5.3	6.5	−1.8	3.3
Other circulatory diseases	1.9	2.7	7.1	1.7	0.2	5.6	4.4
Cancer of lung	24.0	13.5	14.9	20.2	16.8	18.3	13.6
Cancer of oral cavity, oesophagus, larynx	3.3	2.9	2.7	0.2	3.0	2.2	2.2
Other cancer	−0.2	9.8	8.9	6.3	−2.2	7.2	7.6
Bronchitis and emphysema	9.6	1.1	4.0	1.3	5.6	8.2	3.8
Influenza and pneumonia	−2.4	1.6	0.4	2.4	1.5	1.5	1.5
Stomach and duodenal ulcers	2.7	3.1	1.4	−1.7	2.2	2.9	1.3
Cirrhosis of liver	2.9	1.6	2.5	6.9	2.2	0.8	0.9
Accidents, suicides, violence	0.2	1.2	2.0	8.3	3.7	4.6	0.8
All other causes	9.2	3.0	5.8	4.2	12.5	0.4	3.4
All causes	100.0	100.0	100.0	100.0	100.0	100.0	100.0

[†]All cigarette smokers (current and ex-) for the two California and men in 25 States studies; current cigarette smokers only for the remainder.
Source: US Department of Health, Education, and Welfare (1964).

the extreme of life, the epidemiological evidence that smoking-related mortality is *premature* mortality is quite strong. Several lines of inquiry are available to us: One is the calculation by Hammond (1967), utilizing the data of the 25-state study of US males, of the loss in life expectancy among cigarette smokers as compared to the non-smokers in the study. A second is the analyses of excess mortality for several age groups of smokers by Horn (1967) as noted above.

Table 4 presents Hammond's data on the loss of life expectancy among those smoking different amounts of cigarettes per day. The data are in years lost as compared to the life expectancy of non-smokers at the several designated ages and also as a percentage of the total life expectancy of non-smokers. It can be noted that although the percentages of loss of life expectancy increase not only with quantity smoked per day but also with age, the absolute loss in years for any level of smoking is greatest among the younger age groups.

Table 5, modified from Horn's presentation, reveals that the proportions of excess mortality among both male and female smokers of cigarettes are highest

Table 4 Loss of life expectancy (in years and as a percentage of total life expectancy of non-smokers) at various ages for cigarette smokers, Hammond study US, 1967

	Number of cigarettes smoked per day							
	1–9		10–19		20–39		40 and over	
Age	Years lost	per cent	Years lost	per cent	Years lost	per cent	Years lost	per cent
25 years	4.6	9.5	5.5	11.3	6.2	12.8	8.3	17.1
30 years	4.6	10.5	5.5	12.5	6.1	13.9	8.1	18.5
35 years	4.5	11.5	5.4	13.8	6.0	15.3	7.9	20.2
40 years	4.3	12.5	5.2	15.1	5.8	16.8	7.6	22.0
45 years	4.1	13.7	5.0	16.7	5.6	18.7	7.0	23.3
50 years	3.8	14.8	4.6	18.0	5.1	19.9	6.3	24.6
55 years	3.5	16.4	4.0	18.7	4.4	20.6	5.4	25.2
60 years	3.1	17.6	3.5	19.9	3.9	22.2	4.4	25.0
65 years	2.8	19.9	2.9	20.6	3.1	22.0	3.4	24.1

Source: Hammond, E. C. (1967).

Table 5 Excess mortality among cigarette smokers as a percentage of all deaths in the respective age and sex groups. Dorn and Hammond studies (Kahn 1966; Hammond 1966)†

Study	Age				
	35–44	45–54	55–64	65–74	75–84
US veterans: men					
Excess deaths as per cent of total	33	43	21	17	8
Hammond: men					
Excess deaths as per cent of total	33	38	25	13	4
Hammond: women					
Excess deaths as per cent of total	5	9	4	2	—

†Modified from Horn (1967).

among the 45–54 year age group, next highest among the 35–44-year-olds, and then, in descending order of magnitude with increasing age from 55 years onward. For the females who also experienced the highest proportionate excess mortality related to smoking in the 45–54-year age group, the excess was of a lower magnitude, but significant nevertheless.

It was noted earlier that in an analysis of smoking mortality by specific cause of death the greatest contribution to the excess attributable to smoking was made by coronary heart disease. Although some of the large-scale prospective studies of mortality among smokers, such as the earlier Hammond and Horn (1958a, b) study, the Framingham studies by Doyle, Dawber, Kannel, Kinch, and Kahn (1964) and Kannel, Castelli, and McNamara (1968), and the Dorn US Veterans study reported by Kahn (1966), either did not have young enough subjects entering the studies or did not present analyses by age groups, a number of other large prospective studies provided data on coronary heart disease mortality for males and females in the age groups under 50. Notable among these are the Doll and Hill (1964) physicians study, the Best (1966) study in Canada, the 25-state study by Hammond and Garfinkel (1969), the Paffenbarger and Wing (1967) study, and the Weir and Dunn (1970) study in California. In virtually all of these the relative risk of coronary disease mortality for male smokers of cigarettes under the age of 50 and at the several levels of consumption was markedly higher than for the older age groups. In the large cohort of women in the later Hammond study (Hammond and Garfinkel 1969) a similar finding was noted. In a number of studies examining the role of smoking and its interaction with other risk factors for coronary heart disease in relatively younger men, cigarette smoking by itself was deemed a greater risk than the individual risks contributed by high serum cholesterol levels (Stamler *et al.* 1966), elevated systolic or diastolic blood-pressures (Borhani, Hechter, and Breslow 1963), obesity (Borhani *et al.* 1963), physical activity (Shapiro *et al.* 1969), and electro-cardiographic abnormalities (Borhani *et al.* 1963). When smoking is combined with these other factors both additive and synergistic effects on mortality are noted. Thus mortality attributed to cigarette smoking, to which coronary heart disease makes the largest specific contribution, is distinctly a *premature* mortality which impacts itself on the prime years of life and in this period of life smoking is probably the greater risk factor in overall mortality.

Role of other factors

It cannot be denied that other factors influence disparities in mortality rates. It must be recognized that genetic or constitutional make-up plays a role. However, there are strong evidences that despite the influences of such variables the smoking factor exerts its own 'specific' strong effect on mortality. Until the 25-state study, few variables had been examined for this purpose and little information derived. The Hammond study provided data on such variables as longevity of parents and grandparents, religion, educational level, native or foreign birth, residence by size of town, occupational exposure, use of alcohol, use of fried food, use of tranquillizers, presence or absence of prior serious disease, marital status, and degree of exercise. Stratifying on each of these variables, age-adjusted death rates among those who smoked more than a pack of cigarettes a day and those who inhaled moderately or deeply were compared with those of non-smokers. In all instances, death rates were higher among individuals who smoked than those who did not. Several selected variables are presented in Table 6 (US Department of Health, Education, and Welfare 1964; pp. 100–1). Ipsen and Pfaelzer conducted further analyses of seven variables for the Surgeon General's Committee. None of these variables, with the exception of prior serious disease, had a stronger association with mortality than did smoking (US Department of Health, Education, and Welfare 1964; pp. 100–1). Hammond also conducted a special analysis for the Committee (US Department of Health, Education, and Welfare 1964; pp. 100–1) by matching pairs of cigarette smokers and non-smokers on the basis of height, religion, education, drinking habits, residence, and occupation. After 22 months of follow-up, mortality among the smokers was almost twice (1.86) that among non-smokers. Thus, the statement that smoking is a considerably stronger determinant of mortality than the variables tested, including those representative of constitutional differences, is warranted, particularly since adjustment for each of these variables individually

Table 6 Age-adjusted death rates per 1000 men (over approximately 22 months) for variables that may be related to mortality

Type of smoking	Long-lived parents and grandparents	Short-lived parents and grandparents	No previous serious disease	Previous serious disease
None	14.8	21.1	11.5	42.5
Cigarettes†	27.1	44.8	22.3	65.0
	Single	Married	Use tranquillizers	Do not use tranquillizers
None	26.0	18.9	29.1	18.2
Cigarettes†	50.1	33.0	52.4	31.8

			Educational level		
	No high school	Some high school	High school graduate	Some college	College graduate
None	22.7	20.0	16.9	18.3	15.8
Cigarettes†	35.2	34.5	35.5	34.2	20.4

		Degree of exercise‡		
	None	Slight	Moderate	Heavy
None	23.8	14.7	11.0	9.5
Cigarettes†	34.1	25.5	20.8	19.7

†Smokers of more than a pack per day who inhaled moderately or deeply.
‡Confined to men with no history of heart disease, stroke, high blood-pressure or cancer (except skin) who were not sick at the time of entry.
Source: US Department of Health, Education, and Welfare (1964).

produced little, if any, change in the smoker–non-smoker mortality ratios. The implications for improvement of longevity are obvious.

Male vs. female mortality

Significant differences are observed in the overall mortality rates between males and females in the US population (US Department of Health, Education, and Welfare 1979c; Section 1, Part A, pp. 1–100). Such differences are particularly prominent for all of the smoking-related diseases discussed earlier. The disparities, with one exception, are in the direction of male excesses. In Table 7 it will be noted that the only exception to this is mortality ascribed to cerebrovascular disease. Otherwise the differences range from 5-fold for cancer of the larynx, 4-fold for both cancer of the lung and the lip, 3-fold for chronic bronchitis and emphysema, and for cancer of the oesophagus, 2.5-fold for cancers of the bladder and of the buccal cavity and for aortic aneurysm, to almost 1.5-fold for ischaemic heart disease.

Much speculation has attended these differences. To a certain extent sex hormonal differences in well-documented observations may account for a significant amount of the difference at ages prior to the menopause. This protective influence is noted in coronary artery disease, and is not specific since such sex disparities in susceptibility occur in poliomyelitis and hepatitis as well. In lung cancer the evidence is conjectural. Occupational exposures and similar differences in environmental exposure between the sexes may contribute to the disparities. Very often the disparities have been cited in attempts to discredit the basic association between smoking of tobacco and the relevant diseases. Such attempts have failed to take into account the disparities of tobacco exposure between males and females, which disparities have included not only intensity of smoking but history of initiation of smoking. Although some European populations, such

Table 7 Comparison of male and female cause specific mortality rates for selected chronic diseases related to tobacco smoking, US 1975

Diseases	Mortality rates/100 000	
	Male	Female
Causally related:		
Cancer of lung, bronchus, trachea (162)	61.1	17.0
Chronic bronchitis and emphysema (490–2)	17.5	4.9
Cancer of larynx (161)	2.6	0.5
Cancer of lip (140)	0.1	0.0
Probably causally related:		
Ischaemic heart disease (410–13)	348.8	257.0
Cancer of bladder (188)	6.4	2.5
Cancer of buccal cavity and pharynx (140–9)	5.5	2.2
Cancer of oesophagus (150)	5.0	1.6
Possibly causally related:		
Cerebrovascular disease (430–8)	81.3	100.4
Aortic aneurysm (non-syphlitic) (441)	9.4	3.5

Source: Department of Health, Education, and Welfare (1979c), Mortality Part A.

as the Finnish, were already smoking heavily in the 1880s, in the United States the main upsurge of cigarette consumption occurred approximately at the time of America's entry into the First World War. This increase was confined virtually entirely to the male population. The next major increase in cigarette consumption occurred during the Second World War when females began to participate extensively. Not only was the time of initiation of the astronomical rise in lung cancer in the male compatible with an induction period of 20–25 years following the First World War, but the acceleration of the rates in females was consistent with an induction period following their change in life-style in the Second World War and their adoption of the cigarette-smoking habit. A survey of smoking patterns by Haenszel in 1955 (Haenszel, Shimkin, and Miller 1956) noted that, at that time, twice as many males as females were smoking cigarettes, and males smoked considerably more cigarettes per day than females. The drift to younger ages for the initiation of the habit began earlier for males than females and inhalation practices were adopted later by the female. At the time of the survey the male to female ratio of lung cancer mortality was about 5:1. On correction for the disparities in the components of the smoking habits among males and females the ratio was reduced to 1.4:1. This residual may well be consistent with both hormonal protection and disparities in occupational and other environmental exposures between males and females. These data justify the conclusion that, at least for lung cancer and probably for other entities in which the relative risks among smokers are relatively large, sex disparities are predominantly the result of disparities in the smoking habits between the sexes.

Earlier in this paper it was noted that fully one-third of the mortality in our population of men between the ages of 35 and 60 would not have occurred if the non-smoker death rates had prevailed in this population (Horn 1967). The studies upon which these calculations were based were executed at a time when 57 per cent of the male and 28 per cent of the female population were current cigarette smokers. By 1966 smoking of cigarettes in persons 18 years and over had declined to 51 per cent in males and risen to 33 per cent in females (US Department of Health, Education, and Welfare 1970). In Table 8 (US Department of Health, Education, and Welfare 1970, 1971, 1976), the trend in cigarette smoking for males and females through the survey of 1975 can be noted. Male cessation of cigarette smoking has continued and is now true for all age groups over 18. This may, if it continues, be portentous for male survival and hence longevity. Declines in cigarette smoking in the younger age groups are especially noteworthy for those diseases with longer induction periods. For the older age groups, since cessation of smoking needs to have prevailed for 10 or more years to reduce mortality risk from coronary artery disease and lung cancer, little gain in survivorship can be expected here and now. However, improvement in survivorship among those with other entities more readily arrestable or reversible, such as the respiratory diseases associated with cigarette smoking, can be expected (Schuman 1971).

Table 8, however, reveals a gloomy picture for the female. In the 11-year period between 1955 and 1966 cigarette smoking prevalence actually increased

Table 8 Percentage of current smokers of cigarettes by sex and age. US surveys: 1955 and 1966 (Current Population Surveys-CPS) and 1970 and 1975 (Surveys conducted for National Clearinghouse for Smoking and Health-NCSH).

| | Male | | | | Female | | | |
Age	CPS 1955	CPS 1966	NCSH 1970	NCSH 1975	CPS 1955	CPS 1966	NCSH 1970	NCSH 1975
18–24	53.0	48.3	47.0†	41.3‡	33.3	34.7	31.1†	34.0‡
25–34	63.6	58.9	46.8	43.9	39.2	43.2	40.3	35.4
35–44	62.1	57.0	48.6	47.1	35.4	41.1	39.0	36.4
45–54	58.0	53.1	43.1	41.1	25.7	37.3	36.0	32.8
55–64	45.8	46.2	37.4	33.7	13.4	23.0	24.3	25.9
65+	25.8	24.6	23.7	24.2	4.7	8.1	11.8	10.2

†Estimated.
‡21–4 years of age.
Sources: Haenszel *et al.* 1956; Department of Health, Education, and Welfare 1970, 1971.

among females in every age group and in one age group in particular, the 55–64-year-olds, by almost 50 per cent. Although declines in smoking prevalence occurred by 1970, and continued by 1975 in all but the oldest age-groups, the levels achieved did not equal those observed in 1955 except for those under 35 years of age. Increases actually continued to occur in the 55–64 age group. Any recidivism here may be expected to have a deleterious effect on female longevity.

Cessation of smoking and population mortality

The numerous prospective studies of general and cause-specific mortality and the case-control studies of specific smoking-associated diseases have left no doubt as to the benefits to be derived from cessation of cigarette smoking. In a review article, Schuman (1971) summarized these benefits. With specific respect to mortality, remarkable gains in survival were noted among ex-cigarette smokers both in terms of total mortality and by specific causes. Mortality ratios for ex-smokers declined, for example, an average of 63 per cent for lung cancer in 4 studies, 35 per cent for cerebrovascular disease, 33 per cent for coronary heart disease, and 28 per cent for chronic bronchitis and emphysema. In the instance of coronary heart disease this relatively modest gain compared to that of lung cancer is far more significant, since the *absolute excess* number of deaths from coronary heart disease attributable to smoking is far greater than that for lung cancer even though the proportion of lung cancers attributable to smoking is 90 per cent or more of the total load of such cancers.

These data do not take into account the interval since smoking was discontinued. For coronary heart disease, in men in the age group of 50–69 years, cessation of smoking of less than a pack a day yielded reductions in mortality in one to four years and, for a-pack-or-more-a-day smokers, in 5 to 9 years (Hammond 1966).

Public health benefits of cessation

Since, in the United States, declines in the proportion of male smokers over 18 years of age have occurred over the period 1955–75, certain impacts on mortality might be detectable. Several complicating factors must be considered in assessing any changes, however. Since *per capita* consumption of cigarettes declined from 1966 to 1970 following the release of the Report of the Advisory Committee to the Surgeon General and since women, particularly young women, had increased their consumption, the decline signified a marked decrease in consumption by men.

It is of interest that two categories of disease with relatively rapid 'turn-around' properties in relation to tobacco smoking declined significantly. Whereas coronary heart disease in men had been increasing over the previous two decades, in 1966 there began a reversal of this trend which continues. No such decline has been noted in women. It would be tempting to ascribe this reversal to the reduction in smoking, but, as the relative risk for smokers is of far smaller magnitude in coronary heart disease than in lung cancer, the evidence is not clear-cut and it is possible that other causal or risk factors not currently being surveyed in the population may also be declining. However, it would be somewhat difficult to assume a change in the latter factors operating solely in males. The natural experiment invoked by the cessation of smoking among British physicians (Fletcher and Horn 1970) yielded a 6 per cent reduction in total cardiovascular mortality in an eight-year period.†

Similarly male death rates from chronic bronchitis and emphysema have been declining since 1967, whereas female death rates have not declined.

Lung cancer with its high relative risk among smokers would be a sensitively responding disease since more than 90 per cent of all such cancers are attributable to cigarette smoking. However, we are faced with several complicating factors. The induction period being relatively long, response to a decline in smoking would lag significantly. Furthermore, the declines in consumption have been proportionately greater in the younger age groups in which switches to filter cigarettes and those with lower tar and nicotine have also occurred. In these age groups the lung cancer rates are normally low. Further data will be necessary over the next several years for an appraisal of the groups of males born after 1919, which was the last birth cohort to reach the peak of cumulative cigarette exposure. Cumulative exposure for birth cohorts since then has been declining. A suggestive decline in lung cancer among these younger males has already been noted.

Longevity and quality of life

I turn now to what I deem to be the more significant aspect of longevity. The ultimate aim of this Conference on Aging has most appropriately been expressed

---

† In a more recent paper published by Doll and Peto, after this chapter was written, a 25 per cent reduction in ischaemic heart disease mortality was noted for smokers aged 30–54 years discontinuing for more than 15 years.

as the improvement of the quality of life for older people in society. Certainly longevity without productivity, sustained interest, reciprocal appreciation of the life about us, without a contribution to humanity and the joy of living is not life. The saving of life alone is not enough. The prolongation of life without quality is a questionable goal. Thus, life for those whose demise has been postponed, but who suffer the ailments and disabilities induced by smoking is certainly of inadequate quality.

A large number of case-control and cohort studies on morbidity prevalence and incidence in relation to smoking can be found in the literature. As with mortality studies the association of tobacco smoking with a number of cardio-respiratory entities representing serious and disabling states has been well documented and the declines in *morbidity* ratios upon cessation of smoking summarized (Schuman 1971). Parallel with total mortality excesses among smokers, an over-all measure of morbidity is excess disability among smokers as measured by days lost from work, days of restricted activity, and days confined to bed. Information on excess morbidity related to smoking has become available through periodic inquiries on smoking among those in probability samples of the ongoing National Health Survey (Department of Health, Education, and Welfare 1967). This source indicates that for all three types of disability measures noted above and for both men and women, higher morbidity rates, higher morbidity ratios, and higher percentages of excess disability days were recorded for cigarette smokers.

In Table 9, a modification of the data as calculated by Horn (1967), it will again be noted that, as for mortality, the excess disability days among cigarette smokers were found to be proportionately greater in the younger age groups. For males the greatest excess in each of the three disability measures is in the 45–64-year age group. For females it is in an even younger group—17–44 years of age. The same data source provided information on prevalence of chronic conditions. Among smoking men and women, the youngest age groups (17–44 years) showed the highest proportion of excess prevalence. For all these measurements a dose-effect gradient with the number of cigarettes smoked per day was noted. Thus smoking is also related to *prematurely* disabling illness.

Table 9 Excess morbidity among cigarette smokers as a percentage of all disability days in the respective age and sex groups. National Health Survey (US Department of Health, Education, and Welfare 1967)†

Disability measure	Males			Females		
	17–44	45–64	65+	17–44	45–64	65+
Work-loss days	20	28	0‡	18	11	§
Restricted activity days	23	28	8	14	5	2
Bed days	23	28	−1	10	6	0

†Modified from Horn (1967).
‡0 indicates no difference in rates between smokers and non-smokers.
§Too few smokers.

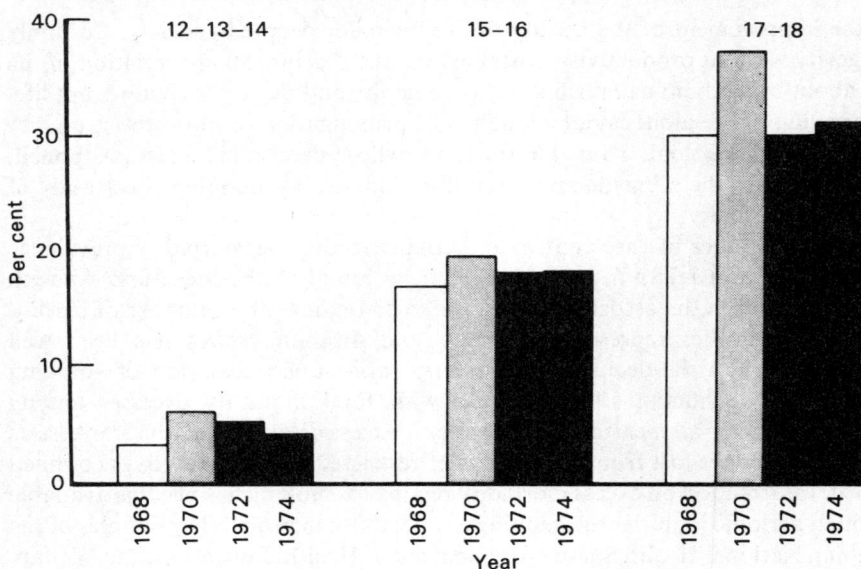

Fig. 2. Per cent current regular smokers—teenage boys, 1968–74.

The literature is also replete with evidence of the reversibility of the pathology of early bronchopulmonary entities (Huhti 1965; Coates, Bower, and Reinstein 1965; Holland 1966; Higgins, Gilson, Ferres, *et al.* 1968; Holland and Elliott 1968; Fletcher 1968; Comstock *et al.* 1970; Wilhelmsen 1967; Peterson *et al.* 1968; Auerbach *et al.* 1962, 1963). Thus, not only will abstinence from smoking prevent both early morbidity and mortality, but cessation of smoking will materially reduce the risks of development of the specific smoking-related diseases in those now smoking, thus increasing longevity and reversing the process in some diseases with elimination of disabling illness.

Unfortunately a note of pessimism must be interjected if only to evoke attention to a social imperative. Very recent surveys on patterns of cigarette smoking in the US population from ages 12 to 18 reveal the disturbing fact that although the percentage of current regular smokers among boys aged 12 to 14 has declined somewhat from 1970 to 1974, the percentages have plateaued at relatively high levels for boys aged 15 to 16 and 17 to 18 (Fig. 2) and for girls at all ages the percentages of smokers have steadily increased in every year between 1968 and 1974 (Fig. 3).† If these are the cohorts of the future, then the risk of thwarting improvements in longevity is great.

To paraphrase a conclusion from the Report on Smoking and Health by the Advisory Committee to the Surgeon General which is just as timely today: 'Cigarette smoking continues to be a health hazard of sufficient importance to warrant appropriate immediate remedial action.'

† Teen-age smoking—national patterns of cigarette smoking, ages 12 through 18, in 1972 and 1974. DHEW Publication No. 76–931.

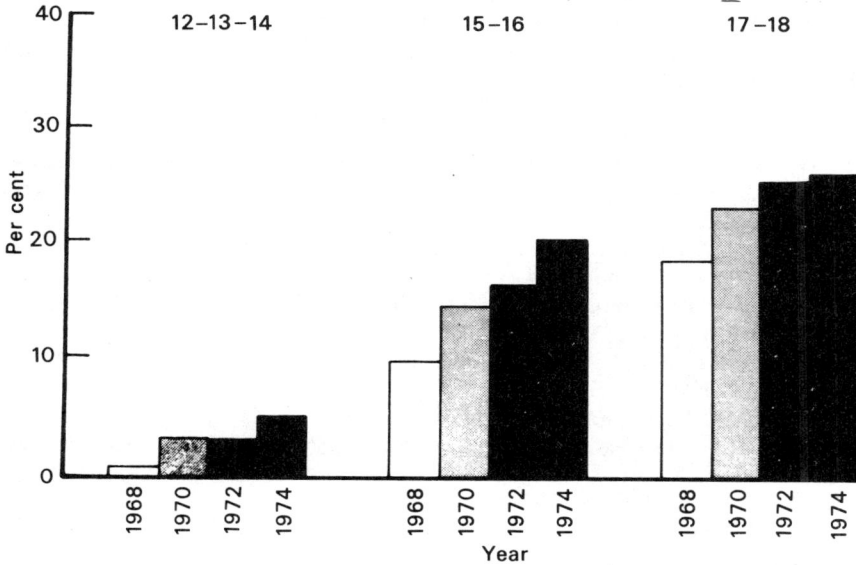

FIG. 3. Per cent current regular current smokers—teenage girls, 1968–74.

References

AUERBACH, O., STOUT, A. P., HAMMOND, E. C., and GARFINKEL, L. (1962). *New Engl. med. J.*, **267**, 111.

——, ——, ——, —— (1963). *New Engl. med. J.*, **269**, 1045.

BEST, E. W. R. (1966). *Canadian study of smoking and health*. Department of National Health and Welfare.

BORHANI, N. O., HECHTER, H. H., and BRESLOW, L. (1963). *J. chron. Dis.*, **16**, 1251.

COATES, E. O., Jr., BOWER, G. C., and REINSTEIN, N. (1965). *J. Amer. med. Assoc.*, **191**, 161.

COMSTOCK, G. W., BROWNLOW, W. J., STONE, R. W., and SARTWELL, P. E. (1970). *Arch. Environ. Hlth*, **21**, 50.

DOLL, R. and HILL, A. B. (1964). *Brit. med. J.*, **1**, 1399.

DORN, H. (1958). *Proc. Soc. Stat. Sec. Am. Stat. Ass.*, p. 34.

DOYLE, J. T., DAWBER, T. R., KANNEL, W. B., KINCH, S. H., and KAHN, H. A. (1964). *J. Amer. med. Assoc.*, **190**, 886.

FLETCHER, C. M. (1968). *J. roy. Coll. Phys. London.*, **2**, 183.

—— and HORN, D. (1970). Smoking and health. *WHO Chron.*, **24**, 345.

HAENSZEL, W., SHIMKIN, M. B., and MILLER, H. P. (1956). *Tobacco smoking patterns in the U.S.* Public Health Monograph No. 45.

HAMMOND, E. C. (1966). In *Epidemiological approaches to the study of cancer and other diseases* (ed. W. Haenszel), p. 127. National Cancer Institute, Monograph No. 19.

—— (1967). In *Summary of the Proceedings of the World Conference on Smoking and Health*, p. 21. National Interagency Council on Smoking and Health, New York City, September 1967.

—— and HORN, D. (1958a). *J. Amer. med. Assoc.*, **166**, 1159.

—— and —— (1958b). *J. Amer. med. Assoc.*, **166**, 1294.

—— and GARFINKEL, L. (1969). *Arch. environ. Hlth*, **19**, 167.
HIGGINS, I. T. T., GILSON, J. C., FERRES, B. G., WATERS, M. E., CAMPBELL, H., and HIGGINS, M. W. (1968). *Amer. J. publ. Hlth*, **58**, 1667.
HOLLAND, W. W. (1966). *J. Coll. gen. Practition.*, Suppl., 2, **11**, 8.
—— and Elliott, A. (1968). *Lancet*, **i**, 41.
HORN, D. (1967). In *The health consequences of smoking. A public health science review:* 1967, pp. 13, 20. Public Health Service Publication 1696. U.S. Gov't. Printing Office, Washington D.C.
HUHTI, E. (1965). *Acta Tuberculosia Pneumologica Scand. Suppl.*, 61.
KAHN, H. A. (1966). In *Epidemiological approaches to the study of cancer and other diseases* (ed. W. Haenzsel), p. 1. National Cancer Institute Monograph No. 19.
KANNEL, W. B., CASTELLI, W. P., and McNAMARA, P. M. (1968). In *Toward a less harmful cigarette* (ed. E. L. Wynder and D. Hoffman), p. 9. National Cancer Institute, Monograph No. 28.
PAFFENBARGER, R. S., Jr. and WING, A. L. (1967). *Amer. J. Epid.*, **90**, 527.
PETERSON, D. I., LONERGAN, L. H., and HARDINGE, M. G. (1968). *Arch. environ. Hlth*, **16**, 215.
SCHUMAN, L. M. (1971). *Chest*, **59**, 421.
SHAPIRO, S., WEINBLATT, E., FRANK, C. W., and SAGER, R. V. (1969). *Amer. J. publ. Hlth*, (*Suppl. June*), **59**.
STAMLER, J., BERKSEN, D. M., LEVINSON, M., LUNDBERG, H. A., MAJONNIER, L. MILLER, W. A., HALL, Y., and ANDELMAN, S. L. (1966). *Arch. environ. Hlth*, **13**, 322.
US DEPARTMENT OF HEALTH, EDUCATION, AND WELFARE (1964). *Smoking and Health. Report of the Advisory Committee to the Surgeon General of the U.S. Public Health Service.* U.S. DHEW.
—— (1967). *Vital and health statistics: Data from the National Health Survey NCHS. Cigarette smoking and Health characteristics.* DHEW Series 10, No. 34.
—— (1970). *Vital and health statistics: Data from the National Health Survey. NCHS. Changes in cigarette smoking habits.* DHEW, Series 10, No. 59.
—— (1971). *Health consequences of smoking. A Report to the Surgeon General:* 1971. DHEW. Publication No. (HSM) 71–7513, p. 6.
—— (1976). *Teen-age smoking*, DHEW Publcation No. (N14) 76–931.
—— (1976). *Adult use of tobacco 1975.* National Clearing House for Smoking and Health, DHEW, June.
—— (1979a). *Vital statistics of the United States 1975*, Vol. II, Part A, Sec. 2 DHEW.
—— (1979b). *Vital statistics of the United States 1975*, Vol. II, Part A, Sec. 5 DHEW.
—— (1979c). *Vital statistics of the United States 1975*, Vol. II, Part A, Sec. 1 DHEW.
WEIR, J. M. and DUNN, J. E. Jr. (1970). *Cancer*, **25**, 105.
WILHELMSEN, L. (1967). *Scand. J. resp. Dis.*, **48**, 407.

Discussion—Session 12 Alexander Leaf

An anonymous prescription for a long life states, 'Choose your parents carefully!' The importance of genetic factors in determining the life span becomes apparent when differences in longevity among species are compared. Rats very rarely exceed four years; cats, thirty years; horses, forty years; elephants, sixty years.

Man is the longest lived of all mammalian species. But in this most interesting species how much the life span is influenced by genetic versus environmental factors is not always clear even when infectious diseases, accidents, warfare, and starvation are not causing premature death.

Several studies of life expectancy of children of long-lived parents indicate a significant advantage over offspring of short-lived parents. The advantage, however, seems to be a modest one. In a detailed study of the inheritance of longevity based upon life insurance records, L. I. Dublin and H. H. Marks (1941) found that offspring of long-lived parents had a life expectancy at age 20 that probably does not exceed by three years the expectancy of a similarly aged group whose parents were short-lived. This was the maximal statistical advantage that Dublin could attribute to heredity from his examination of insurance records. The classic study of Pearl and Pearl on the inheritance of longevity has been reviewed recently (Abbott, Murphy, Bolling, and Abbey 1974) and the original cohort of these investigators reexamined. Though a familial pattern of life span was again noted, the evidence was insufficient to distinguish between genetic factors or family environment as the significant determinant.

Perhaps the best evidence for the presence of genetic factors in longevity in man comes from the long-term study of twins aged sixty years and over commenced by F. J. Kallman and continued by L. F. Jarvik (1971) to evaluate genetic influences on the life span. It has been found by Kallman and associates that the differences between fraternal twins in ages reached at death varied a great deal more than was the case with monozygotic twins. There were greater differences in longevity between fraternal twins than identical twins. On the average monozygotic twins die within 5 years of each other though pairs have been observed in which differences in ages at death exceeded a decade. The difference in age at death for dizygotic twins was much larger.

From such observations on twins it may be concluded that genetic factors do affect longevity. The important fact for us is how much of your health and longevity depends upon environmental factors which are potentially controllable. It gives us as physicians and scientists the possibility to improve health, vigour, and life span. It is embarrassing how little we yet know today regarding the role of specific environmental factors in longevity. In the absence of certain knowledge the field has been exploited by faddists, quacks, and extortionists. Fortunately, the subject is becoming a focus of legitimate scientific study and it can even appear in a volume such as this.

General agreement will support the view that many of the practices common in our society are self-destructive and incompatible with optimal health and longevity. We have had the case against cigarette smoking thoroughly reviewed for us by Professor Schuman. But drug abuse and alcoholism are also clearly suicidal but prevalent. When it comes to positive factors which promote health and longevity our ignorance is overwhelming. Professor Buskirk reviewed some effects of exercise on the elderly and noted (parenthetically) that there are no data from man that indicate that chronic exercise will increase life expectancy; admittedly such data are difficult to obtain. His observations do not, however, include the effects of exercise on cardiopulmonary function. Here the epidemiological evidence seems to me to be compelling that sustained physical exercise reduces the incidence and severity of heart attacks which in our society are the leading cause of death.

We have also read the surprising views of Dr. Andres that obesity promotes longevity—quite a departure from our usual teachings and this again emphasizes the amazing uncertainty and ignorance that shroud the entire subject of positive environmental influences that may promote health and longevity. Other studies have indicated that obesity in the absence of hypertension, diabetes, and hyperlipidaemia was not a risk factor, but to learn that it is a positive factor is indeed surprising.

From my own anecdotal observations (Leaf 1975) on long-lived populations in Vilcabamba, Ecuador; Hunza, West Pakistan; and Abkhasia, USSR, I have concluded that longevity is a multifactorial phenomenon. It is a happy coincidence of several factors, a few of which I think one can identify now, and there are no surprises among my list of four:

1. *Diet*. Although the diet is changing, especially in the affluent Caucasus, it has been basically of low calories and low animal fats and protein. Dr. Guillermo Vela, a nutritionist from Quito who has studied the diet in Vilcabamba, finds that the average daily caloric intake of an elderly person in Vilcabamba is 1200 calories. Protein provided 35–38 g and fat only 12–19 g; 200–250 g of carbohydrate completed the diet.

According to Dr. S. Maqsood Ali, a Pakistani nutritionist who had surveyed the diet of 55 adult males in Hunza, the daily diet averages 1923 calories: 50 g are protein, 36 g fat, and 354 g carbohydrate. Meat and dairy products accounted for only 1 per cent of the total. Land is too precious to be used to support livestock; the few animals that are kept are killed for meat only during the winter or on festive occasions.

Dr. Deli Dzhorbendze and Professor Pitzkhelauri had studied the dietary habits of a large number of persons over the age of 80 in the Caucasus. The old people, they found, consume 1700–1900 calories, which is less than the 2000 calories the Central Institute of Nutrition of Russia recommends for old people. no special diet is eaten by the elderly. Seventy per cent of the calories are of vegetable origin and the remainder from meat and dairy products. 70–90 g protein and 40–60 g fat are included in the average daily diet and, of the latter, 30 per cent is of vegetable origin and the remainder is animal fat. By contrast in the United States the average daily fat ingestion is 157 g. But even the present dietary figures from the Caucasus are surely reflecting the effects of the post-Second World War affluence in this region. When I questioned the elderly about their diets when they were young I was invariably told, 'When we were young life was very difficult. We had only beans and vegetables, but now life is good—we have meat and wine every day!'

As I observed the obesity prevalent among the younger generations, I wondered whether they would maintain the tradition of longevity of their parents.

2. *Physical activity.* All three areas I visited had agrarian cultures. Everyone worked on the farms from earliest days to literally their last. Since all three areas were mountainous, the considerable physical effort of farming was compounded by the hilly terrain. Vilcabamba in the Andes, Hunza in the Karakorum range, and Georgia in the Caucasus all demanded a degree of continued exertion which should have contributed to sustained cardiopulmonary fitness. There is a considerable body of epidemiological evidence to indicate that regular endurance exercise—as represented by walking, bicycling, jogging, rowing, swimming—reduces the incidence of fatal heart attacks. Certainly equivalent physical activity was an unavoidable part of the daily life in each of these areas.

3. *Genetic factors.* The meagreness of the diet and the persistent hard work seemed no different from what one might encounter in any other underdeveloped agrarian community, so what was so special about the three areas I visited? The remoteness and isolation of Vilcabamba and Hunza led us to think that genetic factors might be of prime importance.

There do not seem to be 'good' genes which favour longevity but only 'bad' genes which increase the probability of acquiring a fatal illness. Natural selection has little interest or use for extension of the life span beyond the procreative period. One might speculate, however, that a small number of individuals singularly lacking such 'bad' genes settled these isolated mountainous valleys initially and over the centuries this tendency for longevity manifested itself.

This, of course, is sheer speculation and the possible role of genetic factors seemed less likely in the Caucasus. In Abkhasia on the shores of the Black Sea and in the adjoining low Caucas mountains one encounters many people over 100 who are not only Georgian but also Russian, Jewish, Armenian, and Turkish. With such ethnic diversity the genetic factor would seem to be of lesser importance. Nevertheless, when one inquires of the centenarians in this region, one invariably discovers that each of them has parents, siblings, or close relatives who also had attained great age. The genetic factor, therefore, cannot be dismissed.

4. *Psychological factors.* It became increasingly evident to me in the places I visited that psychological factors were important in affecting longevity. In all three places, the older one becomes, the greater the esteem one merits and the higher the social position one holds. There is no retirement age and the old people continue to participate actively in the economic and social life of their communities. In stable agrarian societies there always are some chores that the elderly can do. Physically the work may become less taxing but nevertheless it provides a stimulus for a feeling of usefulness and of being needed.

We seem to need a *raison d'etre*, a purpose to live, without which our mental and physical faculties deteriorate rapidly. It is unrealistic to believe that our industrial economy will ever re-employ the retired elderly, so we need to explore alternatives to preserve the psychological outlook that can sustain a useful, vigorous, and joyful old age.

I am certain that many other factors play a role in promoting a long and healthy life. I am embarrassed as a physician that our understanding of how to maintain health and prevent disease is at this time so rudimentary. I think it is a great challenge to the medical profession and to science to redirect itself from a preoccupation with the terminal phases of life to learning how to sustain optimal health throughout life with all the benefits to the individual and society that this would entail, for in this pursuit both the individual and society's interests are served. Research into the causes of disease—so that full understanding will lead to rational means of prevention—should be a major responsibility of a national health effort. The other major task—perhaps an even more difficult one—will be to persuade, cajole, or convince people to adopt a life-style which incorporates the tenets of health maintenance. The current public belief that we can pursue any life-style and at the end the medical profession will stand ready with a pill or an operation to absolve us of a lifetime of abuse of our bodies is indeed a myth and its fostering a disservice to mankind. A major responsibility for good health will always remain with the individual but the understanding of how this may be achieved is the responsibility of science and medicine, while society must provide the means and the environment in which optimal health may flourish.

References

ABBOTT, M. H., MURPHY, E. A., BOLLING, D. R., and ABBEY, H. (1974). The familial component in longevity. A study of offspring of nonagenarians. *Johns Hopkins Med. J.*, **134**, 1–16.

DUBLIN, L. I. and MARKS, H. H. (1941). The inheritance of longevity—a study based upon life insurance records. 52nd Annual Meeting of the Association of Life Insurance Medical Directors of America, Oct. 23–4, 1941.

JARVIK, L. F. (1971). Genetic aspects of aging. In *Clinical geriatrics* (ed. I. Rossman) Chapter 4, pp. 85–105. J. B. Lippincott Company, Philadelphia.

LEAF, A. (1975). *Youth in old age*, pp. 1–233. McGraw-Hill Book Co., New York.

CHAPTER III

Session 15

Aging of physiological functions

Age changes in the kidney   Robert D. Lindeman

Introduction

The kidney is responsible for elimination from the body of most of the non-volatile waste products of metabolism. Equally important is its role in the maintenance of a constant internal environment of fluid volume, electrolyte, and hydrogen ion concentrations. By formation of large volumes of an ultrafiltrate of plasma in the glomerular capillary beds followed by selective reabsorption and secretion of electrolytes and other ions in the tubule, the normal kidney possesses an enormous capacity to maintain precisely fluid, electrolyte, and acid–base balances.

Renal mass and function decrease with age. The blood vessels, glomeruli, tubules, and interstitium are potential sites of primary involvement with age as with different renal diseases. Whether the observed decrease in renal function associated with age is the result of intercurrent pathologic processes, e.g. ischaemic, immunological, or infectious injuries, or is the result of some more physiologic involutional process remains undetermined. Regardless of the anatomic structure primarily affected, most chronic processes ultimately evolve with destruction of entire nephron units. The functional decreases with age in all parameters studied, e.g. secretory and reabsorptive tubular maximums, have paralleled the decreases in glomerular filtration rate and renal plasma flow.

Normally, despite the decrease in renal function with age, the integrity of the volume and composition of the body fluids is maintained under basal conditions. However, when disease or environmental stress results in a greater demand on renal function, renal adjustments are slower in older than younger individuals. Most imbalances result not from the loss of renal function, but rather from extrarenal pathology that transmits faulty information, appropriate for that receptor at that time but inappropriate for the total body environment, to renal regulatory mechanisms.

Changes in renal morphology with age

A decline in kidney weight or volume with age has been documented in both the rat (Arataki 1926) and man (Roessle and Roulet 1932; Dunnill and Halley 1973) The loss in renal weight between maturity and old age is in the range 20–30 per cent in both species. In each normal human kidney up to age 40 years, there are approximately one million glomeruli. By the seventh decade, this has decreased to 70 per cent of these numbers (Dunnill and Halley 1973). The size of surviving glomeruli does not appear to change appreciably once the kidney reaches maturity.

Light and electron microscopic studies indicate there is an increase with age in mesangial volume in the glomeruli (Wehner 1968) and glomerular and tubular basement membrane thickness (Farquhar, Vernier, and Good 1957; Darmady, Offer, and Woodhouse 1973). The aged kidney also shows an increased incidence of obsolescent, scarred, and abnormal glomeruli (Sworn and Fox 1972). Oliver (1952) suggested that the senile changes in kidney were the result of ischaemic atrophy developing from vascular pathology associated with aging. Several investigators have described a process of glomerular obsolescence which leaves only a shunt between the afferent and efferent arteriole (McManus and Lupton 1960; Ljungkvist 1963; Takazakura, Sawabu, Handa, Takada, Shinoda, and Takenchi 1972; Reynes, Caulet, and Diebold 1968). A variety of vascular changes have been attributed to aging (collagen deposition between the intima and internal elastic lamina, fraying, splitting, reduplication, and calcification of the elastic lumina, and replacement of muscular cells with collagen without change in luminal diameter (Darmady *et al.* 1973; Oliver 1952)). These changes occur slowly in larger arteries; they develop later and more rapidly in smaller vessels and are accelerated by the development of hypertension.

Changes in renal function with age

The observation has been made repeatedly that the decreases in specific renal functions with age, as well as with various kinds of renal pathology, parallel the decrease in glomerular filtration rate. Bricker, Morrin, and Kime (1960) at first felt this meant that diseased nephrons did not contribute importantly to the development of the final urine ('intact nephron hypothesis'). Later, after Biber, Mylle, Baines, Gottshalk, Oliver, and MacDowell (1968), using micropuncture studies, showed that diseased and damaged nephrons can contribute importantly to the formation of urine, Bricker (1969) revised his hypothesis to incorporate these observations by assuming that the healthy nephrons had to compensate for glomerulotubular imbalances that might develop in the damaged nephrons. Nevertheless, except in specific disease entities, e.g., nephrogenic diabetes insipidus (urine concentrating deficit) or renal tubular acidosis (deficit in tubular secretion of hydrogen ion) where tubular dysfunction exists, changes in other measures of renal function parallel changes in glomerular filtration rate.

Glomerular filtration rate

A number of studies using several measures of glomerular filtration rate have been published showing the decline in renal function with age after the age of 30 years (Lewis and Alving 1938; Davies and Schock 1950; Rowe, Andres, Tobin, Norris, and Shock 1976; Wesson 1969). Wesson (1969) plotted the individual inulin clearances (corrected to 1.73 square meters body surface) of nearly 40 different reports. More males were studied than females. In both sexes there appears to be an acceleration of the rate of decline with advancing age. Rowe *et al.* (1976) recently reported the results of both cross-sectional and longitudinal studies of 'true' creatinine clearances in a large group (884 subjects) followed in a longitudinal study at the Gerontology Research Center, National Institute on Aging and found a similar accelerated rate of decline in creatinine clearance with age. Between the age of 40 and 80, one can estimate the decline as one per cent per year.

Although creatinine clearance rates fell from a mean of 140 cc/min/1.73 m^2 (age 25–34 years) to a mean of 97 cc/min/1/73 m^2 (age 75–84 years), serum creatinine concentrations rose insignificantly from 0.81 to 0.84 mg/100 ml. The proportionate decrease in creatinine production is a reflection of the decrease in body cell mass, and more specifically muscle, that occurs with aging. The practical implication of these observations is that serum creatinine concentrations in older patients have to be interpreted differently when being used to modify the dosages of drugs cleared by the kidney, e.g. aminoglycoside antibiotics and digoxin.

Renal plasma and blood flow

The amount of plasma or blood perfusing the kidney, using the paraaminohippuric acid (PAH) clearances, decreases with age. Davies and Shock (1950), confirming the work of Bradley (1947), showed the extraction ratio for PAH at low arterial PAH concentrations was approximately 92 per cent and was not affected by age. The mean decrease in PAH clearance with age was slightly greater than was the decrease in inulin clearance with age (Davies and Shock 1950; Wesson 1969).

The decrease in renal blood flow with age without a decrease in blood-pressure suggests either vascular obliteration due to intraluminal pathology (sclerosis, atheromata, etc.) or an increase in renal vascular resistance. Since renal blood flow can be increased transiently by administration of pyrogen in both young and old subjects (McDonald, Solomon, and Shock 1951), a reversible or vasoconstrictive component must be important in the regulation of the renal circulation in both age groups. Administration of pyrogen produces a greater vasodilation in the afferent arterioles of the kidney in the older subject suggesting a greater vasoconstriction exists in the resting state in these subjects. The reason for this remains unclear but one might speculate that since cardiac output also decreases with age, the renal vasoconstriction is an attempt to conserve and better maintain the blood supply to other vital organs.

Hollenberg, Adams, and Solomon (1974) observed an increasing filtration fraction with age and, with their xenon wash-out data, felt that the perfusion of outer cortical nephrons fell more with age than did perfusion of the corticomedullary nephrons. They investigated whether this selective decrease in cortical nephron perfusion was due to sclerotic changes in the small arcuate arterioles or represented a selective vasoconstriction of the more peripheral vessels. The vasodilator, acetylcholine, increased renal blood flow in both young and old subjects but the effect was more striking in the younger subjects. In contrast, the vasoconstrictive response to angiotensin was similar in the young and old subjects. Modification of sodium intake also affected renal haemodynamics differently in young and old subjects. In young subjects, renal blood flow varied directly with salt intake while in older subjects, renal blood flow was unaltered by the level of salt intake. These studies suggest that the kidney in the aged patient is in a relatively greater state of baseline vasodilatation or else has less capacity to vasodilate than does the kidney of a young person. These data are in contrast to those published by McDonald, Solomon, and Shock (1951) suggesting a state of resting vasoconstriction in the older patient, so further studies are needed to resolve this discrepancy.

Maximum tubular transport capacity

The tubular maximum of PAH, a measure of the ability of the renal tubules to secrete PAH when the arterial blood level is raised sufficiently to saturate the tubular transport capacity so that all of the PAH cannot be removed from the blood in one passage through the kidney, decreased with age at a rate almost parallel to the decrease in inulin clearance (Davies and Shock 1950). The decrease in the tubular maximum of glucose (TM glucose) with age also matched the decrease in inulin clearance (Miller, McDonald, and Shock 1952).

Although most of the reduction in the secretory and resorptive tubular maximum of the kidney with age can be explained by a progressive loss of nephrons, animal experiments have shown fewer energy-producing mitochondria (Barrows, Falzone, and Shock 1960), lower enzyme concentrations (Barrows *et al.* 1960), lower concentrations of sodium–potassium activated ATPase activity (Beauchene, Fanestil, and Barrows 1965) and diminished tubular transport (Beauchene *et al.* 1965) in old compared to young kidneys. Thus, aging may not only reduce the nephron population but changes in the basic biochemistry may develop at the tubular level.

Concentrating and diluting ability

A decrease in concentrating ability with age has been well documented (Lindeman, Van Buren, and Raisz 1960; Miller and Shock 1953; Lindeman, Lee, Yiengst, and Shock 1966). Maximum ability to dilute urine also decreases significantly with age (Lindeman *et al.* 1966). Whether this is due to a basic defect in tubular function with age or is merely a reflection of the increased solute load in surviving nephrons cannot be answered by the available studies. In order to answer this question, one would need to artificially decrease by dietary manipulation the total solute excretion so that the decrease in solute excretion matched the decrease in glomerular filtration rate in older subjects.

When diluting abilities in young vs. old persons have been compared on the basis of free water clearance (CH_2O) per unit of glomerular filtration rate, there is no defect in diluting ability with age (Lindeman *et al.* 1966). No comparable data are available to evaluate concentrating ability.

Urine acidification

Despite the decrease in renal function with age, the blood pH, pCO_2, and bicarbonate of aged patients without renal disease do not differ from the values observed in young subjects under basal conditions (Shock and Yiengst 1950; Adler, Lindeman, Yiengst, Beard, and Shock 1968). The decreases in blood pH and bicarbonate concentrations of blood are prolonged, however, in elderly persons following ingestion of an acid load (Shock and Yiengst 1948; Hilton, Goodbody, and Kruresi 1955). The minimum urine pH achieved in young vs. old patients is similar but total acid excretion (ammonia + titratable acid minus bicarbonate) decreases at a rate paralleling the decrease in glomerular filtration rate (Adler *et al.* 1968).

Glomerular permeability

Essentially no information exists to suggest that glomerular permeability changes with age. In a population survey of persons over age 65 years, Van Zonneveld (1959) found an increasing incidence of proteinuria with age. Still, by age 85, only a minority (32 per cent) had proteinuria. Glomerular permeability to free haemoglobin, determined by factoring free haemoglobin clearance by inulin clearance in healthy young and old subjects, showed no change with age (Lowenstein, Faulstick, Yiengst, and Shock 1961).

Regeneration and compensatory hypertrophy in the aging kidney

McKay, McKay, and Addis (1932) were the first to report that the aging kidney loses its ability to replace or regenerate injured or destroyed renal cells. They found, after unilateral nephrectomy in rats aged 30, 60, 270, 360, and 540 days, that the gain in kidney weight over a fixed time period was 44, 35, 33, 23, and 23 per cent of control kidney weight. Kennedy (1958) subsequently reported differences in DNA, RNA, and total nitrogen concentrations in surviving kidneys two to six weeks after unilateral nephrectomy in rats of different ages. He showed that in young animals (one month old), there was a striking hyperplasia (increased DNA content) and hypertrophy (increased RNA content). In older rats (6 months old), no hyperplasia occurred and hypertrophy was decreased compared to young rats. Additional studies (Barrows, Roeder, and Olewine 1962; Koniski 1962; Phillips and Leong 1967; Dicker and Shirley 1973; Ogden 1967; Boner, Shelp, Newton, and Rieselback 1973; Galla, Klein-Robbenhaar, and Hayslett 1974) have further documented the greater compensatory hypertrophy in the kidneys of young vs. old animals and man after unilateral nephrectomy. Koniski (1962) showed that a high protein intake will greatly increase compensatory hypertrophy; however, the age differences persist even when this variable is controlled.

Contrary to Kennedy's findings, Barrows *et al.* (1962) found no change in cortical RNA to DNA ratios with age, suggesting the relative contributions of cellular hyperplasia and hypertrophy to renal enlargement do not change with age. Two other studies, however, tend to support the conclusions of Kennedy

(Phillips and Leong 1967; Dicker and Shirley 1973). Phillips and Leong (1967), in the most elaborate studies, measured the rates of DNA synthesis using tritiated thymidine autoradiography and quantified mitotic activity in the remaining kidney of young vs. old rats following unilateral nephrectomy. In both age groups, peak concentrations occurred 36 hours after nephrectomy being three times greater in the young compared to old rats. Although qualitatively the type of response indicative of compensatory hypertrophy is similar in young and old animals, quantitatively the proliferative activity is greatly reduced in older animals. Dicker and Shirley (1973), using techniques similar to those reported by Barrows *et al.* (1962) felt their results provided evidence that cellular hyperplasia was the primary event in younger animals while hypertrophy of existing cells is the principal means for nephron enlargement in older animals. Galla *et al.* (1974) provided evidence that the increase in renal mass is matched by an increase in renal function. Similar age-related differences in ability to increase renal mass and function after unilateral nephrectomy have been reported in man using kidney transplant donors as the study population (Ogden 1967; Boner *et al.* 1973).

In summary, the number of glomeruli does not increase after birth so that compensatory hypertrophy at all ages occurs by enlarging residual nephrons rather than by increasing the number of functional nephrons. In young animals, the kidney enlarges by hyperplasia (cellular division of glomerular and tubular cells); in older animals, the capacity for kidney growth is greatly decreased and is accomplished primarily by hypertrophy of existing cells.

Pathophysiology of the decline in renal function with age

How does kidney function decrease with age in the individual subject? Cross-sectional and longitudinal data collected from 'normal' aging populations demonstrate consistently the decrease in renal function with age which tends to accelerate in the oldest individuals. Is this due to a progressive involutional change with loss of nephron units through the life of the individual, or does renal function remain stable until intermittent pathological processes inflict acute decreases in renal function? Some types of subclinical or silent renal injuries might include undetected glomerulonephritis due to immunological injury, pyelonephritis due to bacterial or viral infectious, acute tubular injury or interstitial nephritis due to drugs, poisons, or acute illnesses, vascular occlusions of small vessels with resultant ischaemic changes, and partial urinary tract obstruction. Since there are no adequate tests to diagnose many of these 'events', they may well go undetected or unappreciated in the selection of 'normal' populations. What role does the decreasing ability to repair and replace injured and destroyed cells in the nephron play in the accelerating decrease in renal function with age? These are all questions which can be answered only partially with the evidence currently in hand.

Friedman, Raizner, Rosen, Solomon, and Sy (1972) utilized scintillation scanning techniques to localize defects in kidney function in elderly persons with no past history of renal disease. They found abnormal scans in 25 of 35 elderly patients (71 per cent) with a mean age of 75 years (range 60 to 93 years) and mean creatinine clearance of 53 ml per minute. Sixteen (46 per cent) showed focal areas of diminished uptake which were felt to represent ischaemic lesions. Significant pyuria was present in 37 per cent of the patients; however, intravenous pyelograms were interpreted as normal in all cases. No significant proteinuria was detected in any patient. These findings are consistent with the hypothesis that focal lesions due to vascular occlusions and/or interstitial infection (pyelonephritis) are contributing to the decrease in renal function observed in aging persons.

Tauchi, Tsuboi, and Okutomi (1971) compared post-mortem renal pathology in elderly Caucasians and Japanese. Arteriosclerotic lesions appeared earlier and were more severe in the small arteries of the kidney in the Japanese compared to Caucasians consistent with the increased severity of the arteriosclerotic lesions found in other parts of the body. Kidney weight, size of glomeruli, number of cells per glomerular tuft, and number of tubular epithelial cells in a given area all decreased significantly with age and the decline was significantly more rapid in the Japanese. The size of the individual epithelial cell nuclei, however, increased significantly with age with the increase more apparent in the Caucasians. The authors concluded that sclerotic and fibrotic changes in the renal vasculature paralleling a generalized arteriosclerotic process were primarily responsible for the senile changes occurring in the kidney.

Asymptomatic bacteriuria also may be an important contributor to the decrease in renal function with age observed in cross-sectional studies. Dontas, Papanayiotou, Marketos, and Papanicolaou (1968) found 24 of 90 clinically healthy residents of the Athens Home for the Aged (27 per cent) had persistent bacteriuria. The mean inulin clearance was significantly lower (70 vs. 81 cc/min) in the bacteriuric group when compared to other residents. Concentrating ability also was decreased more in the bacteriuric residents. Wolfson, Kalmanson, Rubini, and Guze (1965) found asymptomatic bacteriuria in 15 per cent of 521 geriatric male patients (median age 63 years). The age-related incidence of bacteriuria was relatively constant at 9 per cent up to age 60 years; it then increased rapidly reaching 42 per cent in individuals over age 80 years. Although the incidence of prostatic hypertrophy, urinary calculi, previous infection, instrumentation, and surgery increased with age, there were some bacteriuric individuals in whom these predisposing conditions were not found.

In order to determine how the kidney ages in the individual subject, one would need to follow frequently accurate and precise measures of renal function over a period of many years. Studies reported recently from the Gerontology Research Institute at Baltimore City Hospitals (Rowe *et al.* 1976) following endogenous true creatinine clearances longitudinally at 18-month intervals (548 normal male subjects) over a period of ten years document an accelerating decrease in renal function with age. Unfortunately, the determination of endogenous creatinine clearance is insufficiently accurate and precise to answer the posed question on how the individual kidney ages. More accurate and precise measures of glomerular filtration rate using inulin (or I^{125} iothalamate) infusions, requiring much more effort and expense per study, will be necessary to answer this question with confidence.

Ability of the kidney to maintain a constant internal environment of fluid volume and electrolyte concentrations

The kidneys are responsible for maintenance of a constant internal environment of fluid volume and electrolyte concentrations. Imbalances result not from intrinsic renal changes with age, but rather from extrarenal pathology affecting renal regulatory mechanisms. Cohn and Shock (1949) found no change in blood volumes or plasma volumes with age in a large number of male subjects. Shock (1956) showed that extracellular fluid volumes, as measured by determination of thiocyanate space, also fails to change with age. Sodium, potassium, chloride, calcium, and magnesium concentrations in serum are not significantly altered by age under basal conditions (Elkington and Danowski 1955; Shock 1961; Korenchevsky 1961). Acid–base balance also is unaffected by age. Small but significant changes in the serum concentrations of certain trace metals have been observed with age. Serum zinc concentrations decrease (Lindeman, Clark, and Colmore 1971) and serum copper concentrations increase (Yunice, Lindeman, Czerwinski, and Clark 1974) with age in male subjects. It remains unclear whether these serum changes are merely the result of differences in the serum concentrations of metal binding proteins or represent a deficiency (zinc) and excess (copper) of these metals occurring with age.

Changes with age in the response of the kidney to alterations in the internal and external environment

The responses of the kidney with age to changing external and internal conditions and stimuli are more often dependent on different inputs to the kidney through extrarenal regulatory mechanisms than to inherent changes in the kidney itself. The diurnal variations in urinary sodium, potassium, and chloride excretions and glomerular filtration rate appear to be blunted in older subjects when compared to young subjects (Lobban and Tredie 1967; personal observations). One possible explanation might be that the normal daytime increases in electrolyte excretions and glomerular filtration rate might be partially eliminated by an exaggerated response to assumption of an upright position during most of the day. This assumes that older persons decrease electrolyte excretion and glomerular filtration rate more with standing than do younger persons. Actually when the response to tilt is compared in young and old subjects (Lee, Lindeman, Yiengst, and Shock 1966), there is little difference in the per cent change in urinary sodium excretion or glomerular filtration rate at the end of one hour of upright tilting compared to results obtained in the supine position, i.e. no exaggerated antinatriuresis to tilting occurs in older persons.

Little information is available on the ability of the aging kidney to regulate sodium excretion in response to volume contraction and expansion. The aged individual can conserve sodium under conditions of acute dehydration (Sporn, Lancestermere, and Papper 1962), but the efficacy of this conservation has been compared critically only recently in young vs. old subjects. Epstein and Hollenberg (1976) found that older subjects failed to conserve sodium as rapidly and efficiently as did younger subjects. Elderly male subjects are more likely to develop an exaggerated natriuresis after administration of a water or saline load than are younger male subjects (Lindeman, Adler, and Yiengst 1970). Schalekamp, Krauss, and Schalekamp-Kuyken (1971) found that older hypertensive patients, in whom renal vascular resistance and filtration fraction were increased and plasma renin concentrations were suppressed, consistently developed a more marked natriuresis following an intravenous saline load than did young hypertensive patients. The ability of the aged person to eliminate large amounts of sodium when stressed with excessive salt intake remains poorly defined.

Summary

Renal mass and function decrease with age once the individual reaches maturity. The decreases in all functions of the kidney parallel that of glomerular filtration rate. It remains unclear whether this decline in renal function is due to a series of undetected renal injuries resulting from a variety of pathological processes (immunological, infectious, ischaemic, etc.) or is the result of some progressive involutional process. It is clear that the ability to regenerate and repair injured cells decreases with age. This decrease in renal function with age normally is not sufficient to be life-threatening even in those individuals with the longest life span. The aged kidney maintains its ability to eliminate metabolic waste products and maintain fluid and electrolyte balance; only when a demand is placed on the kidney does it take longer for the individual to return the internal environment to the basal state.

References

ADLER, S., LINDEMAN, R. D., YIENGST, M. J., BEARD, E., and SHOCK, N. W. (1968). *J. Lab. clin. Med.*, **72**, 278.

ARATAKI, M. (1926). *Amer. J. Anat.*, **36**, 399.

BARROWS, C. H. Jr., FALZONE, J. A. Jr., and SHOCK, N. W. (1960). *J. Gerontol.*, **15**, 130.

——, ROEDER, L. M., and OLEWINE, D. A. (1962). *J. Gerontol.*, **17**, 148.

BEAUCHENE, R. E., FANESTIL, D. D., and BARROWS, C. H. (1965). *J. Gerontol.*, **20**, 306.

BIBER, T. U. L., MYLLE, M., BAINES, A. D., GOTTSHALK, C. W., OLIVER, J. R., and MacDOWELL, M. C. (1968). *Amer. J. Med.*, **44**, 664.

BONER, G., SHELP, W. D., NEWTON, M., and RIESELBACH, R. E. (1973). *Amer. J. Med.*, **55**, 169.

BRADLEY, S. E. (1947). *Transactions of the first conference on factors regulating blood pressure*, p. 118. Josiah Macy, Jr. Foundation, New York.

BRICKER, N. S. (1969). *Amer. J. Med.*, **46**, 1.

——, MORRIN, P. A. F., and KIME, S. W. Jr. (1960). *Amer. J. Med.*, **28**, 77.

COHN, J. E. and SHOCK, N. W. (1949). *Amer. J. Med., Sci.*, **217**, 388.

DARMADY, E. M., OFFER, J., and WOODHOUSE, M. A. (1973). *J. Pathol.*, **109**, 195.

DAVIES, D. F. and SHOCK, N. W. (1950). *J. clin. Invest.*, **29**, 496.

DICKER, S. E. and SHIRLEY, D. G. (1973). *J. Physiol.*, **228**, 193.

DONTAS, A. S., PAPANAYIOTOU, P., MARKETOS, S. G., and PAPANICOLAOU, N. T. (1968). *Clin. Sci.*, **34**, 73.

DUNNILL, M. S. and HALLEY, W. (1973). *J. Pathol.*, **110**, 113.

ELKINGTON, J. R. and DANOWSKI, T. S. (1955). *The body fluids, basic physiology and practical therapeutics.* Williams and Wilkins Co., Baltimore.

EPSTEIN, M. and HOLLENBERG, N. K. (1976). *J. Lab. clin. Med.*, **87**, 411.

FARQUHAR, M. G., VERNIER, R. L., and GOOD, R. A. (1957). *Schweiz. Med. Wschr.*, **87**, 501.

FRIEDMAN, S. A., RAIZNER, A. E., ROSEN, H., SOLOMEN, N. A., and SY, N. (1972). *Ann. int. Med.*, **76**, 41.

GALLA, J. H., KLEIN-ROBBENHAAR, T., and HAYSLETT, J. P. (1974). *Yale J. Biol. Med.*, **47**, 218.

HILTON, J. G., GOODBODY, M. F. Jr., and KRURESI, O. R. (1955). *J. Amer. Geriat. Soc.*, **3**, 697.

HOLLENBERG, N. K., ADAMS, D. F., and SOLOMON, H. S. (1974). *Circulation Res.*, **34**, 309.

KENNEDY, G. C. (1958). *Water and electrolyte metabolism in relation to age and sex* (ed. G. E. W. Wolstenholme and M. O'Connor), p. 250. Little, Brown and Co., Boston.

KONISKI, F. (1962). *J. Gerontol.*, **17**, 151.

KORENCHEVSKY, V. (1961). *Physiological and pathological aging* (ed. G. H. Bourne), p. 129. Karger, Basel, Switzerland.

LEE, T. D. Jr., LINDEMAN, R. D., YIENGST, M. J., and SHOCK, N. W. (1966). *J. appl. Physiol.*, **21**, 55.

LEWIS, W. H. Jr. and ALVING, A. S. (1938). *Amer. J. Physiol.*, **123**, 500.

LINDEMAN, R. D., VAN BUREN, H. C., and RAISZ, L. G. (1960). *New Engl. J. Med.*, **262**, 1306.

——, LEE, T. D. Jr., YIENGST, M. J., and SHOCK, N. W. (1966). *J. Lab. clin. Med.*, **68**, 206.

——, ADLER, S., and YIENGST, M. J. (1970). *Nephron*, **7**, 289.

——, CLARK, M. L., and COLMORE, J. P. (1971). *J. Gerontol.*, **26**, 358.

LJUNGKVIST, A. (1963). *Acta Pediat.*, **52**, 443.

LOBBAN, M. C. and TREDIE, B. E. (1967). *J. Physiol.*, **188**, 480.

LOWENSTEIN, J., FAULSTICK, D. A., YIENGST, M. A., and SHOCK, N. W. (1961). *J. Clin. Invest.*, **40**, 1172.

MCDONALD, R. K., SOLOMON, D. H., and SHOCK, N. W. (1951). *J. clin. Invest.*, **5**, 457.

MCKAY, E. M., MCKAY, L. L., and ADDIS, T. (1932). *J. exp. Med.*, **56**, 255.

MCMANUS, J. F. A. and LUPTON, C. H. (1960). *Lab. Invest.*, **9**, 413.

MILLER, J. H., MCDONALD, R. K., and SHOCK, N. W. (1952). *J. Gerontol.*, **7**, 196.

—— and SHOCK, N. W. (1953). *J. Gerontol.*, **8**, 446.

OGDEN, D. A. (1967). *Ann. intern. Med.*, **67**, 998.

OLIVER, J. R. (1952). *Cowdry's problems of aging* (3rd ed.) (ed. A. I. Lansing). Williams and Wilkins, Baltimore.

PHILLIPS, T. L. and LEONG, G. F. (1967). *Cancer Res.*, **27**, 286.

REYNES, M., CAULET, T., and DIEBOLD, J. (1968). *Path. Biol. (Paris)*, **16**, 1081.

ROESSLE, R. and ROULET, F. (1932). *Mass und Zahl in der Pathologie*, p. 144. Berlin.

ROWE, J. W., ANDRES, R., TOBIN, J. D., NORRIS, A. H., and SHOCK, N. W. (1976). *J. Gerontol.*, **31**, 155.

SCHALEKAMP, M. A. D. M., KRAUSS, X. H., and SCHALEKAMP-KUYKEN, M. P. A. (1971). *Clin. Sci.*, **41**, 219.

SHOCK, N. W. (1956). *Bull. NY Acad. Med.*, **32**, 268.

—— (1961). *Ann. Rev. Physiol.*, **23**, 97.

—— and YIENGST, M. J. (1948). *Fed. Proc.*, **7**, 114.

—— and —— (1950). *J. Gerontol.*, **5**, 1.

SPORN, I. N., LANCESTERMERE, R. G., and PAPPER, S. (1962). *New Engl. J. Med.*, **267**, 130.

SWORN, M. J. and FOX, M. (1972). *Brit. J. Urol.*, **44**, 377.

TAKAZAKURA, E., SAWABU, N., HANDA, A., TAKADA, A., SHINODA, A., and TAKENCHI, J. (1972). *Kidney International*, **2**, 224.

TAUCHI, H., TSUBOI, K., and OKUTOMI, J. (1971). *Gerontologia*, **17**, 87.

VAN ZONNEVELD, R. J. (1959). *Gerontol. Clin.*, **1**, 167.

WEHNER, H. (1968). *Arch. Virchows Abt. A. Path. Anat.*, **344**, 286.

WESSON, L. G. Jr. (1969). *Physiology of the human kidney*, p. 96. Grune and Stratton, New York.

WOLFSON, S. A., KALMANSON, G. M., RUBINI, M. E., and GUZE, L. B. (1965). *Amer. J. med. Sci.*, **250**, 168.

YUNICE, A. A., LINDEMAN, R. D., CZERWINSKI, A. W., and CLARK, M. (1974). *J. Gerontol.*, **29**, 277.

Aging and endocrine function Edwin L. Bierman

Introduction

Mastery of the glands of internal secretion was once viewed as the key to longevity. Such thinking now seems naive, since it is abundantly clear that aging involves more than simply a failure of the endocrine glands to secrete their hormones. Nevertheless, normal aging in man is associated with a variety of critical effects on hormone production, secretion, and action, resulting in functional alterations that could culminate in age-associated diseases (Gregerman and Bierman 1974).

Hormones can be divided into two broad categories with different functional significance (Table 1). The steroid hormones are produced and stored by endocrine cells at sites distant from specific target cells, circulate bound to specific transport proteins, enter cells to bind to specific intracellular proteins, ultimately to effect modulation of nuclear processes controlling synthesis of certain cell proteins. The polypeptide hormones may be produced and stored by endocrine cells in a similar manner, but they need not be transported to a distant site (may act on neighbouring cells). Furthermore, peptide hormones are soluble in plasma and often circulate in the free (unbound) form. They avidly bind to specific

Table 1 Hormones

		Chemical class	
		Steroid	Polypeptide
	Embryologic origin	mesoderm	neuroectoderm
	Target action	inside cell	cell surface
	Path to target	endocrine	endocrine
			paracrine
			neurocrine

receptors on the surfaces of the target cells and regulate cell function by a few common mechanisms, most often involving activation of cell membrane adenyl cyclase and formation of cyclic AMP.

Despite these differences, the hormones in common are organized into a hierarchy of feedback loop systems. Endocrine homeostasis is maintained by a balance of a number of processes, each in communication with each other. Blood levels of a hormone are determined by synthesis rates, secretion rates, concentration of specific binding carrier proteins (determining the 'free' or metabolically active hormone fraction in plasma), and metabolic degradation rates (which may or may not be related to biological action). Aging can affect one aspect of hormonal balance, leading to compensatory shifts in others such that the concentration of the hormone in the blood is unchanged. Thus a normal hormone level in the blood in an older individual does not mean that a functional change with aging has not occurred.

Endocrine change with aging

Most hormone secretion is episodic or cyclic with periodicities ranging from minutes (insulin) to weeks (oestrogens). The longer endocrine rhythms show the more obvious changes with age (e.g. the menopause), but all frequencies of oscillatory endocrine behaviour may be altered with aging as well. The amplitude of responses to perturbation and counter-regulation may be altered in old age without affecting steady state hormonal levels (Fig. 1, line 1). Alternatively,

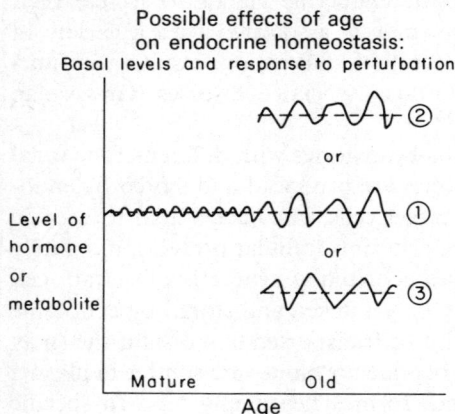

FIG. 1. Hypothetical alterations in basal hormone levels and responses to perturbations during aging in man. See text for detailed explanation.

target tissues may become less responsive to hormones with age (effects on surface receptors, intracellular binding proteins, and other steps related to the expression of hormonal effects) leading to a compensatory increase in hormone production and hormone levels to maintain homeostasis (Fig. 1, line 2). Another possible general type of functional abnormality is an impairment of hormone production, either associated with a compensatory decrease in hormone disposal rate, an increase in tissue sensitivity, or more likely, simply a lower blood level and reduced target tissue effect (Fig. 1, line 3). A few specific examples will serve to illustrate the major general types of endocrine change with aging.

Hormonal changes in the female menopause
The female menopause represents the most clear-cut example of endocrine senescence in which decreased hormone secretion appears to be the primary event. The ovary is the site of failure with a precipitous decline in blood levels and urinary excretion of oestrogen after age forty at a time close to the menopause (Pincus, Romanoff, and Carlo 1954; Longcope 1971). Oestrogen excretion continues to decline further between ages 50 and 60 reaching a level in the elderly of about one-fifth of that before the menopause (Judd, Judd, Lucas *et al.* 1974). While the ovary ceases completely to secrete oestrogens, increased amounts of adrenal androstenedione are converted to oestrogen in the periphery (Hemsell, Grodin, Brenner *et al.* 1974) in partial compensation for ovarian failure.

Other compensatory mechanisms also come into play. Metabolic clearance rates of oestrogen decrease. Negative feedback on the hypothalamic–pituitary axis is relaxed leading to marked increases in pituitary gonadotrophin secretion (Albert, Randall, Smith *et al.* 1974; Taymor, Toshihiro, and Pheteplace 1968). Levels of the hypothalamic releasing factor for luteinizing hormone (LHRF) are reduced in postmenopausal females (Seyler and Reichlin 1973), possibly due to short-loop feedback control of LHRF secretion via increased LH. Thus a cascade of functional endocrine alterations stem from a type of primary hormone production failure with aging.

The thyroid
However, such age-associated primary production failure of hormones is not typical of all endocrine systems. The thyroid axis is illustrative of a probable primary decrease in metabolic disposal rate of thyroid hormone with age (Gregerman 1971), amounting to a loss of about 50 per cent over the entire adult age span. This is attributed largely to a progressive slowing of the rate of cellular degradation of thyroxine. A compensatory decrease in secretion rate by the thyroid results in unchanged levels of circulating thyroxine.

Despite the decrease in thyroidal secretion of hormone with age, the thyroid gland of the elderly has good reserve, as judged by unaltered response to stimulation by thyrotropin (TSH), and acceleration of thyroxine turnover during severe illness in older subjects (Gregerman and Solomon 1967). Plasma thyrotropin levels with or without thyrotropin-releasing hormone stimulation (TRH) are not increased in the elderly, a sensitive indication that primary gland failure does not exist (Snyder and Utiger 1972). The anatomic alterations of the gland often seen with advancing age (multinodular goitre) are apparent compensatory changes associated with the maintenance of adequate function and reserve capacity.

The slowing of the metabolic disposal rate of thyroxine with age does not appear to be associated with a decline in oxygen consumption or basal metabolic rate, when corrected for the change in lean body mass that occurs with aging (Gregerman and Bierman 1974). The peripheral conversion of thyroxine (T4) to triiodothyronine (T3) and its inactive sister molecule, reverse T3, appears to regulate the metabolic effects of thyroid hormone, exerted at the cellular level primarily by T3. Plasma levels of T3 are decreased in the elderly (Snyder and Utiger 1972; Rubenstein, Butler, and Werner 1973), but further studies are needed to elucidate the relationship of that observation to hormone effects. Thus the bulk of evidence supports a primary alteration in the hormone effector mechanism as an explanation for the functional changes in the thyroid axis seen with aging.

Glucose and glucoregulatory hormones
Analagous age-related changes are observed for the most important glucocorticoid of man, cortisol. Thus, the adrenal cortical axis represents another illustration of a primarily slowed metabolic disposal rate and decreased hormone secretion rates resulting in unaltered plasma cortisol concentrations, even at very advanced ages (Gherondache, Romanoff, and Pincus 1967; West, Brown, Simons *et al.* 1961).

Changes in the function of the glucoregulatory peptide hormones with aging at first glance appear to be due to a different mechanism, i.e. changes in effector sensitivity, perhaps related to decreased cell surface receptor function. In the basal state, plasma glucose levels increase with age without changes in the basal concentrations of the three major glucoregulatory hormones, insulin, growth hormone, and pancreatic glucagon. Following intravenous or oral glucose loads, glucose tolerance is progressively impaired with aging (Andres 1971). In association with decreased glucose tolerance, neither glucagon (Dudl and Ensinck 1977) nor growth hormone (Andres and Tobin 1974) release in response to stimulation is altered during aging. However, in some studies, glucose intolerance has been associated with impaired acute insulin responses (Andres, Pozefsky, Swerdloff *et al.* 1976), but in others such changes have not been observed (Dudl and Ensinck 1977) and a summary of such studies has shown a spectrum of discordant results relating insulin responses to aging (Andres and Tobin 1974). Alternatively, decreased sensitivity to insulin has been shown in some older humans (Silverstone, Brandfonbrenner, Shock *et al.* 1957). Glucose and insulin clamp infusion studies have confirmed these findings in some (de Fronzo) 1979) but not all studies (Andres *et al.* 1976).

The crucial problem in interpretation of glucose and glucoregulatory hormone homeostasis during aging relates to the confounding effects of the increase in both absolute and relative adiposity with age (Gregerman and Bierman 1974) (Fig. 2).

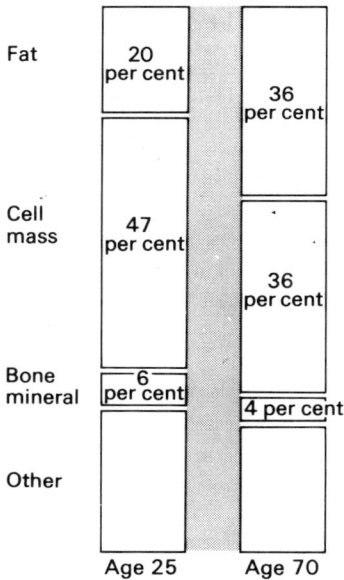

FIG. 2. Idealized representation of the change in body composition during aging in normal males. Comparable age-related increased in relative adiposity occur in females. (Reprinted from Gregerman and Bierman (1974).)

The increase in adipose cell mass is associated with decreased insulin sensitivity (Rabinowitz 1970), perhaps due to a reduction in effective insulin receptors (Archer, Gorden, and Roth 1975) or to postreceptor deficits. Thus aging man, even at constant body weight, would be expected to show a decline in insulin sensitivity. In some individuals, relatively normal glucose homeostasis will be maintained at the expense of higher rates of insulin secretion; in others glucose homeostasis will deteriorate in association with relatively impaired insulin secretory responses. It has also been suggested that insulin secretion might become defective with aging, with a larger proportion of the less biologically active synthetic precursor, proinsulin, appearing in the circulation (Duckworth and Kitabachi 1972).

Thus, indirectly, endocrine homeostasis with aging can be affected by changes in body composition, as illustrated by alterations in insulin–glucose relationships.

Summary

To summarize, aging affects many aspects of endocrine regulation in man, but not all the hormonal systems are affected in the same way or to the same extent (Fig. 3). Hormone production, secretion rates, patterns of secretion, and responses to physiologic or pharmacologic stimuli each may be affected by aging. Diminished hormone secretion may be primary or may be a secondary compensatory response to an age-related decrease in hormone degradation and metabolic clearance. Circulating levels of hormone transport proteins may change with age. Feedback control mechanisms may be altered by age-related

	Hormone concentration in blood	Response to physiologic or pharmacologic stimulation	Metabolism (disposal rate)	End-organ sensitivity
Growth hormone	↔	↓		↓
Gonadotropins	↑*			
Thyrotropin (TSH)	↔	↓		↔
Thyroxine (T4)	↔	↔	↓	↑
Triiodothyronine (T3)	↓			
Parathyroid hormone	↑			↑
Cortisol	↔	↔	↓	
Adrenal androgens	↓	↓		
Aldosterone	↓		↓	
Insulin	↔	↓	↔	↔
Glucagon	↔	↔		
Testosterone	↓		↓	
Oestrogens	↓		↓	

Hormones

	Chemical class	
	Steroid	Polypeptide
Embryologic origin	mesoderm	neuroectoderm
Target action	inside cell	cell surface
Path to target	endocrine	endocrine paracrine neurocrine

FIG. 3. Endocrine changes during aging in man. ↑, increase; ↓, decrease; ↔, no change; *, postmenopausal. Blank spaces indicate that no data are presently available. (Reprinted from Gregerman and Bierman (1974).)

increases or decreases in target tissue sensitivity. Thus evaluation of the endocrine system with age depends on the continued acquisition of knowledge regarding the wide variety of age-related alterations in hormone function that occur in man.

References

ALBERT, A., RANDALL, R. V., SMITH, R. A., and JOHNSON, E. E. (1956). In *Hormones and the aging process* (ed. E. R. Engle and G. Pincus), p. 49. Academic Press, New York.

ANDRES, R. (1971). In *Medical clinics of North America* (ed. P. Felig and P. K. Bondy), pp. 55, 835. W. B. Saunders Co., Philadelphia, London, Toronto.

—— and TOBIN, J. D. (1974). In *Advances in experimental medicine and biology* (ed. V. Cristofalo, T. Roberts, and R. Adelman), Vol. 61, p. 239. Plenum Press, New York.

——, POZEFSKY, T., SWERDLOFF, R. S. *et al.* (1976). In *Advances in metabolic disorders* (ed. R. Levine), Suppl. 1, p. 349. Academic Press, New York.

ARCHER, J. A., GORDEN, P., and ROTH, J. (1975). *J. clin. Invest.*, **55**, 166.

DE FRONZO, R. A. (1979). *Diabetes* **28**, 1095.

DUCKWORTH, W. C. and KITABCHI, A. E. (1972). *Amer. J. Med.*, **53**, 418

DUDL, R. J. and ENSINCK, J. W. (1977). *Metabolism*, **26**, 33.

GHERONDACHE, C. N., ROMANOFF, L. P., and PINCUS, G. (1967). In *Endocrines and aging* (ed. L. Gitman), p. 76. Charles C. Thomas, Springfield, Illinois.

GREGERMAN, R. I. (1971). In *The thyroid: a fundamental and clinical text* (3rd ed.) (ed. S. C. Werner and H. I. Sidney), p. 137. Harper and Row, New York.

—— and SOLOMON, N. (1967). *J. Clin. Endocrinol.*, **27**, 93.

—— and BIERMAN, E. L. (1974). In *Textbook of endocrinology* (5th ed.) (ed. R. H. Williams), p. 1059. W. B. Saunders, Philadelphia.

HEMSELL, D. L., GRODIN, J. M., BRENNER, P. F., SIITERI, P. K., and MACDONALD, D. C. (1974). *J. clin. Endocrinol. Metab.*, **38**, 476.

JUDD, H. L., JUDD, G. E., LUCAS, E. W., and YEN, S. S. C. (1974). *J. clin. Endocrinol. Metab.*, **39**, 1020.

LONGCOPE, C. (1971). *Amer. J. Obstet. Gynec.*, **111**, 778.

PINCUS, G., ROMANOFF, L. P., and CARLO, J. (1954). *J. Gerontol.*, **9**, 113.

RABINOWITZ, D. (1970). *Ann. Rev. Med.*, **21**, 241.

RUBENSTEIN, H. A., BUTLER, V. P. Jr., and WERNER, S. C. (1973). *J. clin. Endocrinol. Metab.*, **37**, 247.

SEYLER, E. L., Jr., and REICHLIN, S. (1973). *J. clin. Endocrinol. Metab.*, **37**, 197.

SILVERSTONE, F. A., BRANDFONBRENER, M., SHOCK, N. W. *et al.* (1957). *J. clin. Invest.*, **36**, 504.

SNYDER, P. J. and UTIGER, R. D. (1972). *J. clin. Endocrinol.*, **34**, 380.

TAYMOR, M. L., TOSHIHIRO, A., and PHETEPLACE, C. (1968). In *Gonadotrophins 1968, Proceedings of the Workshop Conference — Vista Hermosa, Mor., Mexico* (ed. Rosenberg), p. 349. Geron-X Inc., California.

WEST, C. D., BROWN, H., SIMONS, E. L., CARTER, D. E., KUMAGAI, L. F., and ENGLERT, E. (1961). *J. clin. Endocrinol.*, **21**, 1197.

Session 16
Hormone action

Introduction Richard C. Adelman

It is the intent of this session to communicate recent progress in the area of aging and hormone action in its broadest possible sense. In other words, the phrase hormone action will represent the entire spectrum of key endocrinological events, including the following: hormone–receptor interaction in target cell populations; the availability of circulating hormones whose presence is absolutely essential to the integrity of specific adaptive mechanisms in intact animals; the role of the pituitary gland in regulating a vast array of peripheral tissue response; and a probe of genome expression in certain brain regions that probably are crucial to initiation of neuroendocrine cascade mechanisms. The contributors should bare both the potential importance and the crying need for additional studies relating to the role of hormonal regulatory mechanisms in the understanding of biological aging.

Aging and transcription of the rat brain genome Caleb E. Finch

A major issue in the study of aging is the state of genomic function. The key point concerns whether changes are global or, whether they are selective and limited. A great deal of effort by many laboratories has not led to any clear resolution of how extensive the changes are in gene transcription. Studies of response to hormones show that some mechanisms (e.g. the glucocorticoid-mediated induction of tyrosine aminotransferase in the liver) are intact in old rodents, whereas others are impaired (e.g. catecholamine-mediated lipolysis in adipocytes) (reviewed in Finch 1976). Studies by Cutler of the amount of the genome transcribed during aging in the mouse indicate major decreases in liver and brain (Cutler 1973, 1975). Similar studies were undertaken by this laboratory, and as described below, fail to show major transcriptional impairment. The technical factors which may be involved are also discussed.

Our approach to the study of transcription and aging employs the technique of RNA-driven hybridization reaction of brain poly (A) containing RNA with ^{3}H-unique sequence DNA. This approach is currently in extensive use to characterize developmental changes (e.g. Galau, Klein, Davis, Wold, Britten, and Davidson 1976) and tissue differences in gene activity (Ryffel and McCarthy

1975; Bantle and Hahn 1976). Using specific fractions of cellular RNA in which the ribosomal RNA contribution is minimized (e.g. poly (A) Hn RNA, or poly (A) m RNA), it is possible to obtain completion of the RNA driven hybridization reaction during incubation periods of less than 7 days. Hybridization reactions which require a longer incubation period rarely achieve completion because of thermolytic degradation of the RNA and DNA. From the data of Bantle and Hahn (1976) or our data, it can be calculated that whole brain RNA would require 5–10 times longer to achieve saturation of ^{3}H-unique sequence DNA than nuclear or cytoplasmic poly (A) RNA fractions containing 20 per cent or less of the non-hybridizing ribosomal RNA. Thus many of the hybridization values in the past represent incomplete RNA–DNA hybridization reactions.

In our initial studies we chose to use total brain poly (A) RNA for a practical reason: total poly (A) RNA can readily be obtained from frozen brain. This permitted us to obtain RNA from tissues frozen immediately after sacrifice, thereby reducing uncertainties of degradation. The following research represents the laboratory efforts of Drs Janet Allen, Barry Kaplan, Beth Schachter, and Mr Heinz Osterburg.

The poly (A) RNA was extracted at Tris buffers pH 7 and 9 with phenol at 3 °C. Pilot studies showed 95 per cent extraction of pulse-labelled (^{3}H-orotic acid precursor) nuclear RNA. The brain DNA also removed by this procedure was digested by RNA-se free DNA-se 1 and extracted by 3M NaCl. Residual proteins were removed by pronase digestion and chloroform-phenol. Poly (A) RNA was isolated from the total RNA by 2 passages over oligo(dT) cellulose.

During our studies, we improved the techniques for precipitation of RNA by using ammonium acetate (0.24 M) with 2 volumes of cold ethanol. We found that RNA is quantitatively precipitated from solutions as dilute as 5 μg/ml, with less co-precipitation of detergents than in the traditional NaCl, Na acetate approach (Osterburg, Allen, and Finch 1975). The RNA was finally passed over Chelex

Table 1 Complexity of poly(A)RNA from the male rat brain: effect of age

Age–strain	Yield μg poly (A)/g brain	Per cent unique-sequence hybridized saturation values[†]		Average complexity[‡]
		Mean $\pm$ SEM	n	
3 months				
Fisher 344	20.0	11.60 $\pm$ 0.24	5	
	25.3	12.80 $\pm$ 0.24	13	6.7×10^8
10 months				
Fisher 344	18.9	12.35 $\pm$ 1.1	10	
	22.9	13.31 $\pm$ 0.8	13	6.7×10^8
24 months				
Fisher 344	18.5	10.8 $\pm$ 0.5	10	
	23.9	13.1 $\pm$ 1.0	14	6.3×10^8

[†]Corrected for DNA-DNA hybrids in each preparation and non-hybridizable DNA (25 per cent): $R:t$s 18 000 μs.

[‡]Assumes that transcription is asymmetric and that the rat unique-sequence DNA has a complexity of 2.6×10: nucleotides (Kaplan *et al.* 1978).

(Biorad) to remove trace quantities of metal ions which favour thermolytic degradation. Yields of RNA (total or poly (A)) from the brain did not vary appreciably between male rats aged 3 and 24 months (Table 1).

The ^{3}H-unique sequence DNA was obtained from rat Walker carcinoma cells grown with ^{3}H-thymidine. DNA was purified (by chloroform extractions, pronase, and RNA-se treatment), sheared to 400 nucleotides, and reassociated (Fig. 1). The fraction which failed to reassociate after 2 cycles of hybridization to Cot 1500 showed expected kinetics of reassociation with sheared total DNA driver ($k = 3 \times 10^{-4}\,1\,mol^{-1}\,s^{-1}$; $C_0t\frac{1}{2} = 3400\,mol/s^{-1}$) (Fig. 1). Its size on alkaline sucrose gradients was 287 + 24 nucleotides Mean 1 SEM.

In RNA-driven reactions, poly (A) RNA were combined in a capillary with 0.01 μg of ^{3}H-unique sequence DNA at an RNA concentration of 4–5 m/mlg and an RNA/DNA ratio of 750–3500:1 in 0.4M Na$_2$PO$_3$ buffer containing 0.1mM EDTA and 0.2 per cent SDS. Incubations were conducted at 70 °C for up to 5 days. At the end of 5 days of incubation, appreciable degradation of the poly (A) RNA had occurred, although the remaining pieces exceeded 5 s by density gradient sedimentation. The RNA–DNA hybrids, isolated by chromatography on hydroxylapatite (HAP), had thermal elution profiles similar to unique-sequence DNA hybrids (Fig. 2). (For further details, see Kaplan, Schachter, Osterburg, de Vellis, and Finch (1978).)

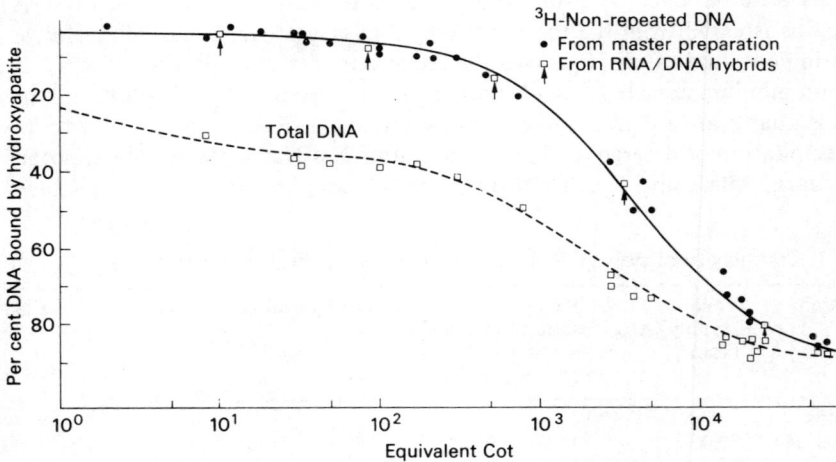

FIG. 1. Total sheared DNA was reassociated with tracer quantities of [^{3}H]non-repetitive sequence in 0.41 MPB to various equivalent Cots at 60°C. The reassociation of DNA was measured by binding to HAP in 0.12 MPB at 60°C. The rate of reassociation conformed to second-order kinetics (eqn 2); indicates a Cot 1/2 of 3100 for ^{3}H-non-repetitive sequence and a K of 0.0032 M^{-1}s^{-1}. The open squares on the curve representing ^{3}H-non-repeated DNA indicate the reassociation of ^{3}H-DNA obtained from the RNA/DNA hybrid fraction at saturation with whole brain poly(A) RNA by RNAse treatment (see Materials and methods). Their reassociation profile is not distinguishable from the original ^{3}H-non-repeated sequence fraction, indicating little or no contamination by repeated ^{3}H-DNA sequences (less than 5 per cent). (From Kaplan *et al.* (1978).)

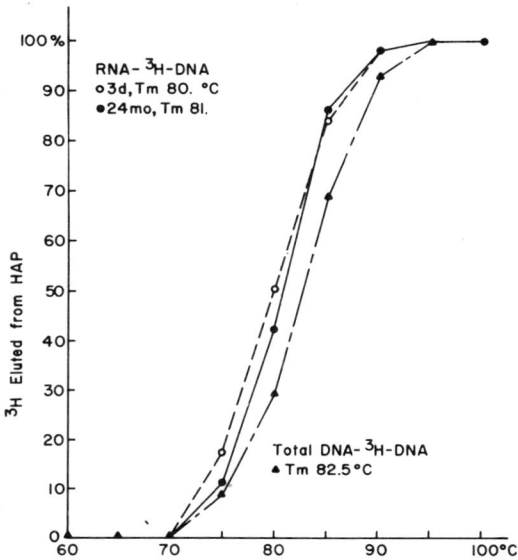

Fig. 2. Thermal elution of DNA/ DNA duplexes and brain RNA/DNA hybrids. Whole, sheared rat liver DNA was incubated at 60°C with [³H]non-repeated DNA (1700 : 1) to a Cot of 21 000 Ms. The sample was passed over a 1-ml HAP column in 0.12 MPB 0.1 per cent SDS, 60°C to remove non-reassociated DNA. The column was equilibrated with 0.10 MPB and the double-stranded DNA denatured and eluted from the column by elevation of temperature in 5°C increments. A 3-ml wash of the column at each temperature was made, and monitored for A_{260} absorbance (total DNA, O——O) and cpm (³H-non-repeated DNA). Brain RNA and [³H]non-repeated DNA (1000 : 1) were incubated at 70°C to a Rot of 21 000 mol l⁻¹s. Elution of the ³H-DNA (O- - -O; O——O) in the hybrids was assayed for as described above. The T_m values were 85.0 for the total DNA, 83.2 for the ³H-non-repetitive DNA in DNA/DNA duplexes and 80.5 for ³H-DNA in RNA/DNA hybrids. (From Kaplan *et al.* (1978).)

The hybridization reaction follows pseudo-first-order kinetics between Rots of 50 to 20 000. The values obtained for 30 and 12-month-old brain poly (A) RNA are shown contained in Fig. 3 and analysed by computer according to the equation

$$\frac{D}{D_0} = e^{-kR_0 t}$$

where D_0 and R_0 are the initial concentrations of DNA and RNA (moles nucleotide/litre), D is the concentration of unhybridized DNA, and t is time in seconds. The appreciable hybrids formed at very low Rots probably represent more abundant classes of RNA as described by many laboratories (Ryffel and McCarthy 1975; Bantle and Hahn 1976; Hastie and Bishop 1976). The fraction of RNA hybridizing slowly as in Fig. 3 has been termed the 'complex' class and contains relatively few copies per cell on the average. At saturation, this RNA corresponds to transcription of 25 per cent of the non-repeated genome. From the observed RNA complexity and the computed reaction rate, it can be calculated that about 4 per cent of the poly (A) RNA is driving the hybridization reaction (Kaplan *et al.* 1978).

The high complexity of the brain total poly (A) RNA predominantly represents nuclear poly (A) RNA species (Bantle and Hahn 1976).

In studying the effect of aging on transcription of the brain, 2 preparations of

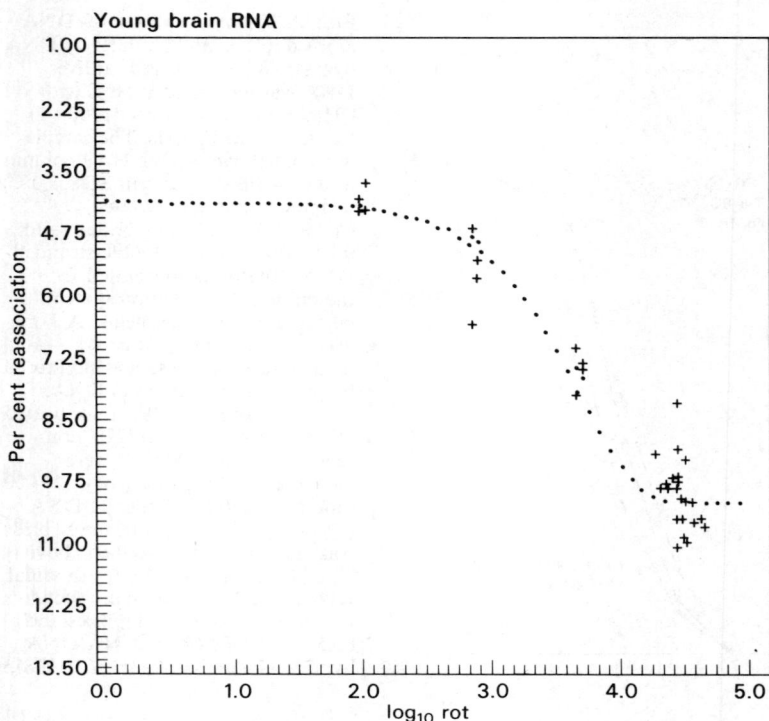

FIG. 3. Whole brain (90-day-old rats) RNA/DNA hybrids analysed according to pseudo-first-order kinetics.

RNA were made from each of 3 age groups: 3, 10, and 24 month-old Fisher 344 male rats. RNA was prepared hybridized and analysed simultaneously to minimize procedural variations. Other preparations of brain RNA from Sprague–Dawley rats gave very similar results (data not shown). There were no age differences in hybrid melting profile (Fig. 2).

Two conclusions can be drawn from saturation values (R_0t's > 18 000) of the RNA/DNA hybridization reaction:

(1) There are small (< 1 per cent net) differences between saturation values obtained from the RNA preparation of each age group.

(2) *If* age differences occur, they are on the order of 0.5 per cent net decrease in transcription and are *smaller* than the differences in the hybridizability between RNA preparations within any age group.

These results differ markedly from the major (~ 30 per cent) decrease in brain RNA complexity in mice of corresponding age groups which was reported by Cutler (1973, 1975). Several factors may be involved: Cutler's study of nuclear RNA may not have achieved completion of the hybridization reaction with unique sequence DNA, since Hahn and others have found that mouse brain nuclear RNA can hybridize to at least 40 per cent higher values of unique sequence (Bantle and Hahn 1976) than Cutler reported (1975). Decreased number of copies of some types of RNA hybridizing to unique-sequence DNA could yield apparent differences in the saturation values, since this would retard the completion of the reaction. This is a very difficult issue to resolve in prolonged RNA-driven hybridization reactions with inevitable breakdown. Alternatively, the absence of major changes in poly (A) RNA complexity observed by us could imply larger decreases in the transcription of poly (A) minus messenger and nuclear RNA, since Cutler's analysis included both poly (A) RNA and non-adenylated RNA. At present, the function of the 3′ polyadenylate tracts in informational RNA is unknown. Subsequent studies of messenger RNA from aging rat brains have also confirmed the absence of major age change (Coleman, Kaplan, Osterburg, and Finch, 1980).

The apparent absence of global changes in poly (A) RNA complexity is consistent with a considerable literature indicating the *qualitative* persistence during aging of all of the biochemical attributes identified in the 3-month-old brain. For example, studies of total RNA content of the major brain regions showed no change, with the exception of the striatum, in which there was a relative decrease of 15–20 per cent (Chaconas and Finch 1973). Similarly, a careful electrophoretic study of soluble brain proteins of the major regions did not reveal any qualitative difference in the mouse brain during aging (Vaughan and Calvin 1977). Similar results were indicated by an earlier study from this lab (Gordon and Finch 1974). Since at best 100–200 individual proteins can be distinguished by one-dimensional gel electrophoresis, the proteins detected by one-dimensional gel electrophoresis constitute a minute fraction of the total brain proteins, which can be predicted from brain messenger RNA complexity to number about 50 000–100 000 different polypeptides (Bantle and Hahn 1976). Most of these proteins are probably present in very small amounts and would not be detected even with two-dimensional gel electrophoresis of whole brain proteins. Two-dimensional gel electrophoresis might be very useful if applied to subcellular fractions of the brain—e.g. the synaptosomal membranes of specific brain regions.

Another approach to the study of aging and brain function is to look at specific neuronal pathways and functions. Recent evidence from this and other laboratories indicates a high degree of selectivity in the systems which are altered. We have developed a highly sensitive radiometric assay for catecholamines which can distinguish 5 pg of dopamine, noradrenalin, or adrenalin (Donahue, Osterburg, Severson, and Finch, in preparation). This assay is based on a modification of the procedures by Coyle and Henry (1973) and Palkovits, Brownstein, Saavedra, and Axelrod (1974), in which ^{3}H-methyl groups are added enzymatically to the C-3 hydroxyl of the catechols from [^{3}H-methyl]-S-adenosyl methione. We have improved the assay by acetylating the ^{3}H-methylated catecholamines and separating them on thin-layer chromatography. Our preliminary results indicate that dopaminergic pathways may be more altered by age than noradrenergic pathways in C57BL6J male mice. The dopamine levels in the striatum and median eminence of the hypothalamus are reduced by 20 per cent, whereas

Table 2 Catecholamine levels and aging in C57BL/6J male mice

Dopamine	Norepinephrine
μg/mg wet weight tissue, mean ± S.E.M.	
Striatum† (Putamen)	
12 mo. 2.32 ± 0.20	
28 mo. 1.7 ± 0.11	
Per cent change–24 per cent ($p < 0.001$)	
Median eminence‡	
11 mo. 19.8 ± 1.9	4.4 ± 0.7
29 mo. 15.5 ± 1.5	5.3 ± 0.8
Per cent change–22 per cent ($p < 0.05$)	
Cerebellum‡	
11 mo.	0.7 < 0.08
29 mo.	0.76 ± 0.13
Brain stem†	
12 mo.	0.75 ± 0.03
28 mo.	0.77 ± 0.03

†Finch (1973).
‡Donahue, Osterburg, Severson, and Finch (in preparation).

noradrenalin levels in the cerebellum, median eminence, and brain stem are not altered during aging (Table 2). These findings could imply a selective impairment of dopamine neurons originating in the substantia nigra, which have recently been shown to project to the hypothalamus (Kizer, Palkovits, and Brownstein 1976) as well as to the striatum (Andén, Carlsson, Dahlstrom, Fuxe, Hillarp, and Larsson 1964).

Reports of decreased dopamine in the basal ganglia of normal aging humans (Carlsson and Winblad 1976; Riederer and Wuketich 1976) strongly suggest that impaired nigral functions may be a general phenomenon of aging in mammals and support the idea that Parkinson's disease represents an accelerated development of a normal aging trend (Finch 1973, 1976). Another age-related change which may be a consequence of impaired catecholamine functions is the loss of regular oestrous cycles in rats. Numerous laboratories have shown that adrenergic drugs, including L-DOPA, reactivate the regular oestrous cycles (reviewed in Finch 1976, 1978) and it is now a serious hypothesis that deficiencies of hypothalamic catecholamines are involved in these phenomena.

In future, given RNA–DNA reactions of greatly increased sensitivity, it may be possible to relate changes of transcription of specific brain regions (e.g. the striatum, which shows a loss of RNA) to neural changes (e.g. the reduced dopamine of the striatum). At present, it seems unlikely that broadly distributed changes in gene function are involved in normal aging. Attention may fruitfully focus on the analysis of the specialized functions of neurotransmitters and their influence on the genome.

Acknowledgements

This research was supported by grants to C.E.F. from the NIH (HD-07359 and AG 00446), the Orentreich Foundation for the Advancement of Science (NYC), and the Glenn Foundation for Medical Research (Manhasset, NY) and by training grants to the Andrus Gerontology Center (University of Southern California) from the NIH (157) and NIMH (5T22MH0070).

This article was written in March, 1979 and therefore is not our updated review of our current information.

We also warmly acknowledge the generous gift of experimental material from R. C. Adelman (Temple University School of Medicine, Philadelphia, Pennsylvania).

References

ANDEN, N. E., CARLSSON, A., DAHLSTROM, A., FUXE, N., HILLARP, A., and LARSSON, K. (1964). *Life Sci.*, **3**, 523–30.

BANTLE, J. A. and HAHN, W. E. (1976). *Cell*, **7**, 24–52.

CARLSSON, A. and WINBLAD, B. (1976). *J. neural Transmiss.*, **38**, 271–6.

CHACONAS, E. and FINCH, C. E. (1973). *J. Neurochem.*, **21**, 1469–73.

COLEMAN, P. D. KAPLAN, B. B., OSTERBURG, H. H., and FINCH, C. E. (980). *J. Neurochen* **34**, 335–40.

COYLE, J. T. and HENRY, D. (1973). *J. Neurochem.*, **21** 61–7.

CUTLER, R. G. (1973). *Adv. Gerontol.*, **4**, 219–31.

—— (1975). *Exp. Gerontol.*, **10**, 37–60.

FINCH, C. E. (1973). *Brain Res.*, **52**, 261–76.

—— (1976). *Quart. Rev. Biol.*, **51**, 49–83.

—— (1978). In *The aging and reproductive system* (ed. E. L. Schneider), pp. 193–212. Raven Press, New York.

GALAU, G. A., KLEIN, W. H., DAVIS, M. M., WOLD, B. J., BRITTEN, R. J., and DAVIDSON, E. H. (1976). *Cell*, **7**, 487–505.

GORDON, S. M. and FINCH, C. E. (1974). *Exp. Gerontol.*, **9**, 269–73.

HASTIE, N. D. and BISHOP, J. O. (1976). *Cell*, **9**, 761–74.

HOLMES, D. S. and BONNER, J. (1974). *Biochem.*, **13**, 841–8.

HOUGH, B. R., SMITH, M. J., BRITTEN, R. J., and DAVIDSON, E. H. (1975). *Cell*, **5**, 291–9.

KAPLAN, B. B., SCHACHTER, B. S., OSTERBURG, H. H., de VELLIS, J. S., and FINCH, C. E. (1978). *Biochemistry*, **17**, 5516–24.

KIZER, J. S., PALKAVITS, M., and BROWNSTEIN, M. J. (1976). *Brain Res.*, **108**, 363–70.

OSTERBURG, H. H., ALLEN, J. K., and FINCH, C. E. (1975). *Biochem. J.*, **147**, 357–8.

PALKOVITS, M., BROWNSTEIN, M., SAAVEDRA, J. M., and AXELROD, J. (1974) *Brain Res.*, **77**, 137–49.

RIEDERER, P. and WUKETICH, St. (1976). *J. neural Transmiss.*, **38**, 277–301.

RYFFEL, G. U. and McCARTHY, B. J. (1975). *Biochemistry*, **14**, 1379–84.

VAUGHAN, W. J. and CALVIN, M. (1977). *Gerontology*, **23**, 110–26.

Pituitary function and aging Arthur V. Everitt

The concept of the pituitary as a regulator of aging had its origin in the work of Simmonds who in 1914 reported senile changes (muscle weakness, baldness, hair-greying, skin wrinkling, loss of sex functions) in a patient suffering from severe pituitary deficiency. In the 1920s similar observations were made by Pribram (1927) on another patient and by Smith (1926) on hypophysectomized rats. At that time pituitary graft experiments (Zondek and Aschheim 1927; Hoffman 1931; Romeis 1931) indicated that the senile changes in the ovary of rodents leading to loss of oestrous cycles were due to a lack of pituitary hormones (see Aschheim 1976). Thus by the 1930s it appeared that an age-related deficiency of hormones secreted by the pituitary and its target glands could account for some of the involutional changes seen in old age. However with the development of techniques for assaying hormones it has become apparent by the 1970s that overt hormone deficiency states (such as oestrogen- and progesterone-lack in postmenopausal women and gonadotrophin deficiency in old female rats) are the exception rather than the rule in old age (Gregerman and Bierman 1974).

The idea that pituitary hormones like ACTH may have an aging action developed in the 1930s. Among Cushing's (1932) collection of 12 patients one is described as 'a man older than his age' and all patients exhibit one or more features of premature senescence such as hypertension, hypercholesterolaemia, atherosclerosis, and hyperglycaemia. However, it was Raab (1936) who first drew attention to the premature aging of patients with Cushing's syndrome. Other workers have associated the hypersecretion of ACTH and adrenocortical steroids with accelerated aging in patients with Cushing's syndrome (Cantillo 1938; Herman 1967; Wexler 1976) in repeatedly bred rats (Wexler 1964, 1976), and spawning salmon (Robertson, Krupp, Thomas, Favour, Hane, and Wexler 1961; Wexler 1976).

Thus both in man and in experimental animals an increased rate of aging or a premature onset of aging has been associated with both hypo- and hypersecretion of pituitary hormones. If the pituitary gland regulates aging processes then its removal should influence the rate of aging. Therefore in my laboratory we are using hypophysectomized rats to study the relationship between pituitary function and aging. Male Wistar rats are surgically hypophysectomized when young at age 50 to 60 days by the intra-aural technique of Koyama (1962) and the course of aging is followed throughout life. We have examined the effects of long-term hormone replacement therapy with cortisone, growth hormone, and thyroxine and investigated the role of food intake in aging. Our work indicates that the pituitary of the male rat secretes both 'aging' and 'life-maintaining' factors.

Acute effects of hypophysectomy

Within a few weeks after removing the pituitary there is a marked decline in metabolic parameters (viz. food intake, heart rate, creatinine excretion), cessation of growth, failure of reproduction, and diminished renal and cardiovascular function (Everitt and Cavanagh 1965; Everitt 1976a). These functions, once reduced, are maintained at low levels throughout life, and for this reason one would expect hypophysectomized animals to have a reduced rate of aging on the basis of the wear and tear hypothesis.

Collagen aging in tail tendon

The strongest evidence for the anti-aging action of hypophysectomy comes from measurements of collagen fibre aging in rat tail tendon. In 1955 Verzár devised the first test of biological age in which he showed that the tension developed during the thermal contraction of an isolated collagen fibre at 65 °C increased with age. In my laboratory we use a modification (Boros-Farkas and Everitt 1967) of a test developed by Elden and Boucek (1962), in which one measures the time-to-break an isolated collagen fibre under a load of 2 g when immersed in 7 M urea solution at 40 °C.

Life-long studies show that hypophysectomy retards the aging or cohesion of collagen fibres in tail tendon both by the thermal contraction test (Verzár and Spichtin 1966) and the time-to-break test (Olsen and Everitt 1965; Everitt, Olsen, and Burrows 1968; Everitt 1971; Everitt and Delbridge 1972). However, short-term studies demonstrate a phase of accelerated aging during the first month after hypophysectomy in young rats aged 35–50 days (Steinetz, Beach, and Elden 1966; Everitt *et al.* 1968) but not in older rats aged 9 months (Elden 1969). This transient increase in collagen aging is probably due to the failure of collagen synthesis after hypophysectomy (Everitt and Delbridge 1972), and it may involve the adrenal corticosteroids (Elden 1969).

The reduced food intake of hypophysectomized rats (7 g per day compared with 20 g per day in intact controls) is a major factor in the long-term retarded aging of collagen fibres (Olsen and Everitt 1965). Nevertheless, our studies show that hypophysectomy has a significantly greater anti-aging action than food restriction (Everitt 1971; Everitt and Delbridge 1976). At a chronological age of 750 days the 'collagen age' of tail tendon collagen fibres from the hypophysectomized rat is approximately 400 days compared with 500 days in the food-restricted rat eating the same amount of food (Fig. 1). Thus there is residual pituitary hormonal effect on collagen fibre aging, after correcting for food intake. This effect appears to be due in part to the pituitary adrenocorticotrophic hormone (ACTH) which stimulates corticosteroid secretion by the adrenal cortex. Our data show that physiological doses of corticosteroid (1 mg cortisone acetate per week, subcutaneously) increase the aging of tail tendon collagen in hypophysectomized rats although not to the food restriction level (Everitt 1973). It must be appreciated that food-restricted rats are chronically subjected to the stress of partial starvation, which increases corticosteroid secretion and thereby raises the 'collagen age'.

The food-intake-dependent factor is apparently the thyroid hormone (controlled by the pituitary thyroid stimulating hormone, TSH), since thyroxine increases collagen aging in rat tail tendon in direct proportion to its action in raising food intake (Giles and Everitt 1967). Long-term thyroidectomy was found to retard collagen aging in the same manner as long-term hypophysectomy, and its effects were completely reversed by long-term replacement therapy with thyroxine (Giles and Everitt 1967).

Pituitary growth hormone was found in our studies (Everitt 1973) to retard the

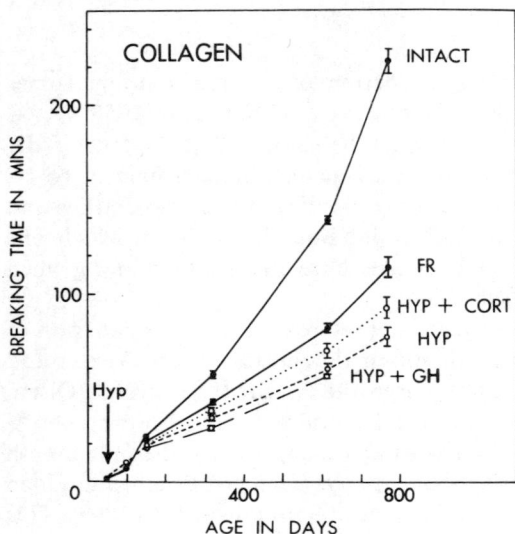

FIG. 1. The effects of hypophysectomy (HYP) and food restriction (FR) in retarding the aging of collagen fibres in rat tail tendon. Life-long cortisone replacement therapy (HYP+CORT) increased collagen aging, whereas growth hormone (HYP+GH) reduced it. Collagen age was measured as the time-to-break an isolated collagen fibre under a load of 2 g when immersed in 7 M urea at 40°C.

aging of collagen as measured by the time-to-break test. This apparent anti-aging effect of growth hormone is probably due to its well known action in stimulating the synthesis of collagen (Aer, Halme, Kivirikko, and Laitinen 1968; Valavaara, Heikkinen, and Kulonen 1968). As the result of increased collagen synthesis, the collagen fibre of the growth-hormone-treated rat contains more 'young' or newly synthesized collagen, and therefore behaves as a younger fibre in the time-to-break test.

Hypophysectomy retards collagen aging because it interferes with cross-linking. Shoshan, Finkelstein, Kushner, and Weinreb (1972) showed that the cross-linking of collagen implants was inhibited in hypophysectomized rats. They postulated that hypophysectomy inhibits the first step in intermolecular cross-linking by diminishing the production and/or activity of lysyl oxidase. Our studies (Delbridge and Everitt 1972) show that hypophysectomy inhibits the conversion of the intermediate labile cross-link described by Bailey (1969) to the stabilized form. As the intact rat ages the labile intermediate bond (which is cleaved by NaH_2PO_4) becomes stabilized in middle age, but this does not occur in hypophysectomized rats (Delbridge and Everitt 1972). Hypophysectomy also prevents the fall in collagen solubility with age, and so the youthful property of high collagen solubility is preserved even in old age (Everitt and Delbridge 1972). Collagen solubility was measured in water at 65 °C for 10 min using fibres previously washed in NaH_2PO_4.

Collagen aging in other tissues

It is generally assumed that age changes in tail tendon collagen mirror age changes in collagen in other organs, such as arteries, bone, and skin. This has been shown by Verzár to be true for skin. Verzár (1960) measured aging in skin collagen by determining the quantity of hydroxyproline released at 65 °C in Ringer solution, and using this test showed that hypophysectomy retarded collagen aging in the dorsal skin of the rat as in tail tendon (Verzár and Spichtin 1966).

Renal aging

Hypophysectomy (Everitt and Duvall 1965; Everitt 1976a) like food-restriction (Saxton and Kimball 1941; Berg and Simms 1960; Bras and Ross 1964) markedly delays the development of age-related kidney disease (variously called nephrosis, glomerulonephritis, glomerulonephrosis, glomerulosclerosis) which occurs in all male Wistar rats in old age. This disease is believed to be of immunological origin (Couser and Stilmant 1976). Its development can be assessed in the living animal by measuring protein excretion (Everitt 1958) since Berg (1965) showed that the degree of proteinuria corresponds to the severity of renal lesions. We are currently measuring protein in 24-hour urine specimens using the trichloracetic acid—Ponceau S reagent (Pesce and Strande 1973). In the hypophysectomized rat protein excretion increases only slowly with age, compared with the rapid rise in the intact rat (Fig. 2). Thus pituitary hormones are necessary for the development of this age-related disease. The male sex hormone (testosterone) also plays a role because in female rats the renal disease is milder (Boorman and Hollander 1973; Hirokawa 1975; Berg 1976), develops later (Berg 1976), and the protein excretion (Sellers, Goodman, Marmorston, and Smith 1960; Perry 1965; Rümke, Breekveldt-Kielich, and Van Den Broecke-Siddré 1970) is considerably less than in the male.

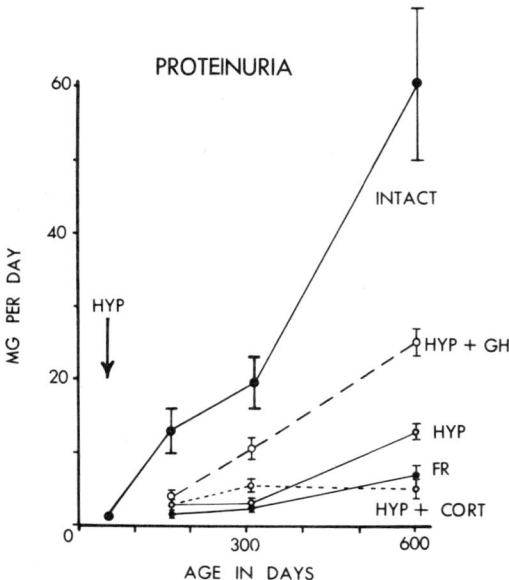

FIG. 2. The effects of hypophysectomy (HYP) and food restriction (FR) in retarding the development of renal disease in the male rat as measured by the 24-hour excretion of protein in urine. Life-long growth hormone replacement therapy (HYP +GH) significantly increased protein excretion, while cortisone therapy (HYP+CORT) significantly reduced it.

In old hypophysectomized rats the histopathological age changes in the kidney are minimal compared with intact rats (Everitt 1976a). Age-associated kidney disease has recently been described by Bras (1969), Hirokawa (1975), and Berg (1976). The kidneys are grossly enlarged in old age and have a light tan colour. Histologically the most obvious change in advanced renal disease is a marked cystic dilatation of tubules containing PAS positive proteinaceous casts. With increasing age glomeruli and tubules are progressively replaced by these cysts and connective tissue. The glomerular count falls with age (Arataki 1926) and the diameter of remaining glomeruli increase (Arataki 1926; Andrew and Pruett 1957). Lymphocytic infiltration is often found. Most workers (Guttman and Kohn 1960; Berg 1965; Striker and Nagel 1969; Elema, Koudstaal, Lamberts, and Arenda 1971) now believe that the primary change is more subtle and occurs in the basement membrane of the glomerulus. Hirokawa (1975) has described the glomerular changes as an increase in mesangial PAS positivity at 3 months, followed by thickening of the capillary basement membrane, fibrous thickening of Bowman's capsule, proliferation of epithelial cells, crescent formation, and hyalinization. Such histopathological changes are less marked in hypophysectomized rats and develop more slowly. In the light microscope the kidney of the old hypophysectomized rat resembles histologically that of the young intact rat. Glomerular diameter does not increase with age and there is significantly less thickening of the basement membranes of the glomerulus and the proximal tubule compared with the control. Grossly the increase in kidney weight with age is significantly less in the hypophysectomized rat.

Important factors affecting the development of age-related renal pathology and proteinuria in the male Wistar rat are the food intake (Saxton and Kimball 1941; Berg and Simms 1960; Bras and Ross 1964; Everitt 1976c), the metabolic rate (Linkswiler, Reynolds, and Bauman 1952; Everitt 1976c) and the hormones which regulate these processes. Presumably these factors are acting on the immune system by affecting the production or action of the immunoglobulin which damages the glomerulus. In hypophysectomized and thyroidectomized rats food intake is reduced and the development of proteinuria and renal pathology are minimal. Age changes in proteinuria are almost independent of food intake up to about 14 g per day (the food consumption of the thyroidectomized rat) and then rise sharply as more food is consumed (Everitt 1976c). Thyroxine raises food intake above this level and increases protein excretion in proportion to the rise in food consumption. Pituitary TSH controls thyroxine secretion and for this reason is considered to be the most significant pituitary factor influencing renal aging. Proteinuria in the hypophysectomized rat is also increased by growth hormone and testosterone (Goodman, Marmorston, Sellers, Smith and Manders 1951). Long-term growth hormone replacement therapy increased renal aging in the hypophysectomized rat but not to the level seen in the intact rat. Growth hormone caused significant increases in glomerular diameter, thickening of Bowman's capsule, thickening of the tubular basement membrane, tubular dilatation, number of proteinaceous casts in the tubules, atrophy of tubules, lymphocytic infiltration, and protein excretion. On the other hand long-term corticosteroid replacement therapy reduced protein excretion but did not affect the histological pattern.

Cardiovascular aging

The heart undergoes hypertrophy in the old rat. This age change develops at a significantly slower rate if the rat is hypophysectomized early in life (Everitt 1976b). Clearly a pituitary factor accelerates this age change. Our studies showed that long-term replacement therapy with either growth hormone or cortisone in physiological amounts did not promote cardiac hypertrophy. However the earlier work of Beznák (1963) indicated that both growth hormone and thyroxine are necessary for experimental cardiac hypertrophy in the young rat.

Age changes in the aorta of the rat are considerably less marked than in man. Spontaneous atherosclerosis is extremely rare in the rat and age changes in elastic properties of the aorta are minimal (Band, Goedhard, and Knoop 1972; Everitt 1976b). However the thickness of the wall of the thoracic aorta increases from 0.20 mm in the young adult rat at 300 days to 0.30 mm in the old rat at 900 days. In the hypophysectomized rat there is only a small increase with age in wall thickness. In a similar manner the diameter of the thoracic aorta increases with age (1.2 mm at 300 days, 1.8 mm at 900 days) in intact rats but not significantly in hypophysectomized animals.

Histological age changes in the aortic tunica media are found to be considerably less severe in the hypophysectomized rat (Everitt 1976b). In the old intact rat Cliff (1970) describes the principal changes as narrowing and branching of the elastic laminae, reduced number and hypertrophy of muscle cells, increased numbers of collagen fibrils, and collections of debris.

The work of Wexler (1976) has shown that hypersecretion of corticosteroids in repeatedly bred rats produces accelerated aging of arteries with an early onset of arteriosclerotic changes. The pituitary glands are enlarged in arteriosclerotic breeder rats (Wexler 1969). The severity of the arterial lesions is increased in breeder rats chronically treated with cortisone (Wexler 1969).

Brain aging

Our preliminary studies show that the weight of the rat's brain increases during growth and declines in old age. The brains of rats hypophysectomized early in life or food restricted from the same time did not show any significant changes with age, after the initial growth to 85 per cent of the control weight.

Skeletal aging

Following hypophysectomy there is almost complete cessation of skeletal and body growth in the rat. In 1954 Ray and co-workers showed that skeletal maturation continues for a very limited period after hypophysectomy, the actual advance being equal to three weeks of normal differentiation. Thyroxine probably accounts for this advance in skeletal age (Ray, Asling, Walker, Simpson, Li, and Evans 1954). In a 508-day-old rat hypophysectomized at 28 days epiphyseal plates which normally close between 85 and 120 days (proximal radius, distal tibia, metacarpals, medial epicondyle of the humerus) had failed to fuse (Simpson, Asling, and Evans 1950). After reviewing the literature Silberberg (1976) concluded that skeletal aging is accelerated by growth hormone and thyroxine and retarded by the corticosteroids.

Skeletal muscle degeneration develops in the hind leg of old rats causing them to drag their hind legs. There is 70 per cent incidence of this disease in 1000-day-old controls. However the hypophysectomized rat of 1000 days is completely free of this disease and can walk normally.

Ovarian aging

In the old female rat oestrous cycles become irregular and there is a loss of fertility even though the ovaries contain large numbers of oocytes (Mandl 1959). Such age changes are not due to ovarian deficiency (as in the human female) because normal cycles can be restored by the administration of pituitary extract (Everitt 1939) or gonadotrophin (Aschheim 1965) and ovulation can be induced by electric stimulation of the preoptic area of the hypothalamus (Clemens, Amenomori, Jenkins, and Meites 1969). Furthermore Aschheim (1964/1965) showed that the ovaries from senile rats, when transplanted into young adult spayed rats, restore normal cycles, but young rat ovaries do not cycle after transplantation to an old host. Aschheim (1976) believes that the primary failure resides in the hypothalamus. Hypophysectomy in the rat changes the ovarian interstitial cells into deficiency cells which are normally seen only in the senile ovary (Aschheim 1976) and such changes can be reversed with pituitary gonadotrophic hormone. Here is one example of an age change brought on by hormonal deficiency.

In the CBA mouse Jones and Krohn (1961) showed that hypophysectomy significantly retards, but does not prevent, the normal progressive loss of oocytes from the ovary with age. The ovaries of mice hypophysectomized 300 days previously when grafted into young ovariectomized recipients lead to normal pregnancies, whereas the ovaries of the intact mice are sterile. One ovarian graft from a hypophysectomized CBA mouse gave birth to its last litter at 502 days. In the normal CBA mouse oocytes have disappeared completely at age 430 days. Ingram (1953) in an earlier study on the rat also reported a slower disappearance of oocytes after hypophysectomy but his data were not statistically significant.

Metabolic aging

Denckla (1974) has shown a 75 per cent decline with age (from 3 to 52 weeks) in the minimal oxygen consumption of the female rat (ml O_2 at STP/min/100 g fat-free body weight) measured under pentobarbitone anaesthesia at the thermo-neutral temperature (Denckla and Marcum 1973). A considerable part of this metabolic decline, according to Denckla (1974), is due to a pituitary factor (called DECO) which decreases the responsiveness of peripheral tissues to thyroid hormones. He finds that immature rats are three times more responsive to thyroxine than adults and hypophysectomy arrests the normal age-associated decrease in responsiveness to thyroxine (Denckla 1974). In adult rats hypophysectomy partly restores the tissue responsiveness to thyroxine (Denckla 1974).

Immune aging

Denckla (1976) has shown that hypophysectomy in the female rat has a delayed effect in restoring immune competence which normally decreases with age. Immune function was measured by the rejection of mouse skin grafts and phagocytosis of colloidal carbon. The loss of competence with age in these two defence systems of the body is reversed to juvenile levels 16 to 40 weeks after hypophysectomy in rats receiving thyroxine and corticosterone replacement therapy. Thyroxine appears to be the critical hormone required to restore competence. More recently Scott, Bolla, and Denckla (1979) found that long-term hypophysectomy with minimal hormone replacement therapy delayed the age-related decline in the immune response of rats to sheep erythrocytes.

Tumour incidence

It has been known for many years that hypophysectomy will suppress experimental tumourigenesis in the rat (Moon, Simpson, Li, and Evans 1951; Moon and Simpson 1955; Dodge, O'Neal, Chang, and Griffin 1961; Isler 1967; Nadler, Mandavia, and Goldberg 1970). In a similar way destruction of the pituitary in the rat by deuteron irradiation was found to suppress the development of spontaneous tumours in pituitary-dependent endocrine glands of the male rat, 27 months after irradiation (Van Dyke, Simpson, Koneff, and Tobias 1959).

In my laboratory gross examination of 40 old male (800 to 1312 days) hypophysectomized rats revealed only 3 rats with tumours, compared with 22 in a randomly chosen series of age-matched intact male rats, excluding three rats which had only a pituitary tumour. Hypophysectomy obviously eliminates pituitary tumours which are found at autopsy in 26 per cent of intact males 800 days or older. About 70 per cent of tumours grossly seen at autopsy occurred in the pituitary, adrenals, or testes.

Life duration

An intact pituitary gland is essential for a normal life span in the male Wistar rat, since hypophysectomy significantly shortens the duration of life (Fig. 3). Corticosteroid replacement therapy (1 mg cortisone acetate per week subcutaneously) restored the life duration of hypophysectomized rats to normal when housed at 28 °C and fed a commercial rat chow. The mode of action of cortisone in preventing deaths in hypophysectomized rats was difficult to identify, since most hypophysectomized rats die without obvious signs of disease. The

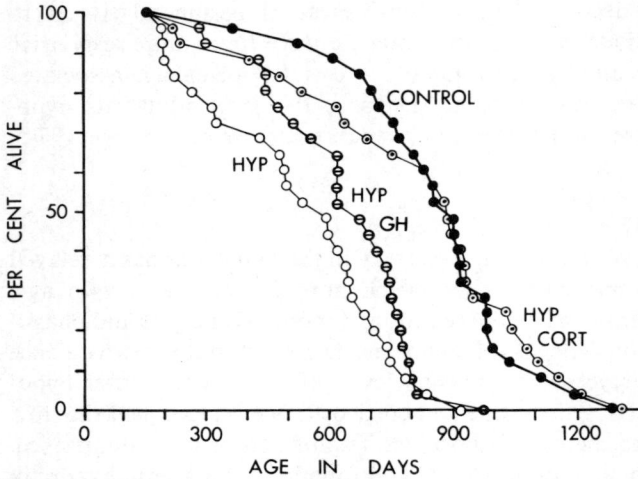

FIG. 3. Survival curves of male Wistar rats showing the life-shortening action of hypophy-sectomy (HYP) and the restoration of normal life expectancy by life-long cortisone acetate replacement therapy (HYP+CORT). Growth hormone therapy (HYP+GH) did not significantly increase life duration.

tissues of old hypophysectomized rats are remarkably free of pathological lesions. However, it was discovered that hypophysectomized rats had very low blood sugar levels when near death. It is now believed that cortisone increases survival because it prevents the development of hypoglycaemia which is a common cause of death in our hypophysectomized rats (Everitt 1976a). Boros-Farkas and Verzár (1967) found that 5 per cent glucose as drinking water significantly prolongs the life of the hypophysectomized rat. Growth hormone replacement therapy (1 unit hog (Raben-type) growth hormone per day) reduced early mortality but did not significantly increase life duration (Everitt and Burgess 1976).

Discussion

It is quite apparent from the data presented here that the pituitary affects aging processes in collagen, kidney, heart, aorta, skeleton, ovary, tissue metabolism, and the immune system. It influences tumourigenesis and is a determinant of the life duration. Obviously, the course of aging, the development of the diseases of old age, and the duration of life are strongly influenced by pituitary hormones. I propose that the pituitary regulates not only the process of aging, but also the onset of terminal pathology which determines the duration of life (Everitt 1973, 1976d), and that it does this by mediation of its hormones and the hormones secreted by its target glands.

We can now identify four types of pituitary factor which affect aging and the duration of life: 1. life-maintaining factors; 2. life-shortening factors; 3. aging factors; and 4. anti-aging factors.

1. *Life-maintaining factors.* Since corticosteroid replacement therapy restores the life duration of the hypophysectomized rat to normal (Fig. 3) the pituitary life-maintaining factor thus identified must be ACTH which controls the secretion of corticosteroids (Everitt 1973, 1976d). Corticosteroids may increase survival by either a metabolic action affecting the blood sugar level as discussed earlier, or by increasing immunity to infectious diseases (Beisel and Rappoport 1969).

Temperature regulation is not a problem for these rats since the temperature of the rat quarters is maintained at 28 °C, which is in the thermoneutral zone of the rat. However, if the ambient temperature were lower rats would have to increase their heat production with the aid of thyroid hormones in order to maintain body temperature. Thus at lower temperatures thyroid hormones and hence pituitary TSH would become important determinants of survival. There may be other pituitary life-maintaining factors, for example, Friedman and Friedman (1963) have shown that posterior pituitary hormones increase the life span of old rats.

2. *Life-shortening factors.* Direct evidence for a life-shortening factor comes from the study of Larsen (1973) who showed that the life span of the lamprey is increased by hypophysectomy. Further evidence comes from Silberberg (1972) who has reported that hypo-pituitary dwarf mice are long-lived. The pituitary can shorten life by either pathological or hormonal mechanisms.

The pituitary of the old female Wistar (WAG/Rij) rat has a life-shortening action because it develops chromophobe adenoma in 69 per cent of animals. This tumour compresses the brain and appears to be the most common factor limiting life span in these rats over one year of age (Boorman and Hollander 1973). However this is not true for all rats since there are large sex and strain differences in the incidence of pituitary tumours (Saxton and Graham 1944).

Denckla (1975) postulates that the pituitary factor DECO (decreasing oxygen consumption hormone) reduces the response of peripheral tissues to thyroxine and so leads to the decline and failure of the immune and circulatory systems resulting in death. Thus the pituitary may also shorten life by secreting one or more hormones which accelerate the rate of aging, and so shorten life.

3. *Aging and anti-aging factors.* Hypophysectomy as we have seen retards aging processes in tail tendon collagen, skin collagen, kidney, heart, aorta, skeleton, ovary, and the immune system, and reduces the frequency of tumours and other pathological processes in the old rat. Thus the pituitary must secrete one or more aging factors. However, there is little evidence for the existence of a general pituitary aging hormone which would accelerate physiological aging and increase the incidence of age-related pathology. Instead each hormone exhibits specific effects; it may have an aging action in one tissue and retard aging in another. For example ACTH and the adrenocortical hormones inhibit skeletal aging (Silberberg 1976), but accelerate the aging of the tail tendon (Árvay and Takács 1965), and in large amounts lead to a premature onset of cardiovascular (Wexler 1976) and renal (Christian 1976) disease. Thyroid hormones accelerate collagen (Giles and Everitt 1967; Everitt *et al.* 1969), skeletal (Silberberg 1976),

and renal aging (Everitt 1976c), but appear to have inhibitory actions on atherosclerosis (Everitt 1976c), aging of the immune system (Denckla 1975), and tumourigenesis (Everitt 1976c). Growth hormone appears to inhibit the aging of tail tendon collagen (Everitt and Delbridge 1976) accelerate skeletal aging (Silberberg 1976), promote cardiovascular and renal disease (Everitt and Burgess 1976), and increase the incidence of tumours in rats (Moon, Simpson, Li, and Evans 1950). As mentioned earlier, Denckla (1975) has presented evidence suggesting that the pituitary factor DECO accelerates aging in the immune and circulatory systems.

4. *Pituitary hyposecretion.* We have seen that a reduction in hormone output as in the hypophysectomized rat retards aging in many systems. A similar pattern of retarded aging is seen in the food-restricted rat (Everitt and Porter 1976). It has been shown by many workers that in the chronically underfed rat the secretion of almost all pituitary and target gland hormones is reduced (a condition which Mulinos and Pomerantz (1940) called pseudohypophysectomy, see review Everitt and Porter 1976), the principal exception being ACTH and the adrenocortical hormones. It was therefore postulated that the hypophysectomized rat receiving corticosterone would have a long life duration like the food-restricted rat. Our data show that the life duration of the hypophysectomized rat is increased but is less than that of the food-restricted control. Perhaps a larger dose of corticosteroid is needed or possibly other hormones need replacing as in Denckla's studies.

Nevertheless it must not be forgotten that a lack of pituitary hormones can produce aging changes as in the case of gonadotrophin deficiency accelerating ovarian aging in the old female rat (Aschheim 1976). However, this age change is a life-prolonging mechanism since by preventing pregnancy it reduces mortality in old age.

5. *Pituitary hypersecretion.* What happens to the aging process under conditions of pituitary hypersecretion? Pregnancy in the repeatedly bred rat increases the secretion of most pituitary hormones including ACTH which by mediation of the adrenocortical hormones accelerates cardiovascular (Wexler 1976) and collagen (Árvay and Takács 1965) aging. The life-long exposure of rats to low temperature (9 °C) has an aging and life-shortening action which apparently is mediated through the hypothalamic–pituitary–thyroid axis (Johnson, Kintner, and Kibler 1963; Johnson, Kibler, and Silsby 1964; Everitt 1976c). Continuous exposure to stress which augments pituitary hormone secretion increases physiological aging, accelerates the onset of age-related pathology, and shortens life (Selye and Tuchweber 1976). Dilman (1976) has proposed that age-related elevation of the hypothalamic threshold to feedback inhibition increases the secretion of pituitary and other hormones leading to an early onset of age-specific pathology.

6. *Hypothalamic factors and aging centre.* The hypothalamus dominates and drives the pituitary by means of specific releasing hormones. There are also input signals to the hypothalamus from other parts of the brain conveyed by biogenic amines including the catecholamines which according to Finch (1975) play an

important role in aging. Consequently when we speak of the pituitary as a regulator of aging we must also include the hypothalamus and higher centres which control its function. Environmental factors both internal (peripheral aging, pregnancy, disease) and external (stress, food supply, temperature, bacteria, viruses) which affect the rate of aging are probably acting to a large extent by mediation of the hypothalamic–pituitary–peripheral endocrine axis. It has been postulated (Everitt 1976d) that many environmental factors act on a genetically controlled 'aging clock' or centre located in the hypothalamus, which precisely times events in the life programme. The hormones are seen as the effectors or chemical messengers which relay the signal from the aging centre to the tissues, which as a result of long-continued hormonal action undergo cell damage or aging by a variety of mechanisms (metabolic, immunological, or genetic) as suggested in Fig. 4. Collagen aging apparently is influenced mainly by metabolic processes via lysyl oxidase, whereas age-related renal disease seems to be due to immunological damage. Adelman (1976) has discussed the role of hormones in regulating gene expression in aging phenomena.

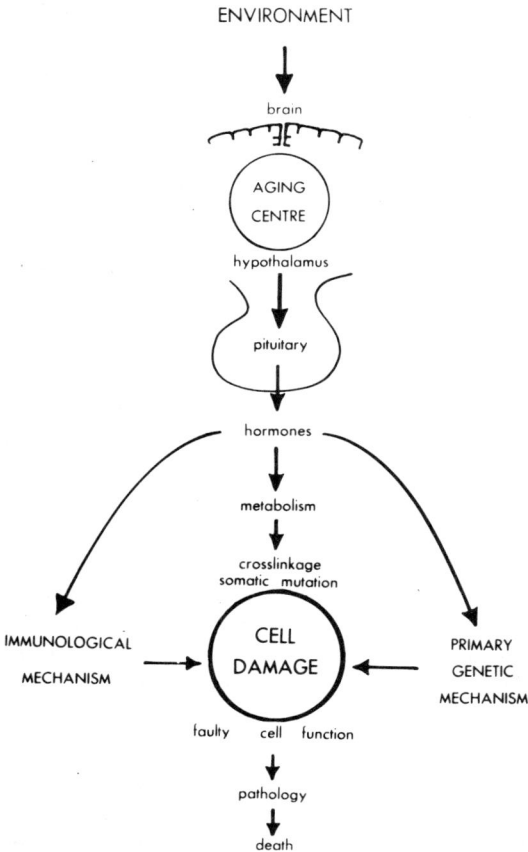

FIG. 4. The role of the pituitary in regulating aging processes. The rate of aging (or cell damage) is primarily under genetic control, but is modified by environmental factors acting via neuroendocrine mechanisms. It is postulated that information from the environment (both internal and external) is relayed to an aging centre in the hypothalamus which regulates the rate of aging by altering the secretion of pituitary and other hormones. The hormones interact with metabolic, immunological, and genetic mechanisms of aging.

Conclusions

Our studies show that the pituitary gland is essential for a normal life span in the male Wistar rat. In its absence the life span is shortened, but may be restored to normal by life-long replacement therapy with cortisone, if the animals are housed in a warm room at 28 °C. For this reason the corticosteroids and pituitary ACTH which controls their secretion are termed life-maintaining hormones.

Most hormones of the anterior pituitary and its target glands (thyroid, adrenal, and gonads) accelerate physiological aging and increase the incidence of age-related pathology in the kidney and cardiovascular system. Therefore hypophysectomy in the rat retards aging processes in tail tendon collagen, skin collagen, kidney, heart, aorta, skeleton, and the immune system, and reduces the frequency of tumours and many other pathological processes in old age.

Many external and internal environmental factors (viz. stress, temperature, food supply, pregnancy) which alter the rate of aging act on the hypothalamic–pituitary–peripheral endocrine system. It is proposed that information from the environment is relayed to an aging centre in the hypothalamus which modifies the secretion of pituitary and other hormones affecting the rate of aging.

Addendum

1. *Effects of hypophysectomy in middle age*

Hypophysectomy performed on male Wistar rats at 400 days retards the aging of both tail tendon collagen and the kidney as measured by protein excretion. After removal of the pituitary moderate levels of proteinuria in middle age fall progressively to low levels in old age. Middle-age hypophysectomy produced considerably less retardation of collagen aging than hypophysectomy in youth. Unfortunately middle-aged rats are less able to withstand the effects of hypophysectomy than young rats. Even with cortisone replacement therapy, life duration is significantly shortened. Apparently other hormones such as thyroxine as used by Denckla in his hormone cocktail are necessary for long-term survival after hypophysectomy in middle age (Everitt, Seedsman, and Jones, 1980).

2. *Effects of hypothatamic lesions*

Recently we found that ventromedial hypothalamic lesions in young male rats aged 70 days doubled the food intake, but did not increase the rate of aging of collagen nor raise the excretion of protein throughout the life span. This study suggests that the anti-aging action of hypophysectomy is due to loss of pituitary hormones rather than the fall in food intake (Everitt, in preparation).

Acknowledgements

I am especially grateful to Frank Jones, who performed most of the hypophysectomies. The studies reported here were supported in part by grants from the Consolidated Medical Research Fund of the University of Sydney and the University Research Grant. Cortisone acetate was generously supplied by Roussel Pharmaceuticals, Sydney. Figures 1, 3, and 4 are reproduced, with modifications and additions, from Everitt and Burgess (eds) *Hypothalamus, pituitary, and aging* with permission of the publisher, Charles C. Thomas, Springfield, Ill., USA.

References

ADELMAN, R. C. (1976). In *Hypothalamus, pituitary and aging* (ed. A. V. Everitt and J. A. Burgess), p. 668. Thomas, Springfield, Illinois.

AER, J., HALME, J., KIVIRIKKO, K. I., and LAITINEN, O. (1968). *Biochem. Pharmacol.*, **17**, 1173.

ANDREW, W. and PRUETT, D. (1957). *Amer. J. Anat.*, **100**, 51.

ARATAKI, M. (1926). *Amer. J. Anat.*, **36**, 399.

ARVÁY, A. and TAKACS, I. (1965). *Gerontologia*, **11**, 188.

ASCHHEIM, P. (1964/1965). *Gerontologia*, **10**, 65.

—— (1965). *C.R. Acad. Sci. (Paris)*, **260**, 5627.

—— (1976). In *Hypothalamus, pituitary and aging* (ed. A. V. Everitt and J. A. Burgess), p. 390. Thomas, Springfield, Illinois.

BAILEY, A. J. (1969). *Gerontologia*, **15**, 65.

BAND, W., GOEDHARD, W. J. A., and KNOOP, A. A. (1972). *Pflüger's Archiv*, **331**, 357

BEISEL, W. R. and RAPPOPORT, M. I. (1969). *New Engl. J. Med.*, **280**, 541.

BERG, B. N. (1965). *Proc. Soc. exp. Biol. Med.*, **119**, 417.

—— (1976). In *Hypothalamus, pituitary and aging* (ed. A. V. Everitt and J. A. Burgess), p. 43. Thomas, Springfield, Illinois.

—— and SIMMS, H. S. (1960). *J. Nutr.*, **71**, 255.

BEZNÁK, M. (1963). *Amer. J. Physiol.*, **204**, 279.

BOORMAN, G. A. and HOLLANDER, C. F. (1973). *J. Geront.*, **28**, 152.

BOROS-FARKAS, M. and EVERITT, A. V. (1967). *Gerontologia*, **13**, 37.

—— and VERZÁR, F. (1967). *Gerontologia*, **13**, 50.

BRAS, G. (1969). *J. infect. Dis.*, **120**, 131.

—— and ROSS, M. H. (1964). *Toxicol. appl. Pharmacol.*, **6**, 247.

CANTILLO, E. (1938). *Presse med.*, **46**, 1900.

CHRISTIAN, J. J. (1976). In *Hypothalamus, pituitary and aging* (ed. A. V. Everitt and J. A. Burgess), p. 297. Thomas, Springfield, Illinois.

CLEMENS, J. A., AMENOMORI, Y., JENKINS, T., and MEITES, J. (1969). *Proc. Soc. exp. Biol. Med.*, **132**, 561.

CLIFF, W. J. (1970). *Exp. mol. Pathol.*, **13**, 172.

COUSER, W. G. and STILMANT, M. M. (1976). *J. Geront.*, **31**, 13

CUSHING, H. (1932). *Bull. Johns Hopkins Hosp.*, **50**, 137.

DELBRIDGE, L. and EVERITT, A. V. (1972). *Exp. Gerontol.*, **7**, 413.

DENCKLA, W. D. (1974). *J. clin. Invest.*, **53**, 572.

—— (1975). *Life Sci.*, **16**, 31.

—— (1976). In *Hypothalamus, pituitary and aging* (ed. A. V. Everitt and J. A. Burgess), p. 703. Thomas, Springfield, Illinois.

—— and MARCUM, E. (1973). *Endocrinol.*, **93**, 61.

DILMAN, V. M. (1976). In *Hypothalamus, pituitary and aging* (ed. A. V. Everitt and J. A. Burgess), p. 634. Thomas, Springfield, Illinois.

DODGE, B. G., O'NEAL, M. A., CHANG, J. P., and GRIFFIN, A. C. (1961). *J. nat. cancer. Inst.*, **27**, 817.

ELDEN, H. R. (1969). *Trans. NY Acad. Sci.*, **31**, 855.

—— and BOUCEK, R. J. (1962). In *Biological aspects of aging* (eds. N. W. Shock), p. 334. Columbia University Press, New York.

ELEMA, J. D., KOUDSTAAL, J., LAMBERTS, H. B., and ARENDA, A. (1971). *Arch. Path.*, **91**, 418.

EVERETT, J. W. (1939). *Endocrinology*, **25**, 123.

EVERITT, A. V. (1958). *Gerontologia*, **2**, 33.

—— (1971). *Proc. Aust. Assoc. Geront.*, **1**, 127.

—— (1973). *Exp. Geront.*, **8**, 265.

—— (1976a). In *Hypothalamus, pituitary and aging* (ed. A. V. Everitt and J. A. Burgess), p. 68. Thomas, Springfield, Illinois.

—— (1976b). In *Hypothalamus, pituitary and aging* (ed. A. V. Everitt and J. A. Burgess), p. 262. Thomas, Sprinfield, Illinois.

—— (1976c). In *Hypothalamus, pituitary and aging* (ed. A. V. Everitt and J. A. Burgess), p. 511. Thomas, Springfield, Illinois.

—— (1976d). In *Hypothalamus, pituitary and aging* (ed. A. V. Everitt and J. A. Burgess), p. 676. Thomas, Springfield, Illinois.

—— and BURGESS, J. A. (1976). In *Hypothalamus, pituitary and aging* (ed. A. V. Everitt and J. A. Burgess), p. 464. Thomas, Springfield, Illinois.

—— and CAVANAGH, L. M. (1965). *Gerontologia*, **11**, 198.

—— and DELBRIDGE, L. (1972). *Exp. Gerontol.*, **7**, 45.

—— and —— (1976). In *Hypothalamus, pituitary and aging* (ed. A. V. Everitt and J. A Burgess), p. 193. Thomas, Springfield, Illinois.

—— and DUVALL, L. K. (1965). *Nature (Lond.)*, **205**, 1015.

——, GILES, J. S., and GAL, A. (1969). *Gerontologia*, **15**, 366.

——, OLSEN, G. G., and BURROWS, G. R. (1968). *J. Gerontol.*, **23**, 333.

—— and PORTER, B. (1976). In *Hypothalamus, pituitary and aging* (ed. A. V. Everitt and J. A. Burgess), p. 570. Thomas, Springfield, Illinois.

——, SEEDSMAN, N., and JONES, F. (1980). The effects of hypophysectomy and continuous food restriction, began at ages 70 and 400 days, on collagen aging, proteinuria, incidence of pathology and longevity in the male rat. *Mech. Age Devl.*, **12**, 161.

FINCH, C. E. (1975). *Adv. exp. Med. Biol.*, **61**, 229.

FRIEDMAN, S. M. and FRIEDMAN, C. L. (1963). *Nature (Lond.)*, **200**, 237.

GILES, J. S. and EVERITT, A. V. (1967). *Gerontologia*, **13**, 65.

GOODMAN, H. C., MARMORSTON, J., SELLERS, A. L., SMITH, S., and MANDERS, J. (1951). *Endocrinology*, **49**, 490.

GREGERMAN, R. I. and BIERMAN, E. L. (1974). In *Textbook of endocrinology* (ed. R. H. Williams), p. 1059. Saunders, Philadelphia.

GUTTMAN, P. H. and KOHN, H. I. (1960). *Amer. J. Path.*, **37**, 293.

HERMAN, E. (1967). *J. neur. Sci.*, **4**, 101.

HIROKAWA, K. (1975). *Mech. Age Dev.*, **4**, 301.

HOFFMAN, J. (1931). *Amer. J. Obstet. Gynec.*, **22**, 231.

INGRAM, D. L. (1953). *J. Endocrinol.*, **9**, 307.

ISLER, H. (1967). *Anat. Rec.*, **157**, 263.

JOHNSON, H. D., KIBLER, H. H., and SILSBY, H. (1964). *Gerontologia*, **9**, 18.

——, KINTNER, L. D., and KIBLER, H. H. (1963). *J. Gerontol.*, **18**, 29.
JONES, E. C. and KROHN, P. L. (1961). *J. Endocrinol.*, **21**, 497.
KOYAMA, R. (1962). *Endocrinol. Jap.*, **9**, 321.
LARSEN, L. O. (1973). *Development in adult freshwater lampreys and its hormonal control.* University of Copenhagen.
LINKSWILER, H., REYNOLDS, M. S., and BAUMAN, C. A. (1952). *Amer. J. Physiol.*, **168**, 504.
MANDL, A. L. (1959). *J. Endocrinol.*, **18**, 444.
MOON, H. D. and SIMPSON, M. E. (1955). *Cancer Res.*, **15**, 403.
——, ——, LI, C. H., and EVANS, H. M. (1950). *Cancer Res.*, **10**, 297, 364, 549.
——, ——, ——, and —— (1951). *Cancer Res.*, **11**, 535.
MULINOS, M. G. and POMERANTZ, L. (1940). *J. Nutr.*, **19**, 493.
NADLER, N. J., MANDAVIA, M., and GOLDBERG, M. (1970). *Cancer Res.*, **30**, 1909.
OLSEN, G. G. and EVERITT, A. V. (1965). *Nature (Lond.)*, **206**, 307.
PERRY, S. W. (1965). *J. Path. Bact.*, **89**, 729.
PESCE, M. A. and STRANDE, C. S. (1973). *Clin. Chem.*, **19**, 1265.
PRIBRAM, B. O. (1927). *Virchows Arch. Path. Anat.*, **264**, 498.
RAAB, W. (1936). *Wien Klin. Woch.*, **49**, 112.
RAY, R. D., ASLING, C. W., WALKER, D. G., SIMPSON, M. E., LI, C. H., and EVANS, H. M. (1954). *J. bone joint Surg.*, **36A**, 94.
ROBERTSON, O. H., KRUPP, M. A., THOMAS, S. F., FAVOUR, C. B., HANE, S., and WEXLER, B. C. (1961). *J. comp. Endocrinol.*, **1**, 473.
ROMEIS, B. (1931). In *Handbuch der inneren Sekretion* (ed. M. Hirsch), Vol. 2, p. 1960. Kabisch, Leipzig. (Cited by Aschheim (1976).)
RÜMKE, P., BREEKVELDT-KIELICH, J. C., and VAN DEN BROECKE-SIDDRÉ, A. (1970). *Biochim. biophys. Acta (Amst.)*, **200**, 275.
SAXTON, J. A. and GRAHAM, J. B. (1944). *Cancer Res.*, **4**, 168.
—— and KIMBALL, G. C. (1941). *Arch. Path.*, **32**, 951.
SCOTT, M., BOLLA, R., and DENCKLA, W. D. (1979), *Mech. Age Devl.*, **11**, 127.
SELLERS, A. L., GOODMAN, H. C., MARMORSTON, J., and SMITH, M. (1950). *Amer. J. Physiol.*, **163**, 662.
SELYE, H. and TUCHWEBER, B. (1976). *In Hypothalamus, pituitary and aging* (ed. A. V. Everitt and J. A. Burgess), p. 553. Thomas, Springfield, Illinois.
SHOSHAN, S., FINKELSTEIN, S., KUSHNER, W., and WEINREB, M. M. (1972). *Conn. Tissue Res.*, **1**, 47.
SILBERBERG, R. (1972). *Path. Microbiol.*, **38**, 417.
—— (1976). In *Hypothalamus, pituitary and aging* (ed. A. V. Everitt and J. A. Burgess), p. 209. Thomas, Springfield, Illinois.
SIMMONDS, M. (1914). *Dtsch. med. Woch.*, **40**, 322.
SIMPSON, M. E., ASLING, C. W., and EVANS, H. M. (1950), *Yale J. Biol. Med.*, **23**, 1.
SMITH, P. E. (1926). *Anat. Rec.*, **32**, 221.
STEINETZ, B. G., BEACH, V. L., and ELDEN, H. R. (1966). *Endocrinol.*, **79**, 1047.
STRIKER, G. E. and NAGEL, R. B. (1969). *Arch. Path.*, **87**, 439.
VALAVAARA, M., HEIKKINEN, E., and KULONEN, E. (1968). *Experientia*, **24**, 779.
VAN DYKE, D. C., SIMPSON, M. E., KONEFF, A. A., and TOBIAS, C. A. (1959). *Endocrinol.*, **64**, 240.
VERZÁR, F. (1955). *Experientia*, **11**, 230.
—— (1960). *Gerontologia*, **4**, 104.
—— and SPICHTIN, H. (1966). *Gerontologia*, **12**, 48.

WEXLER, B. C. (1964). *Acta Endocrinol. (kbh.)*, **46**, 613.

—— (1969). *J. atheroscl. Res.*, **9**, 267.

—— (1976). In *Hypothalamus, pituitary and aging* (ed. A. V. Everitt and J. A. Burgess), p. 333. Thomas, Springfield, Illinois.

ZONDEK, B. and ASCHHEIM, S. (1927). *Arch. f. Gynäk.*, **130**, 35.

CHAPTER IV

Session 17

Indices of physiological age

Introduction F. Bourlière

For a long time experimental gerontologists and demographers have been confusing mortality rate with rate of aging. Aging itself has been sometimes defined as an increase of a so-called 'force of mortality'. This was to confuse somewhat causes and consequences.

Very quickly, however, it has become clear that mortality and aging were not obligatorily correlated. Animals seldom die of old age in natural conditions — predation, parasitism, and accidents being the major causes of death. A very similar situation prevails in many human populations, outside the industrialized world. Even in our own society the steep and temporary increase in mortality rate which occurs in young males between 18 and 25 years of age has nothing to do with aging, but with a higher incidence of traffic accidents.

The 'quality' of life, on the other hand, does not remain the same throughout the so-called adult period of life. The level of performance of many of our functions is obviously very different at 20, 40, 60, and 80 years of age—even in clinically healthy individuals followed longitudinally, though the decline in performance is often less obvious than in cross-sectional studies.

The three contributors to this session, all belonging to the Baltimore Gerontology Center, will thoroughly review the present state of knowledge on indices of biological age. They will attempt to define the conditions in which some of these indices can be used to quantify the decline in performance of the aging organism.

They will also, I hope, discuss the possible *predictive value* of some of them— a domain of practical importance for those concerned with the identification of 'high risk groups' among adults. This is not an easy task, because all age changes are not obligatorily due to aging processes; some of them are the consequence of specific diseases, and others have an obvious adaptive value as shown by some speakers of yesterday afternoon's session. During the so called 'adult life' the control mechanisms of our body have to adapt to the changes in body composition, lean body mass, etc., taking place throughout our life span, in order to maintain the homeostasis of the organism.

Last, but not least, it must be mentioned that physiological and biochemical tests have a great advantage over the psychometric tests so often used to appreciate functional age. They are *'culture-free'*, can be repeatedly used in the same individual, and are not open to the kind of criticisms some psychometric tests are. They enable the gerontologist to compare various human populations differing by their genetic constitution and their environmental conditions, in a very objective way. They are therefore an unique tool for those concerned with the causal analysis of differential aging in man.

Indices of functional age N. W. Shock

Casual observation indicates that there are wide individual differences in the effects of age on all human performances. Each of us has concluded that some adults seem 'young for their age', recognizing that there are often discrepancies between the progression of changes in an individual with the passage of time and his chronological age. These discrepancies have led to the expression of dissatisfaction with the use of chronological age as the sole criterion for retirement. Furthermore, if we are to test the efficacy of regimes designed to minimize the effects of aging (Comfort 1969), valid indices of functional age are essential.

As early as 1963 the European Bureau of the World Health Organization during a seminar held in Kiev recommended that methods be developed for the determination of biological age (Ries 1974) in order to provide a more rational basis for dealing with retirement and employment of older workers. In 1970 the World Health Organization sponsored a detailed report on *The assessment of biological age in man* which was prepared by Professor Bourlière (1970). In this report, Professor Bourlière summarized much of the data available on changes in physiological functions with age and made recommendations about possible approaches to the development of an index of biological age.

It is, therefore, clear that in addition to its theoretical importance to gerontology†, the identification of a reliable and valid index of biological or functional age is of great practical importance. It is a primary challenge to gerontologists.

The purpose of this paper is to examine:
(1) possible approaches to the problem;
(2) the essential characteristics of an index of functional age and criteria for the tests to be included;
(3) the current status of research;
(4) potentials for the future.

Approaches to the problem

If functional or biological age is to be substituted for chronological age for administrative decisions relating to retirement, employment, or current health status, it is clear that a single index number should be derived for each individual.

---

† It is recognized that, from a theoretical standpoint, indices of 'functional age' are needed for different animal species, such as the rat, mouse, dog, etc., as well. However, this presentation will be limited to a discussion of indices for humans.

This approach makes the implicit assumption that 'functional age' is a single characteristic which can be quantified. Conceptually, it may be regarded as similar to 'mental age' which was first developed by Binet on the basis of performance scores on a battery of tests involving a variety of mental performances. However, it must be remembered that the combination of tests was validated against a rating of 'intelligence' as estimated by teachers who had observed the performance of each child in school classes. Following this model would require the assignment of some estimate of 'functional age' to each individual based on judgements other than chronological age. At present, no such criterion is available for adults and it is doubtful whether similar ratings could be obtained since few judges could be found who would be able to observe an adult subject over a broad spectrum of adult activities.

In view of these difficulties in establishing a 'criterion score' we are faced with having to use chronological age as a basis for judging the validity of any index of functional age. At first this seems to be nonsensical—since, if the index correlated perfectly with chronological age, it would not provide any additional information about the performance status of the individual.

However, one may assume that ideally functional age and chronological age should be the same and that discrepancies between the two represent the meaningful statistic in evaluating deviations in the performance of the individual. In fact, the high degree of variance in physiological and psychological performances shown among individuals of a given chronological age indicates the applicability of this idea (Fig. 1) (Brandfonbrener, Landowne, and Shock 1955). It is clear from Fig. 1 that some 70-year-old subjects have resting cardiac outputs as good as the average for subjects 20 years their junior.

On the average, changes over time in the performances of different organ systems (Fig. 2) proceed at different rates (Shock 1972). Thus nerve conduction velocity diminishes only 10 per cent between the ages of 30 and 70 (Fig. 2(b)) in contrast to renal function which falls by 50 per cent over the same age span (Fig. 2(d)). Furthermore the same individual may show different rates of change with time among different organ systems. Thus a 60-year-old subject may have a cardiac output equivalent to the average value for 60-year-olds, but a kidney blood flow equal to the average value for 40-year-olds. These differences in organ performance indicate clearly that each subject must be evaluated on a variety of performances. One approach to the problem would be to prepare a profile on each subject which indicates his percentile rank among his age peers for each performance. Figures 3 and 4 represent examples of how a subject's percentile rank can be assessed with respect to kidney function (Rowe, Andres, Tobin, Norris, and Shock 1976) and glucose tolerance (Andres 1972).

A straight line drawn between the subject's age and his creatinine clearance (or glucose tolerance) will intersect the percentile rank scale at his percentile rank. Subjects with high percentile ranks have performances better than the average of the subject's age peers.

Thus it is possible to derive a percentile rank score for each individual with respect to a variety of performances, providing test data are available for a

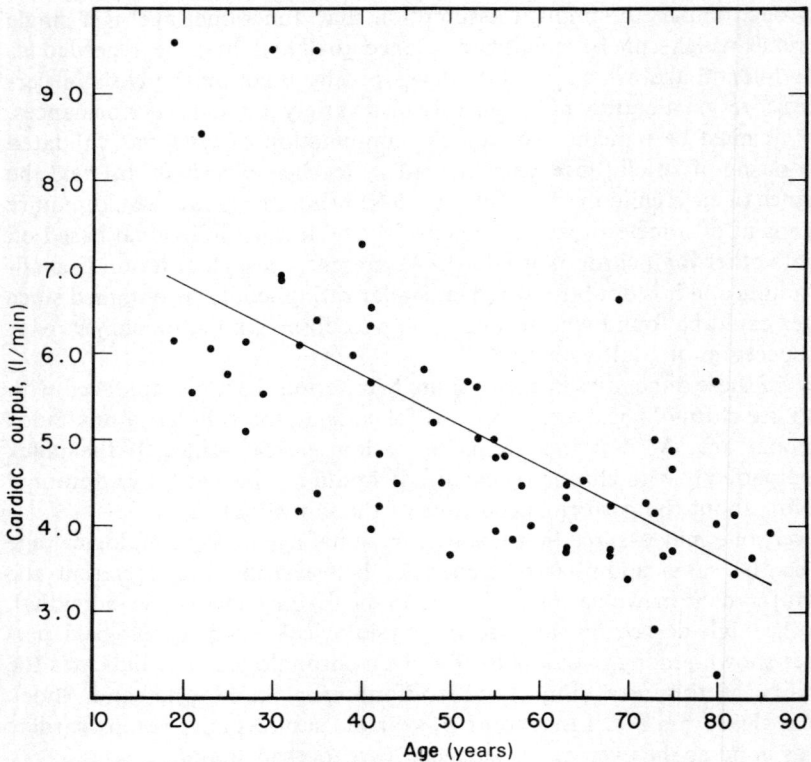

FIG. 1. The relation between resting cardiac output and age in 67 males without circulatory disorders. The line represents the linear regression on age. (From Brandfonbrener *et al.* 1955.)

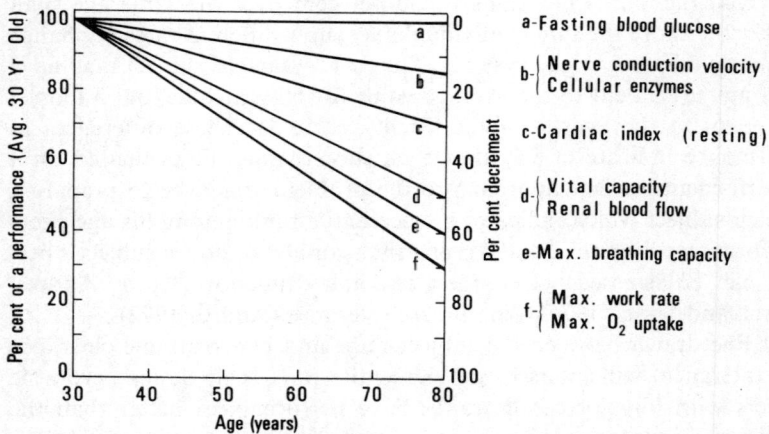

FIG. 2. Age decrements in physiological functions in males. Mean values for 20 to 35-year-old subjects are taken as 100 per cent. Decrements shown are schematic linear projections. (From Shock 1972.)

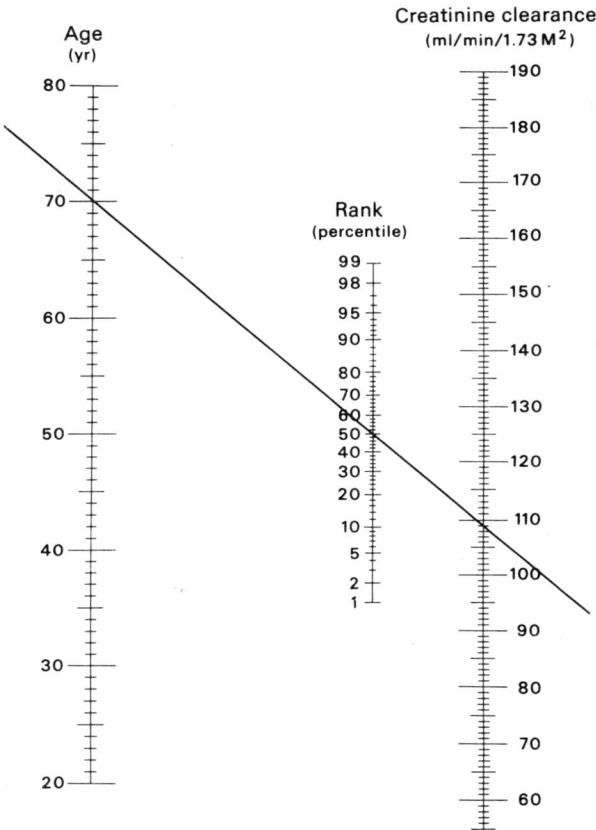

FIG. 3. Nomogram for determination of age-adjusted percentile rank in true creatinine clearance. Clearances based on total chromogen creatinine determinations using Auto Analyzer technique may be multiplied by 1.25 to obtain equivalent true creatinine clearance for use on the nomogram. (From Rowe *et al.* 1976.)

substantial number of normal subjects within each age decade. At present, such data are available on only a few performances. However, the assembly of observations on other types of performances is an important area for gerontological research. The limitation of this approach is that it yields a multiplicity of scores. No single index of 'functional age' can be derived, since there is no way to determine the relative importance of different functions tested in determining overall performance of an individual.

Another approach is to calculate the age of an individual from the regression equation of age on each of a number of variables (Damon 1972). However, because of the marked variability between subjects and the increase in variance with age in many variables, the calculated age for an individual is not very

Age

Two-hour
blood glucose
(mg per 100 ml)

Percentile
rank

Oral glucose tolerance test

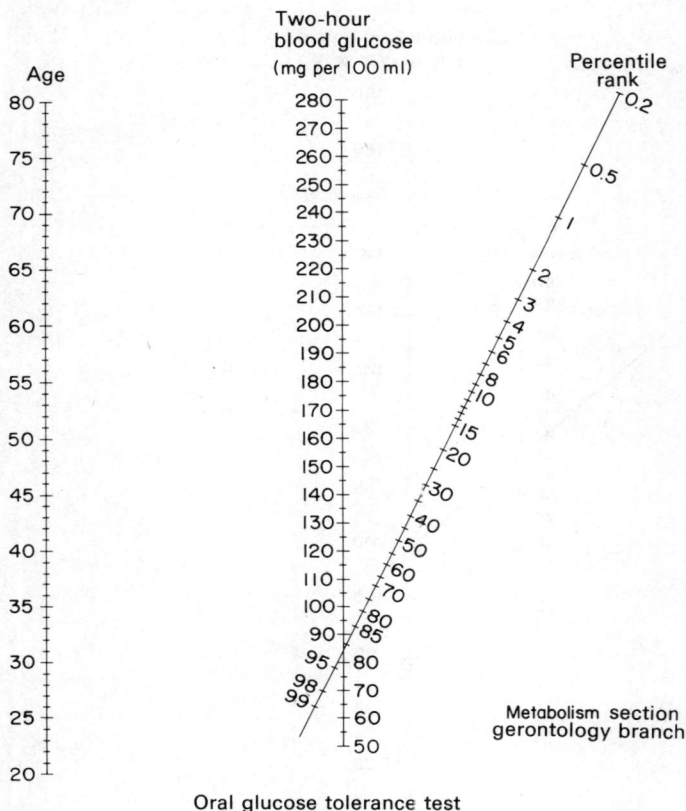

FIG. 4. Nomogram for judging percentile rank on oral glucose tolerance test. Glucose dose is 1.75 grams per kg body weight. 'True' glucose concentration is measured in whole venous blood. (From Andres 1972.)

precise. In fact, the error of the calculated age may be as much as ± 10 years (Young and Rickert 1973).

One way out of this dilemma is to derive a multiple regression equation to predict chronological age on the basis of scores on a variety of tests administered to the same subject. This approach has been used by Heikkinen, Kiiskinen, Käyhty, Rimpelä, and Vuori (1974), Furukawa, Inone, Kajiya, Inada, Takasagi, Fukui, Takeda, and Abe (1975), and Dirken (1972). Although this approach suffers from the logical limitation of using chronological age as the criterion, it has the advantages of making it possible to determine by appropriate analysis of the regression coefficients the relative importance of the tests included in the test battery in determining the calculated chronological age. This approach is, no doubt, the one which will be most effective in the future development of an index of functional age.

On the assumption that cellular processes reflect the basic rate of aging (and performance) in an individual, another approach is to utilize tests of cellular function, such as the rate and duration of cell division in fibroblasts which Schneider and Mitsui (1976) have described.

Tests which require autopsy material have not been regarded as appropriate for this presentation (bone histology, Singh and Gunberg 1970; collagenase digestion of collagen, Hamlin and Kohn 1972, Rickert and Forbes 1972; age pigment accumulation in tissues, Strehler, Mark, Mildvan, and Gee 1959; DNA repair, Samis, 1966; collagen content of heart tissue, Lenkiewicz, Davies, and Rosen 1972).

Forbes and his co-workers have published a number of papers dealing with the estimation of biological age (Brown and Forbes 1974a, b, 1975, 1976; Forbes, Sprott, Feldstein, and Dounce 1970). The approach has been the development of a rational theoretical model from which mortality curves could be derived.

These authors believe that an index of biological age must reflect the probability of death at any chronological age and that individuals who die must have an abnormal level of such an index relative to living individuals of the same chronological age. These criteria are applicable only if the index is to estimate the years of life remaining for the subject. Although this is a possible goal, it is quite different from attempting to identify the performance status of an individual with respect to his age peers. Furthermore, people die of diseases rather than age itself. Consequently, the index relates to a specific end-point (death) rather than the process of aging. Furthermore, any test of the validity of the index can be made only after each subject dies. Since the focus of the discussion is the assessment of aging (rather than death) I do not believe that these criteria are pertinent.

I believe that any battery of tests designed to develop an index of functional age should meet the following criteria:

1. The tests should sample a broad spectrum of performances that have *a priori* significance. Although greying of the hair is highly correlated with age, it probably has little to do with performance, and hence has little to contribute to an index of functional age.

2. Each test should yield reliable quantitative results, i.e., repeated testing of the same individual over short time intervals should yield comparable results. This requirement raises serious doubts about including items which depend on single clinical impressions. On the other hand, ratings made by a number of observers on the same subjects might be appropriate.

3. Each test in the battery should be reasonably correlated with age in a linear fashion. Since some characteristics do not show a linear regression on age, adjustments in scores from these tests will need to be made. In some cases, where age differences do not appear systematically until age 40 or 50, subjects below these ages may need to be excluded.

4. Some tests in the battery should evaluate the individual's response to a measurable physiological stress. Examples of such tests include responses to standardized exercise, rate of removal of excess glucose from the blood, the introduction of standardized distractions during problem-solving or learning tasks.

5. The test must be applicable to subjects of all ages.

6. The tests must be relatively painless with minimal dependence on motivation of the subject.

7. Tests should not require long periods for testing, or elaborate procedures available only in a hospital environment. Although tests, such as measurements of cardiac output, renal clearance, might be useful in relatively small samples for purposes of standardization, they are not applicable for general surveys on large populations.

Methodological problems

A major limitation in attempts to develop an index of functional age is the relatively restricted range of performances which have been measured. Most studies have dealt with anthropometric measurements, sensory and perceptual tests, pulmonary measurements, strength tests, blood-pressure, blood cholesterol, reaction time, immediate memory tests, and questionnaires designed to identify personality characteristics. It seems evident that a broader spectrum of functional tests needs to be explored.

Another methodological problem is the selection of an adequate sample of subjects for evaluation. With the exception of Dirken, most of the present studies have been conducted on small samples (around 10 Ss per decade). Many of the current studies could well be repeated on larger samples of subjects.

In order to completely validate an index of functional age, it will be necessary to collect repeated observations in subjects until they die. Although we may be able to identify subjects who are 'young for their age' we cannot know whether or not the apparent delay in age changes in middle or early old age is a reflection of a slower rate of aging in the individual. Longitudinal observations, or at least an indication of the age of death of the subject, is essential. Thus, until a substantial number of the subjects who have been tested early in life actually die, our basic question must remain unanswered.

Current status of research

Time will not permit a detailed review of all the studies which have attempted to devise an index of functional age. Instead I shall try to present generalizations based on my examination of data from the studies which have used a multiple regression or factor analysis of data derived from quantitative tests of normal subjects covering the age span from 20 to 70 years. These studies include the following: Hollingsworth, Hashizume, and Jablon (1965); Clark (1960);

Morgan and Fevans (1972); Heikkinen *et al.* (1974); Furukawa *et al.* (1975); Bourlière (1963, 1970); Dirken (1972); Heron and Chown (1967); Javalvisto, Lindquist, and Makkonen (1964); and Murray (1951). Reports by Ries (1974, 1976a, b) and Ciucâ and Jucovski (1965) were not considered since the proposed indices were based on clinical judgements or on calculations which involved a subjective judgement.

There is general agreement that the combination of a number of tests will predict chronological age more closely than will any single test. Multiple correlation coefficients of 0.80 to 0.90 have been reported in contrast to correlations of 0.3 to 0.7 for individual tests. It is, therefore, clear that some combination of tests can be formed which may serve as an index of physiological age.

The critical question is 'which tests should be included in computing an index?' Unfortunately, we cannot at the present time answer this question definitively. This is because each investigator has used a different battery of tests, often administered under different circumstances using different techniques. Table 1 summarizes the tests used with their correlation with chronological age. It may be seen that no single test was included in all of the studies. Some studies have placed primary emphasis on tests of mental performance and personality (Clark 1960; Heron and Chown 1967) while others have been

Table 1 Tests used by different investigators for calculation of functional age— correlations with chronological age

Furukawa *et al.* (1975)	Normals aged 21–83 (111 Ss)	Health clinic aged 26–70 (53 Ss)	Workers aged 21–71 (110 Ss)
Accommodation (l. eye)	−0.886		
Accommodation (r. eye)	−0.884		
Vibratory sensitivity (r. hand)	0.830		
Vibratory sensitivity (l. hand)	0.821		
Vital capacity	−0.771		
Height	−0.685		−0.091
PSP excretion (15 min)	−0.637		
Systolic BP	0.634	0.263	0.467
Weight	0.556		−0.004
Diastolic BP	0.542	0.324	0.512
GFR		−0.412	
RPF		−0.672	
Cholesterol		0.573	
Hb		0.285	
Tapping			−0.434
Strength			−0.433
Anteflexion			0.673
Retroflexion			0.624
Side flexion			0.768
Heart rate, resting			0.022
Heart rate 30 seconds after exercise			0.156
Heart rate after exercise		NS	

Table 1 *continued*

Dirken (1972)	Male factory workers, $N = 316$, aged 30–69
Aerobic capacity	0.72
Maximum energy load	0.71
1 s. expiratory volume	0.67
Pitch ceiling	0.66
Vital capacity	−0.55
Picture recognition	0.49
Hand strength	0.49
Choice reaction time	0.49
Visual acuity	0.44
Per cent hearing loss	0.42
Categorization	0.39
Maximum breathing frequency	0.33
Positioning	0.30
Reaction time	0.26
Concentrating ability (mental)	−0.25
Tapping	−0.18
Systolic BP	0.16
Diastolic BP	0.12

Heikkinen *et al.* (1974)	Randomly sampled Finnish males, $N = 456$, aged 25–57
*Vital capacity	−0.596
Vibratory sensitivity (wrist)	0.593
Vibratory sensitivity (ankle)	0.618
Digit symbol	−0.588
*Hearing loss	0.563
Simple reaction time	0.329
Bone cortex thickness	−0.299

*Used in multiple regression equation—$R = 0.785$.

Hollingsworth *et al.* (1965)	Japanese sample, $N = 437$ (169 males, 268 females), aged 20–70+
Skin elasticity	−0.604
Hearing loss (4000 cps)	0.596
Vibratory sensitivity (finger)	0.537
Systolic BP	0.519
Simple reaction time	0.488
Visual acuity	−0.423
Diastolic BP	0.409
Vital capacity	−0.402
Strength—hand grip	−0.323
Blood cholesterol	0.234

Clark (1960)	Male and female community volunteesr, 102 Ss, aged 20–70
Accommodation of the eye	0.67
Systolic BP	0.65
Hearing loss	0.57
Memory for pictures	−0.55
Vital capacity	0.54
Reaction time	−0.52
Reasoning ability	−0.49
Letter comprehension	−0.45
Spatial ability	−0.42
Word association latency	0.42
Immediate recall	−0.40
Maze learning	0.34
Strength—hand grip	−0.21

Table 1 *continued*

Jalavisto (1965)	130 women volunteers, aged 40–93
Memory for pictures	−0.55
Hearing loss (4000 cps)	0.55
Vital capacity	−0.54
Flicker fusion frequency	—0.48
Reaction time	0.48
Retinal rivalry	−0.47
Abstracting ability	−0.44
Maximum tapping speed	−0.44
Memory for numbers	−0.41
Pulse pressure	0.34
Reaction time—light	0.35
Systolic BP	0.35
Height	−0.30
Familial longevity	−0.24
Diastolic BP	0.10
Per cent overweight	0.07

Dequeker *et al.* (1969)	Patients in psychiatric hospital, 140 females, aged 30–94
Metacarpal osteoporotic index	−0.786
Osteoarthritic index, hand joints	0.667
Height/arm span ratio	−0.532
Skinfold thickness—hand	−0.274
Weight	−0.148
Weight/height ratio	0.091
Arm span	0.036

Morgan and Fevens (1972)	Paid community volunteers, Nova Scotia $N = 50$, aged 20–70
Systolic BP	0.69
Hearing loss	0.66
Near vision (accommodation)	0.57
Multiple $R = 0.81$	

Murray (1951)	Male community volunteers, $N = 38$, aged 21–84
Hearing loss (64 to 11 548 cps)	0.829
Range of visual accommodation	−0.758
Visual threshold—dark adapted eye	0.720
Strength—hand grip	−0.662
Systolic BP	0.483

Heron and Chown (1967)	Community volunteers, aged 24–70	
	300 men	240 women
Forced expiratory volume (1 s)	−0.699	−0.696
Non-verbal intelligence	−0.638	−0.508
Perceptual mazes	−0.545	−0.281
Grip strength	−0.523	−0.478·
Trail making test	−0.517	−0.495
Digit coding (unspeeded)	−0.509	−0.48
Systolic BP	0.502	0.525
Hearing loss (1000 cps)	0.449	0.489
Pulse pressure	0.433	0.382
Visual acuity (both eyes)	−0.420	−0.444
Sitting height	−0.333	−0.477
Liking detailed work	0.301	0.353
Liking for habit	0.275	0.247
Digit span—auditory	−0 273	−0.194
Bicep circumference	−0.265	0.150

Table 1 *continued*

Webster and Logie (1976)	1080 females, aged 21–83, from health screening centre
Forced expiratory volume (1 s)	−0.58
Systolic BP	0.43
Alkaline phosphatase ($\log_1 s$)	0.43
Blood cholesterol	0.37
Blood urea	0.36
Erythrocyte sedimentation rate ($\log_{10}$)	0.24
Blood triglycerides	0.12
Fozard and Thomas (1975)	969 'healthy' males, aged 25–81
Greyness of hair	0.63
Disassemble test score	−0.45
Hearing loss (8000 cps)	0.38
Forced expiratory volume	−0.38
Speech reception loss	0.35
Length of ear	0.30
Per cent haemoglobin	−0.17

primarily concerned with physiological measurements (Furukawa *et al.* 1975; Hollingsworth *et al.* 1965). The most common areas of tests used in a number of different studies are perception, psychomotor functions, blood-pressure, anthropometric measurements, and pulmonary function tests. Only Furukawa *et al.* (1975) and Dirken (1972) have included the response to exercise within their test batteries. Furukawa measured heart rate at 30 s, 1, 1½, 2, 3, and 4 min. after exercise. Even though the correlations with age were not significant, the test results were included in the multiple regression equations derived for the prediction of chronological age. Dirken found high correlations with age for measurement of maximum work output and maximum O_2 uptake. Dirken's (1972) study is outstanding because of the relatively large number of industrial workers tested (316) and the assessment of many variables (35) covering both physiological and psychological variables. The primary limitation of this study from the standpoint of gerontology is the fact that the maximum age of the subjects was 69 years.

In order to examine in more detail the potential usefulness of various tests in estimating functional age Table 2 lists all tests in rank order according to their correlation with age. Tests which have been used in a number of studies are entered in the table according to the highest correlation reported. The correlations reported by Murray (1951) as listed in Table 1 are omitted from Table 2 since they are based on only 38 subjects, and are much higher than values reported on the same tests by other investigators.

According to Table 2 an index of metacarpal osteoporosis (Dequeker, Baeyens, and Claessens 1969) and general flexibility of the body (Furukawa *et al.* 1975) are highly correlated with age. Unfortunately, no confirmation of these high correlations has been published by other investigators. However, both these measurements should be seriously considered in future studies. In addition, the test of mobility of carpal joints, as proposed by Emmrich and Schwarz (1963), should be included.

Table 2 Correlations of tests with chronological age

Test	Correlation with age	Investigator
Accommodation of the eye	0.880	Furukawa *et al.* (1975)
	0.670	Clark (1960)
	0.57	Morgan & Fevens (1972)
Vibratory sensitivity—finger	−0.83	Furukawa *et al.* (1975)
	−0.537	Hollingsworth *et al.* (1965)
Metacarpal osteoporotic index	−0.780	Dequeker *et al.* (1969) (females)
Vital capacity	−0.77	Furukawa *et al.* (1975)
	−0.596	Heikkinen *et al.* (1974)
	−0.550	Dirken (1972)
	−0.54	Jalavisto (1965)
	−0.540	Clark (1960)
	−0.402	Hollingsworth *et al.* (1965)
Side flexion	−0.768	Furukawa *et al.* (1975)
Aerobic capacity	−0.720	Dirken (1972)
Maximum energy load	−0.710	Dirken (1972)
Forced expiratory volume (1 s)	−0.699	Heron & Chown (1967)
	−0.670	Dirken (1972)
	−0.580	Webster & Logie (1976)
	−0.38	Fozard & Thomas (1965)
Systolic blood-pressure	0.690	Morgan & Fevens (1972)
	0.643	Furukawa *et al.* (1975)
	0.650	Clark (1960)
	0.519	Hollingsworth *et al.* (1965)
	0.502	Heron & Chown (1967)
	0.467	Furukawa *et al.* (1975)
	0.430	Webster & Logie (1976)
	0.35	Jalavisto (1965)
	0.160	Dirken (1972)
Height	−0.68	Furukawa *et al.* (1975) (111 normal Ss)
	−0.09	Furukawa *et al.* (1975) (110 workers)
	−0.38	Dequeker *et al.* (1969)
	−0.30	Jalavisto (1965)
Anteflexion	0.673	Furukawa *et al.* (1975)
Renal plasma flow	0.672	Furukawa *et al.* (1975)
Pitch ceiling	−0.66	Dirken (1972)
Hearing loss (4000 cps)	0.66	Morgan & Fevens (1972)
	0.596	Hollingsworth *et al.* (1965)
	0.57	Clark (1960)
	0.55	Jalavisto (1965)
	0.563	Heikkinen *et al.* (1974)
	0.449	Heron & Chown (1967)
	0.42	Dirken (1972)
(8000 cps)	0.38	Fozard & Thomas (1975)
Phenolsulfonphthalein excretion—15 min	−0.637	Furukawa *et al.* (1975)
Retroflexion	0.624	Furukawa *et al.* (1975)
Vibratory sensitivity—ankle	−0.618	Heikkinen *et al.* (1974)
Skin elasticity	−0.604	Hollingsworth *et al.* (1965)
Vibratory sensitivity—wrist	−0.593	Heikkinen *et al.* (1974)
Digit symbol	−0.588	Heikkinen *et al.* (1974)
	−0.509	Heron & Chown (1967)
Blood cholesterol	0.573	Furukawa *et al.* (1975)
	0.37	Webster & Logie (1976)
	0.234	Hollingsworth *et al.* (1965)
Weight	0.556	Furukawa *et al.* (1975)

Table 2 *continued*

Test	Correlation with age	Investigator
	0.004	Furukawa *et al.* (1975)
	−0.148	Dequeker *et al.* (1969)
Memory for pictures	−0.550	Clark (1960)
	−0.55	Jalavisto (1965)
Diastolic blood-pressure	0.542	Furukawa *et al.* (1975)
	0.512	Furukawa *et al.* (1975)
	0.409	Hollingsworth *et al.* (1965)
	0.10	Jalavisto (1965)
	0.12	Dirken (1972)
Reaction time (simple)	0.52	Clark (1960)
	0.488	Hollingsworth *et al.* (1965)
	0.48	Jalavisto (1965)
	0.329	Heikkinen *et al.* (1974)
	0.26	Dirken (1972)
Reaction time (4 choices)	0.49	Dirken (1972)
Picture recognition	−0.49	Dirken (1972)
Reasoning ability	−0.49	Clark (1960)
	−0.44	Jalavisto (1965)
Grip strength	−0.523	Heron & Chown (1967)
	−0.49	Dirken (1972)
	−0.433	Furukawa *et al.* (1975)
	−0.323	Hollingsworth *et al.* (1965)
	−0.21	Clark (1960)
Flicker fusion frequency	−0.48	Jalavisto (1965)
Letter comprehension	−0.45	Clark (1960)
Tapping rate	−0.44	Jalavisto (1965)
	−0.434	Furukawa *et al.* (1975)
	−0.18	Dirken (1972)
Spatial ability	−0.42	Clark (1960
Word association latency	0.42	Clark (1960)
Glomerular filtration rate	−0.412	Furukawa *et al.* (1975)
Immediate recall	−0.40	Clark (1960)
Categorization	−0.39	Dirken (1972)
Maze learning	−0.34	Clark (1960)
Maximum breathing frequency	−0.33	Dirken (1972)
Positioning	−0.30	Dirken (1972)
Bone cortex thickness	−0.299	Heikkenen *et al.* (1974)
Blood haemoglobin	−0.285	Furukawa *et al.* (1975)
Concentrating ability (mental)	−0.25	Dirken (1972)

The high correlations of tests of work performances and maximum oxygen uptake reported by Dirken (1972) show clearly the advantages of including stress tests. However, such tests may not be possible in surveys of large numbers of subjects because of the time and technical skills required in their administration. Nevertheless, they should be incorporated in studies where maximum precision in the estimate of functional age is required.

Although systolic blood-pressure may be significantly correlated with age, its inclusion in a test battery for assessing functional age may be debated, because of its use in diagnosing a disease—hypertension—and because high blood-pressure may be reduced by drug therapy. However, I believe that blood-pressure measurements are legitimate for inclusion in an index of physiological age.

Tests which correlate 0.5 to 0.6 with chronological age include most of the perceptual tests (visual acuity, accommodation of the eye, hearing loss, maximum frequency perceived, and vibratory sensitivity) as well as skin elasticity. These tests are relatively simple to apply and should be included in any index of functional age.

Although kidney function tests (renal plasma flow and glomerular filtration rate) correlate well with age, the methods are involved so that they cannot be applied to large numbers of subjects. The excretion of intravenously administered phenolsulfonphthalein as used by Furukawa *et al.* (1975), which correlated 0.637 with age, deserves further exploration.

Tests of vital capacity, tapping rate, strength of hand grip, and choice reaction time seem worthy of consideration for inclusion in the test battery, even though their correlations with age are only 0.4 to 0.2.

Similarly tests of mental performances, such as memory for pictures, picture recognition, reasoning ability, spatial ability, word association latency, immediate recall, and categorization ability, should be included because of their intrinsic interest.

Although personality characteristics may have an important impact on performance, attempts to include such variables in estimates of functional age have thus far failed (Fozard and Thomas 1975). This is because the responses to questionnaires designed to measure personality characteristics have shown very low correlations with age. This may be because personality characteristics change very little with age, or because the tests used are not valid measures. This is an area which still needs extensive work.

Table 3 lists those tests which have been used in three or more studies with the range of correlations with chronological age as reported by different investigators. It may be seen that systolic blood-pressure (9 studies), hearing loss (8 studies), vital capacity (6 studies), reaction time and strength of hand grip

Table 3 Tests used in more than two studies

Variable	No. studies used	Correlation with chronological age
Systolic blood-pressure	9	0.69 – 0.16
Hearing loss	8	0.66 – 0.42
Vital capacity	6	−0.77 – −0.40
Reaction time	5	0.52 – 0.26
Grip strength	5	−0.52 – −0.21
Diastolic blood-pressure	4	0.51 – 0.10
Height	4	−0.68 – −0.09
Visual acuity	4	−0.57 – −0.42
Forced expiratory volume (1 s)	4	−0.699 – −0.380
Accommodation of the eye	3	0.88 – 0.57
Tapping	3	−0.44 – −0.18
Weight	3	0.556 – 0.004

(5 studies) head the list. There is, however, a wide range of correlation coefficients with age among the different studies. At least part of this variability may be a reflection of sample difference in the population tested. For example, correlations for systolic blood-pressure with age vary between 0.69 (Morgan and Fevans 1972) to 0.16 (Dirken 1972). Since the incidence of hypertension increases with age, high correlations may be only a reflection of the incidence of hypertension in the population tested. In other instances, the range in correlation coefficients may reflect differences in measurement techniques and the extent to which subjects were motivated to maximum effort (grip strength, vital capacity, tapping).

Future projections

Although no single index of functional age is yet available, analysis of studies that have been done point the directions for future research.

It is clear that for many tests, a score can be derived which will characterize the deviation of the performance of an individual from the mean value of a group of his age peers. It is also clear that when a number of tests are combined, the chronological age calculated from a multiple regression equation will correlated more highly with chronological age than will any of the individual tests. We know that attempts to derive an overall estimate of functional age is not a gesture of futility.

In order to make significant progress, the following needs to be done:

1. A substantial number of different tests must be administered to a large population of normal subjects living in the community.

2. A broad spectrum of performances should be tested. It is still not clear whether separate indices for physiological and psychological performances should be developed or whether a single index is possible. Research efforts should be directed toward this question.

3. Any test battery should include those tests which have been useful in deriving a functional age in previous studies. These tests include: hearing loss at high frequencies, vital capacity, vibratory sensitivity, accommodation of the eye, visual acuity, reaction time (choice), grip strength, tapping rate, and, perhaps, blood-pressure.

4. Other tests which have shown promise in the hands of some investigators should be included, such as metacarpal osteoporotic index, body flexion, maximum energy load, aerobic capacity, flicker fusion frequency, maximum breathing capacity.

5. Some estimate of body composition should be included. Estimates of body composition may be made from selected anthropometric measurements (Behnke 1961; Bourlière 1963). Other possibilities include basal metabolism, K^{40}, or creatinine excretion.

6. In addition to exercise, other physiological stress tests should be applied.

7. Stepwise regression analyses should be carried out in all studies in order

to evaluate the relative contribution of each test to the calculated index of functional age.

8. Validation studies should be planned in which the calculated index of functional age could be compared for groups of industrial and other workers who are rated as 'outstanding performers' and 'poor performers'.

9. The tests should be incorporated into longitudinal studies that will eventually permit comparison of scores for subjects who die early in life with those who are long-lived.

In conclusion, it may be said that the advances made in gerontological research over the past decade now make it possible to develop valid indices of functional age. With adequate resources to support research the problem can be solved.

References

ANDRES, R. (1972). In *Nutrition in old age* (10th Symposium of the Swedish Nutrition Fdn. (ed. L. A. Carlson), p. 24. Almqvist and Wiksell, Uppsala.

BEHNKE, A. R. (1961). *J. appl. Physiol.*, **16**, 960.

BOURLIÈRE, F. (1963). In *Social and psychological perspectives*, Vol. 1 (ed. R. H. Williams, C. Tibbitts, and W. Donahue), p. 184. Atherton Press, New York.

—— (1970). *The assessment of biological age in man.* Public Health Papers No. 37. World Health Organization, Geneva.

BRANDFONBRENER, M., LANDOWNE, M., and SHOCK, N. W. (1955). *Circulation*, **12**, 557.

BROWN, K. S. and FORBES, W. F. (1974a). *J. Gerontol.*, **29**, 46.

—— and —— (1974b). *J. Gerontol.*, **29**, 401.

—— and —— (1975). *J. Gerontol.*, **30**, 513.

—— and —— (1976). *Gerontology*, **22**, 428.

CIUCA, A. and JUCOVSKI, Vl. (1965). *Münch. med. Wochenschr.*, **107**, 1507.

CLARK, J. W. (1960). *J. Gerontol.*, **15**, 183.

COMFORT, A. (1969). *Lancet*, **ii**, 1411.

DAMON, A. (1972). *Aging and hum. develop.*, **3**, 169.

DEQUEKER, J. V., BAEYENS, J. P., and CLAESSENS, J. (1969). *J. Amer. Geriat. Soc.*, **17**, 169.

DIRKEN, J. M. (ed.) (1972). *Functional age of industrial workers.* Wolters-Noordhoff Publishing, Groningen.

EMMRICH, R. and SCHWARZ, J. (1963). *Z. Alternsforsch.*, **16**, 297.

FORBES, W. F., SPROTT, D. A., FELDSTEIN, M., and DOUNCE, A. L. (1970). *J. theoret. Biol.*, **29**, 293.

FOZARD, J. L. and THOMAS, J. C., Jr (1975). In *Modern perspectives in the psychiatry of old age* (ed. J. G. Howells), p. 107. Brunner/Mazel, New York.

FURUKAWA, T., INOUE, M., KAJIYA, F., INADA, H., TAKASUGI, S., FUKUI, S., TAKEDA, H., and ABE, H. (1975). *J. Gerontol.*, **30**, 422.

HAMLIN, C. R. and KOHN, R. R. (1972). *Exp. Gerontol.*, **7**, 377.

HEIKKINEN, A., KIISKINNEN, A., KÄYTHY, B., RIMPELÄ, M. and VUORI, I. (1974). *Gerontologia*, **20**, 33.

HERON, A. and CHOWN, S. (1967). *Age and function.* Little, Brown and Co., Boston.

HOLLINGSWORTH, J. W., HASHIZUME, A., and JABLON, S. (1965). *Yale J. Biol. Med.*, **38**, 11.

JALAVISTO, E. (1965). In *Behavior, aging, and the nervous system* (ed. A. T. Welford and J. E. Birren), p. 353. Charles C. Thomas, Springfield, Illinois.

——, LINDQVIST, C., and MAKKONEN, T. (1964). Assessment of biological age. III. Mental and neural factors in longevity. *Ann. Acad. Sci. Fenn. A, V Med.*, **106**, 1–20.

LENKIEWICZ, J. E., DAVIES, M. J., and ROSEN, D. (1972) *Cardiovasc. Res.*, **6**, 549.

MORGAN, R. F. and FEVENS, S. K. (1972). *Percept. mot. skills*, **34**, 415.

MURRAY, I. M. (1951). *J. Gerontol.*, **6**, 120.

RICKERT, W. S. and FORBES, W. F. (1972). *Exp. Gerontol.*, **7**, 387.

RIES, W. (1974). *Exp. Gerontol.*, **9**, 145.

—— (1976a). *Totus Homo*, **7**, 39.

—— (1976b). *Z. gesamt. inn. Med. Grenz.*, **31**, 109.

ROWE, J. W., ANDRES, R., TOBIN, J. D., NORRIS, A. H., and SHOCK, N. W. (1976). *J. Gerontol.*, **31**, 155.

SAMIS, H. V., Jr (1966). *J. theor. Biol.*, **13**, 236.

SCHNEIDER, E. L. and MITSUI, Y. (1976). *Proc. nat. Acad. Sci.*, **73**, 3584.

SHOCK, N. W. (1972). In *Nutrition in old age* (10th Symposium of the Swedish Nutrition Fdn.) (ed. L. A. Carlson), p. 12. Almqvist and Wiksell, Uppsala.

SINGH, I. J. and GUNBERG, D. L. (1970). *Amer. J. Phys. Anthropol.*, **33**, 373.

STREHLER, B. L., MARK, D. D., MILDVAN, A. S., and GEE, M. V. (1959). *J. Gerontol.*, **14**, 430.

WEBSTER, I. W. and LOGIE, A. R. (1976). *J. Gerontol.*, **31**, 546.

YOUNG, J. C. and RICKERT, W. S. (1973). *Exp. Gerontol.*, **8**, 337.

Physiological indices of aging   Jordan D. Tobin

The concept of a physiological index of age is intuitively appealing since we have often said that someone 'looks younger than his age' or 'performs better than people his age'. Inherent in these statements is the implicit notion that we know how someone of a given age should look or perform, that we know what is normative or standard. Within the discipline of human physiology, this determination is frequently difficult. In addition to the problems of subject selection, applicability of a given sample to another population, standardization of test conditions, and the choice of which physiological system to study, there is the almost philosophical question of the interrelationships of age, physiology, and disease.

Previous studies, as recently reviewed by Shock (1978) and Costa (1977) have attempted to develop a physiological or functional age for individuals using a multiple regression model. The variables used have included physiological, anthropometric, physical, and biochemical indices. Performances on these tests were used to predict a 'functional' age.

A different approach has been taken for this study. Four physiological variables which are considered clinically important in that they measure functions which are related to the health of an individual were examined. These included the respiratory system (forced expiratory volume in 1.0 second), the renal system (standard creatinine clearance), the cardiovascular system (systolic blood-pressure), and metabolism (oral glucose tolerance). Each of these variables not only is influenced by age but in addition is associated with a disease (chronic obstructive pulmonary disease, renal failure, hypertension, and diabetes). Normative data were derived from individuals who were free of diseases or medications known to influence the system being studied. Age-adjusted standard T-scores were then calculated for all individuals. In order to judge the importance of each variable, the age-adjusted T-scores for these individuals who have died were compared to those who lived.

Population
The data on this study were derived from tests on the volunteers of the Baltimore Longitudinal Study of Aging conducted within the National Institute on Aging under the direction of Dr. Nathan Shock and Dr. Reuben Andres. The study had its inception in 1958 when a retired Public Health Service physician came to Dr. Shock and suggested that researchers on aging of humans should not be studying only the residents of nursing homes and chronic disease hospitals, who represent a minority of the aged population, but should also be looking at the 'healthy' aged. Towards this aim, he offered himself for study and agreed to recruit his friends as well. Thus was formed the nucleus of the study population which has continued to be a self-recruited group of males ranging in age from 18 to 103, with over 1100 men having been seen once, and a currently active group of 650 community-dwelling volunteers.

The characteristics of the group have been previously described (Stone and Norris 1966): briefly, they are predominantly highly educated, upper middle class, white, Protestant, and in academic, managerial, or government positions. No subject is excluded from the study for health reasons. They are admitted for $2\frac{1}{2}$ days to the Baltimore City Hospitals and undergo a series of more than 40 medical, physiological, and psychological tests. They have agreed to return to be retested at 2-year intervals until they are 60 years old, at 18-month intervals until they are 70 years old, and then to return yearly for the remainder of their lives. These dedicated volunteers form the data base for the results to be presented and, obviously, we owe them a great deal of thanks.

We have mentioned that no subject is excluded from the study on the basis of health. However, when we are analysing the effect of *age* on a physiological variable, for instance, the glucose tolerance test, we would not want to include in the group of normal individuals those with the disease diabetes mellitus. These diabetics would have poor performance on this test of metabolism, which would not be a function of their age but of their disease. Similarly, we would not include anyone taking drugs known to influence carbohydrate metabolism or having other diseases which influence it. Thus, for each variable studied a clinical 'clean-up' is necessary in order to ascertain the effect of age *per se*, rather than disease.

Glucose metabolism

The oral glucose tolerance test is a physiological test of metabolism. A blood sample for analysis of glucose is taken after an overnight fast under basal conditions. The subject then drinks a solution of glucose (1.75 grams per kg of body weight) which represents a challenge to the metabolic system and, in part, simulates what each of us does during the day as we eat. Performance on this test is judged by how efficiently the subject metabolizes the load of glucose and returns his blood glucose concentration towards the fasting level. Towards this aim, the blood glucose concentration at two hours is clinically used to categorize people as 'normal', 'borderline', or 'diabetic'.

Results in a 'clinically clean' group of subjects indicate that there is no effect of age on the fasting (unstressed) glucose level. After the stress of the glucose load, initially there is no age effect discernible as the glucose is absorbed from the gut and the blood glucose rises equally in all age groups for the first 40 minutes. By one hour, the 20-year-old subjects have already started to lower their glucose level, and by two hours, there is a clear age-ordering of concentration. The 20-year-olds have the lowest glucose, the 30-year-olds next, the 40-year-olds have not performed as well as the 30-year-olds, but they are better than the 50-year olds, etc with the 80-year-olds having the highest glucose level and, therefore, the poorest performance. The two-hour plasma glucose concentrations for each decade are shown in Fig. 1. These results are mean values;

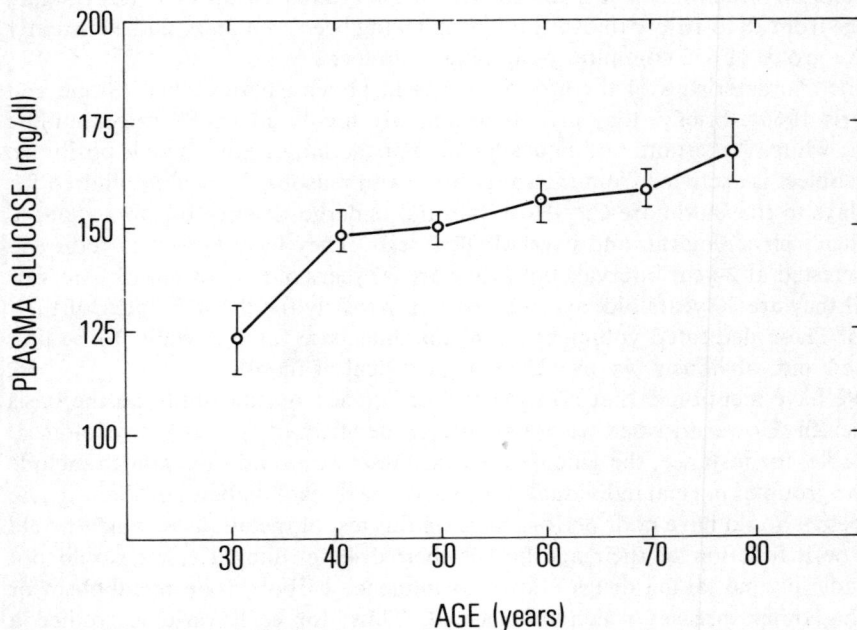

FIG. 1. Effect of age on plasma glucose concentration 2 hours after oral glucose. Clean group. The *N*s for each decade from 30–80 were 14, 50, 82, 67, 53, and 33.

there is a large variance at any age, and there are clearly some superior 70-year-old subjects who behave as well or better than the *average* 20-year-olds. Since these are cross-sectional results, we do not know if these super-performers were even better performers when they were younger and have, in fact, deteriorated as they aged or if they have maintained the same level of performance throughout their life span.

Were the usually accepted criteria of performance on this test (derived from young people) applied to this health group of subjects, more than 50 per cent of the men over the age of 60 would be classified as 'diabetic'. It is worth emphasizing once again that these subjects represent a 'clean' group. They have no family history of diabetes, no diseases known to influence carbohydrate metabolism, and are taking no medications that would influence their performance. They are active, healthy, and, by dietary diary, taking adequate amounts of carbohydrate in their diet. The finding of such a high prevalence of 'abnormal' results on glucose tolerance testing is not in keeping with the known prevalence of the disease, diabetes.

We have chosen (Andres 1971) to judge performance on this test using an age-adjusted monogram constructed from these data. With this technique, a subject can be judged against his age peers, and a percentile rank can be assigned to his performance. An exactly average performance at any age will have a 50 per cent rank; a 5 per cent rank indicates that only 5 per cent of subjects of that age perform that poorly. The actual glucose level that determines a rank of, for example 5 per cent, is of course higher in the 70-year-olds than in the 20-year-olds. The nomogram does not indicate what is normal and what is abnormal but does allow more flexible and appropriate (but equally arbitrary) judgements than one arbitrary diagnostic cut-off level for all ages.

In order to determine which percentile ranking at different ages is significant in terms of predicting future health problems, prospective longitudinal studies are required. A variety of 'end-points' need to be examined, end-points known to be associated with diabetes mellitus. Thus, since mortality rates are markedly increased in diabetics, various levels of glucose tolerance performance should be examined for correlation with mortality. Similarly, the development of the known complication of diabetes, such as coronary heart disease and the micro-angiopathies (eye, peripheral nerve, and kidney problems) should be analysed. Finally, the development of florid diabetes is an essential end-point to be analysed.

Pulmonary function

The functions of the lung in terms of gas exchange, ridding the body of carbon dioxide, and supplying oxygen, show no age effects in the basal state. There are no differences in the content of oxygen, carbon dioxide, or electrolytes in the blood. There are marked age effects, however, on tests of the ability of the lung to perform when stressed. The amount of air that can be forcibly expelled in one second (Forced Expiratory Volume, FEV 1.0) has been found useful as a

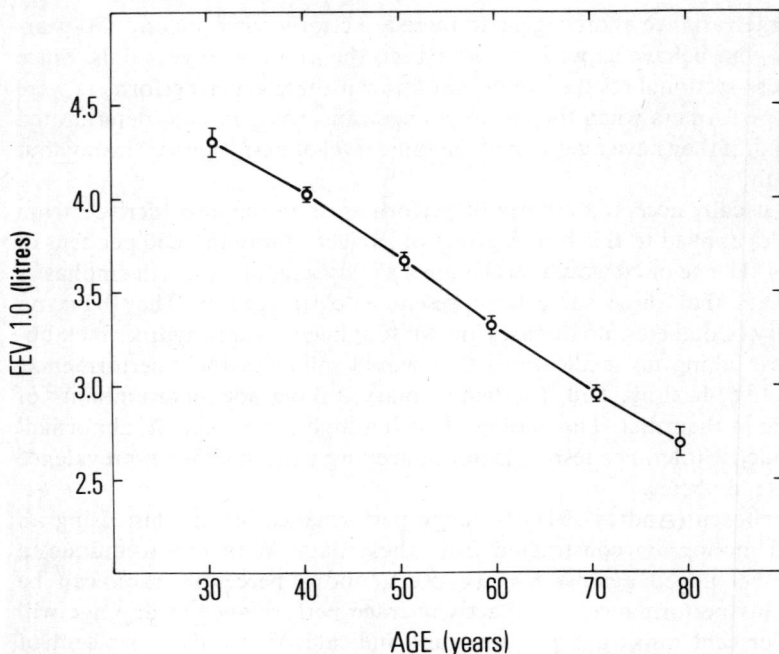

FIG. 2. Effect of age on forced expiratory volume at one second. Clean group. The *N*s for each decade from 30–80 were 97, 107, 151, 114, 115, and 45.

clinical test of respiratory performance. Results of these tests are profoundly influenced by diseases of the lung (bronchitis) and by smoking. In order to assess the effect of age on this test, therefore, another 'clinical clean-up' was necessary. Individuals who were free of overt pulmonary disease, were non-smokers, and who had no other diseases or who were taking no drugs which might affect performance, formed the group of healthy subjects in this analysis. They showed a progressive decrease in performance across the age span, with each successive age decade performing less well than the younger decades (Fig. 2). Again, it is not clear whether the poorer average performance of the older subjects on this test of pulmonary performance is a physiological age effect on all subjects or if it is indicative of the development in some of the subjects of subclinical disease.

Blood-pressure

The control of the blood-pressure level is a complex interrelationship of anatomical, hormonal, neural, renal, and cardiovascular factors. We are examining the summation of these factors when we measure this variable, and this must be kept in mind. The systolic blood-pressures reported here were obtained on our volunteers during their physical examinations. All subjects were screened

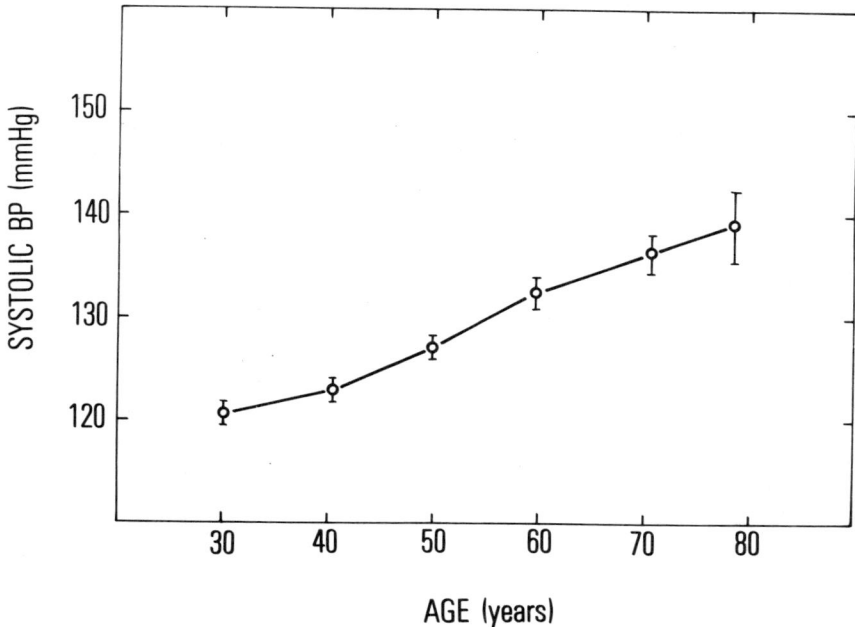

FIG. 3. Effect of age on systolic blood-pressure. Clean group. The *N*s for each decade from 30–80 were 82, 151, 184, 119, 103, and 35.

and any with cardiovascular, renal, or metabolic diseases were excluded from this analysis, as were those on any medications (diuretics, antihypertensives, etc.) known to influence blood-pressure.

There was a significant increase of systolic blood-pressure with age, with each succeeding decade having a higher average pressure than the preceding one (Fig. 3).

Renal function

One measure of the ability of the kidney to function is the creatinine clearance, which is an estimate of the glomerular filtration rate. It measures how many millilitres of plasma are 'cleared' of nitrogenous wastes each minute, with higher numbers (adjusted for body size) indicating better function and lower numbers poorer function. The results of a cross-sectional and longitudinal analysis of creatinine clearance have been presented (Rowe, Andres, Tobin, Norris, and Shock 1976). There is a highly significant decrease in clearance across the age span, with each succeeding decade being lower than the preceding one (Fig. 4). These results are on a clinically clean group who have no diseases known to influence renal function, are on no medications which would influence performance, have not had prostatectomies, and who have a normal urine analysis and no history of renal disease.

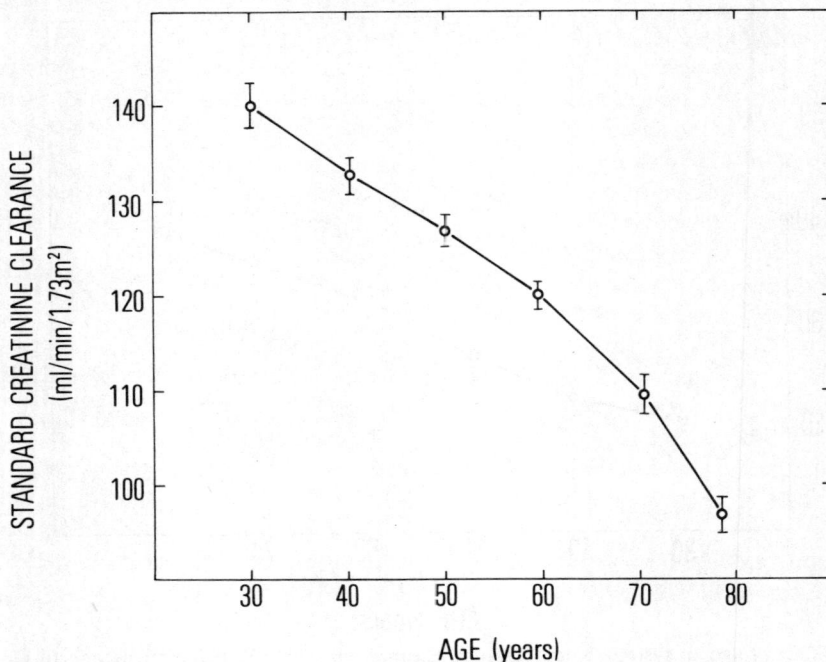

FIG. 4. Effect of age on creatinine clearance. Clean group. The Ns for each decade from 30–80 were 73, 122, 152, 94, 68, and 29.

Analysis

In these four examples of physiological variables which are considered to be clinically important in medicine, there was a decrement in function with age. This was in a group of individuals who were thought to be free of significant disease within the limits of medical judgement; and the decline cannot simply be ascribed to 'sick old men'. The importance of this decline, however, remains a question. Should two individuals who have the same level of performance be considered to be equivalent in a functional sense, even though one of them (a young man) reached this low level because of a disease, while the other (an old man) appears free of disease and has reached this level because of a physiological decrement with age? One approach to this question is to use an age-adjusted score for the subject, and to test whether performance is related to the future health or survival of the individual. An age-adjusted T-score was calculated for each individual. The mean value for each decade was assigned a value of 50 with a standard deviation of 10. Thus, an individual who was one SD above the mean for his age group would have a T-score of 60 (50 + 10), while someone one and one-half SDs below the mean would have a T-score of 35 (50 − 15). For convenience, good performance was always expressed as a T-score above 50 (for BP and glucose tolerance, the better performers, in fact, have been lower absolute values and these were reversed). The T-score thus serves two functions: (1) it removes dimensions from consideration and expresses different variables in the same units, and (2) it age-adjusts performance since each individual is judged against the mean and standard deviation of the performance of those clinically 'clean' individuals in his own age decade.

Since the initiation of the Baltimore Longitudinal Study, 162 of the volunteers are known to have died. T-scores were calculated for each individual's performance on each variable and the scores for those individuals who subsequently died were compared to those who lived. Fig. 5 graphically shows this comparison for each variable.

For the first three variables, blood-pressure, FEV 1.0, and creatinine clearance, the T-score of those volunteers who lived was not significantly different from a score of 50.0 (the mean score of the clean group). The T-scores of those who died, however, were all significantly lower, and represent a poorer age-adjusted performance on the average for those variables (Table 1). There was no significant difference between the group that lived and the group that died on the fourth variable, the glucose concentration at two hours of a glucose tolerance test. Both groups, however, had mean T-scores lower than 50. This difference (which was not observed in the other three variables) probably represents the

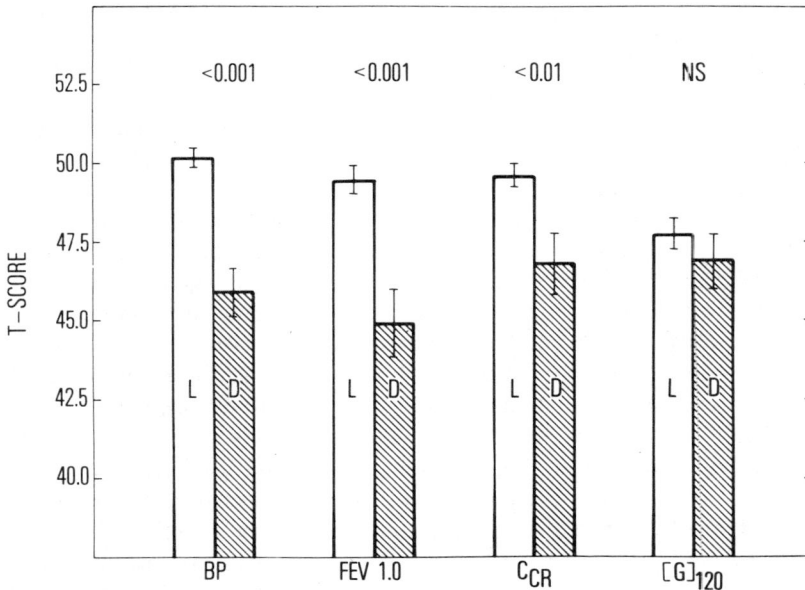

FIG. 5. Relation of performance level on four physiological tests to survival. Cross-hatched bars (D) are results on those subjects who have died; open bars (L) are results on the survivors. BP = systolic blood-pressure on physical examination. FEV 1.0 = forced expiratorycapacity in one second. C_{cr} = creatinine clearance. $[G]_1{}^6{}_0$ = glucose concentration 120 minutes after oral glucose. T-score (see text).

Table 1 T-scores for live and dead groups

		BP	$FEV_{1.0}$	C_{cr}	Glucose
Live					
	Mean	50.2	49.4	49.6	47.8
	SEM	0.33	0.37	0.35	0.46
	N	860	813	772	676
Dead					
	Mean	45.9	44.9	46.8	46.9
	SEM	0.77	1.08	1.01	1.20
	N	162	135	155	100
p		<0.001	<0.001	<0.01	NS

greater sensitivity of the glucose tolerance test to those factors, especially medications, used to exclude subjects from the clean group.

Conclusion

Normative data were derived on men who were free of diseases which might influence the results. The decrements of physiological functioning of the four variables studied (representing four different systems) are not a result of diseases or medications, and must be considered a function of age. Thus, kidney function decreases with age, not because there is more clinical renal disease in the elderly but because of age and the passage of time. The actual mechanism of the decline of a system, be it loss of nephrons in the kidney or a decreased sensitivity of the pancreas to respond to glucose and secrete insulin in the decline of glucose tolerance with age, is under investigation. There may be a central, uniting aging factor with different expression in each organ system but, at the present time, this must be considered speculative.

Just as the mechanisms responsible for the demonstrated age changes are unclear and require future research, the resultant effects of the decline in a practical sense also need further study. In three of the four variables reported, those volunteers who have died had significantly poorer age-adjusted performance than those who lived. Total mortality is, however, a crude (though definitive) end-point. In this population, the bulk of the deaths were, as expected, due to cardiovascular and malignant disease. As the study progresses, more specific mortality data will be available and allow comparison of age changes in function with disease entities. The relationship of poor performance to the development of disease is not a simple one. Does the decreased function and the decreased reserve capacity to respond to stress serve as a fertile soil for disease to seed and grow? Do the organ systems progressively lose more and more function until some critical point is passed and they are, in effect, worn out? The list of questions goes on and, hopefully, the list of answers will grow. The answers will serve not only to increase the body of knowledge about the physiology of aging but, also, an understanding of the processes of health and function in the elderly.

References

ANDRES, R. A. (1971). *Med. Clin. N. Amer.*, **55**, 835.

COSTA, P. J. *Proceedings of the Second Conference on Epidemiology of Aging*, DHEW Publication. (In press.)

ROWE, J. W., ANDRES, R., TOBIN, J. D., NORRIS, A. H., and SHOCK, N. W. (1976). *J. Gerontol.*, **31**, 55.

SHOCK, N. W. (1980). This volume.

STONE, J. L. and NORRIS, A. H. (1966). *J. Gerontol.*, **21**, 575.

A new approach to measuring human biological age: studies on human skin fibroblasts in tissue culture
Edward L. Schneider

Introduction

The contributions to this volume by Shock and Tobin have indicated the complexities and difficulties of formulating indices of human biological or functional age. Most of the physiological tests that have been outlined involve the complex interaction of several organ systems. An example would be blood-pressure which is regulated by the condition of the heart, kidney, and vascular beds as well as by the hormonal and neural systems which act on these organs. Even within these organs, there are several cell-types with unequal contributions to the over-all response.

We would like to offer an alternative approach to measuring human biological age. It involves examining populations of a single cell-type removed from both endocrine and neural control mechanisms. The cell that we are studying is the human skin fibroblast and the setting for our studies is a tissue culture facility. Skin fibroblast cell cultures are established from skin biopsies obtained from members of the Baltimore Longitudinal Study. From a two-millimetre punch biopsy, up to one billion cells can be obtained after a brief time in tissue culture. This is sufficient for a wide number of biological and chemical analyses. In this chapter, we will briefly present some of the results of our preliminary studies on cell cultures obtained from human volunteers and discuss possible future applications of this approach to the study of human biological aging.

Establishment of cell cultures

Since this study was of a preliminary nature and there had been considerable doubt expressed as to whether cells in tissue culture would demonstrate any age effects (Kohn 1975; Schneider and Chase 1976), biopsies were obtained from subjects at the two extremes of the adult age range, a young group (aged 20 to 35) and an old group (aged 65 and above). To minimize differences related to biopsy site, all biopsies were obtained from the inner aspect of the left upper arm. This site was chosen for its minimum exposure to light and other forms of radiation. Although a skin biopsy can be classified as an invasive technique, we have performed over 400 of these procedures without any adverse reactions.

Because of the known variability of tissue culture conditions, all skin explants were treated identically and all tissue culture manipulations were carried out under standard protocols. Equal numbers of old and young cultures were examined in parallel and all cultures were coded by number with the code broken only after data collection was completed. Based on previous evidence that cell replication might be related to donor age (Goldstein, Littlefield, and Soeldner 1969; Martin, Sprague and Epstein 1970), we focused on several *in vitro* expressions of this parameter; the total replicative ability of the cell culture, the cell population replication rate, the percentage of replicating cells in the culture, and the replicating behaviour of individual cloned cells.

Total replicative potential

To measure total replication potential, cells were subcultured weekly. The initial confluent flask was arbitrarily designated as cell population doubling (CPD) 1. At early passage, a split ratio of 1 to 4 usually produced a confluent monolayer at one week. For each 1:4 split, the cell culture would have accumulated two additional cumulative population doublings. If confluency was not reached by one week, the culture was considered to have entered the senescent phase of its *in vitro* life span. Media was then changed weekly and, if the culture did not reach confluency by one month, the culture was termed senesced and the *in vitro* life-span was recorded.

Although cell cultures from young donors replicated rapidly during their initial 20 CPDs, three of the 24 cultures derived from older donors senesced during their first five CPDs (Table 1). The remaining 21 cultures derived from the old donor group also had a significantly earlier onset of cell culture senescence than the cultures derived from young donors (Schneider and Mitsui 1976).

Table 1 Characteristics of skin explants and cell cultures derived from young and old human donors

	Young donors	Old donors
Age of fibroblast donor (years)	28.1 ± 1.0 (23)†	78.9 ± 1.7 (24)
Onset of senescent phase (CPD)	35.2 ± 2.1 (23)	20.0 ± 2.0 (24)
In vitro life span (CPD)	44.6 ± 2.5 (23)	29.8 ± 2.9 (24)
Per cent replicating cells‡	87.7 ± 1.6 (7)	79.6 ± 2.5 (7)
Cell population doubling time (hours)	20.8 ± 0.8 (18)	24.3 ± 0.9 (18)
Cell number at confluency (10^4/cm^2)	7.31 ± 0.42 (18)	5.06 ± 0.52 (17)
Colony size distribution§	69.0 ± 3.3 (9)	48.0 ± 4.4 (8)

†Values are expressed as the mean ± standard error of the mean. The numbers within parentheses are the cell cultures examined.
‡Labelled nuclei after 24-h ^{3}H-thymidine incubation.
§Number of colonies with $\geqslant 16$ cells two weeks after inoculation of dilute cell suspension.

In vitro life span defined as either cumulative cell population doublings or days in culture was also considerably reduced in the cell cultures derived from the old donor group (Schneider and Mitsui 1976).

Measurements of acute cell replication

The percentage of replicating cells in the cell population was determined by measuring the frequency of labelled nuclei after three separate incubation times with tritiated thymidine. The per cent ^{3}H-thymidine-labelled nuclei in old and young donor cell cultures is seen in Fig. 1. Since the cell population doubling times of old and young donor skin fibroblast cultures range from 17 to 31 hours, the 24-hour measurements of percentage of replicating cells are probably the most informative (Table 1). At this time point, a statistically significant increase in the percentage of replicating cells is seen in the young donor cultures when compared with old donor cultures (Schneider and Mitsui 1976).

Cell population replication was assessed by examining growth curves of young and old donor cell cultures at equal levels of early passage (Fig. 2). Cells were inoculated at equal concentrations into a series of 35-mm Petri dishes, and on each of the following days replicate dishes were harvested and cell number counted. After an initial drop in cell number, there was a rapid growth phase, followed by a plateau as the culture became confluent. The initial drop in cell number after transfer, often referred to as the plating efficiency, was not significantly different between young and old donor cell cultures. Cell population doubling times measured during the period of logarithmic growth were increased in old donor cultures reflecting diminished cell population replication (Schneider and Mitsui 1976). Although the difference was small, it was statistically significant. However, the most consistent difference between old and young donor cell cultures was the decreased cell number at confluency observed in the old donor

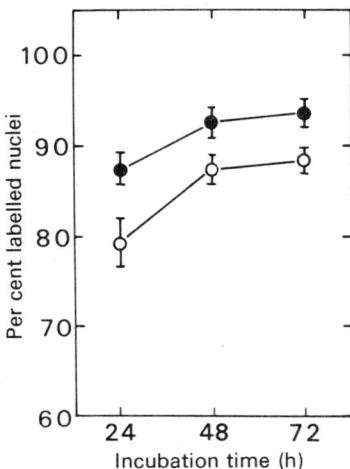

FIG. 1. Percentage of rapidly replicating cells, measured as the frequency of labelled nuclei after 24- to 74-hour incubations with ^{3}H -thymidine. Old (○) and young (●) donor cell cultures. (From Schneider and Mitsui (1976).)

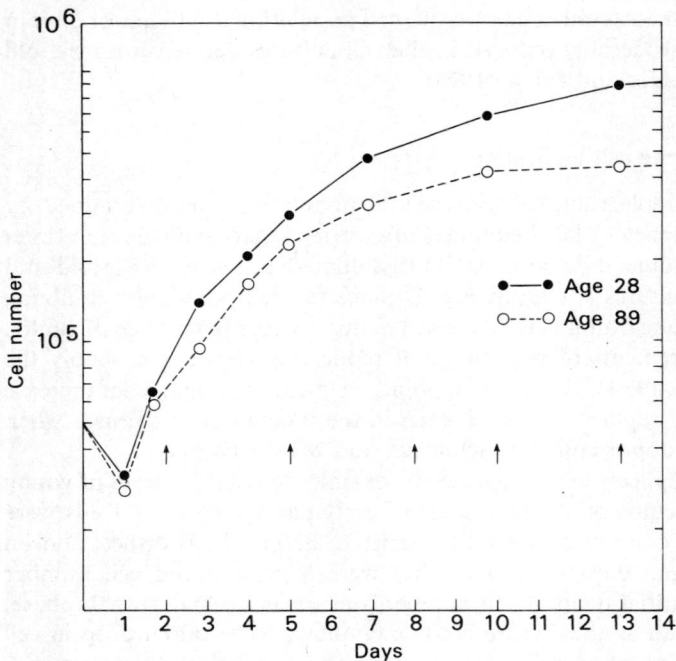

Fig. 2. Typical growth cruves of cell cultures derived from a young (———●———) and old
(– – –○– – –) donor. Arrows indicate addition of fresh media. (From Schneider and Mitsuit
(1976).)

cell cultures. Although cell volumes were also increased in old donor cell cultures,
volume does not seem to be the sole basis for this difference in cell number at
confluency. We feel that it is likely that increased sensitivity to cell-to-cell contact
may play an important role in the lower cell number at confluency exhibited by
the old donor cell cultures.

Examination of individual cells

The last analysis of cell replication involved the examination of the replicative
abilities of single cells derived from young and old human donor cell cultures
(Smith, Schneider, and Smith, 1978). This study was performed in collaboration with James Smith of the W. Alton Jones Cell Science Center. After
plating human skin fibroblasts into Petri dishes at low cell densities, colonies are
formed ranging in size from one cell to 1000 cells. The relative proportion of
small to large colonies appears to be closely related to the age of the donor of the
cell culture. To quantify the replicative capacity of individual cloned cells, the
number of progeny cells are counted two weeks after plating. Colony sizes are
tabulated as the number of population doublings that the original cell must have
undergone to attain the observed cell count. Typical colony size distributions
obtained from a young and an old human donor cell culture are seen in Fig. 3.

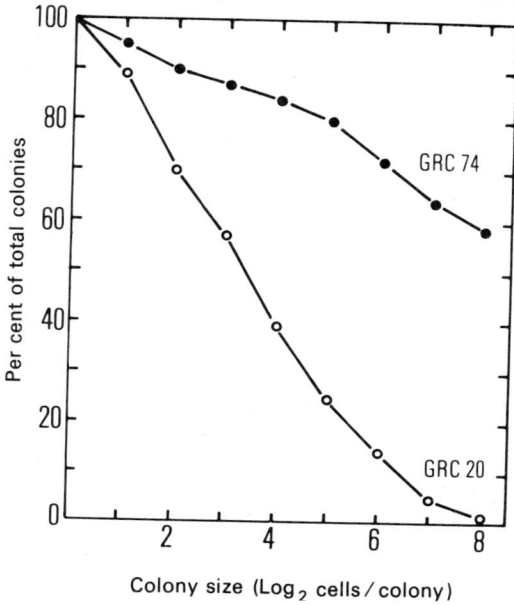

FIG. 3. Colony size distributions of old (GRC 20, O---O) and young (GRC 74, ●——●) donor cell culture. (From Smith *et al.*, unpublished.)

Colony size distributions are expressed as the per cent cloned cells able to attain a specific colony size. Note that while 60 per cent of the young donor cells are able to replicate eight or more times during this period, only two per cent of the old donor cells are able to achieve this level of cell replication. Even at a modest replication level such as four doublings (16 or more cells), a significant decline is observed in the percentage of old donor cells. In fact, we have found the most significant difference between young and old donor cell cultures at this level of four or more CPDs. The results of measurement of colony size distributions on 17 cell cultures are summarized in Table 1. Once again, a highly significant decrease in replicative capabilities was observed in cell cultures derived from old volunteers (Smith *et al.*, 1978).

Discussion

To briefly summarize the results of our preliminary studies, we have found statistically significant differences in a variety of tissue culture measurements related to the chronological age of the subject from which the culture was derived. All of these measurements have involved examinations of replicative capability. However, these cells are equally amenable to a wide number of biochemical, morphological, and physiological investigations.

Our ability to obtain statistically significant data may well have been related to the emphasis placed on standardization of skin biopsy procedures, explanation and subcultivation protocols, utilization of the same media, and the performance of all determinations on parallel old and young donor cell cultures. The importance of obtaining cell cultures from a non-hospitalized, normal population should also be emphasized since disorders such as diabetes have been known to alter *in vitro* life span as well as other *in vitro* parameters (Goldstein *et al*. 1969).

It is likely that in a cross-sectional study of this nature, we have selected a relatively vigorous old population (less vigorous individuals having been removed by death before age 65). Therefore, the results obtained by the above studies may be conservative underestimates of the *in vitro* alterations which may occur as a function of *in vivo* aging.

The results of these preliminary studies have been most encouraging and have led us to undertake a more extensive analysis of the relationship between *in vitro* measurements of cell replication and human aging. We will focus on a single parameter which we have found to be relatively easy to measure and which has demonstrated a significant relationship with chronological age, the colony size distribution. This test will be performed on cell cultures established from 400 unselected members of the Baltimore Longitudinal Study. This should provide sufficient data for correlative analysis with physiological and psychological data collected from the same individuals. It is hoped that this study may result in the formulation of an *in vitro* index of human aging.

One of the important by-products of our studies on the subjects of the Baltimore Longitudinal Study is the establishment of a cell culture bank. Skin fibroblast cultures derived from over 60 subjects are stored in liquid nitrogen at −270 °C. Under these conditions, these cells will remain preserved indefinitely. At any future time, these cells can be thawed and returned to tissue culture for further studies. During the next two years, cell cultures will be established from over 400 members of this Baltimore Longitudinal Study, and these cells will be added to our cell bank.

It is hoped that these cells will provide an invaluable resource for studies of cellular aging. We have initiated collaborative studies with a number of outside laboratories and would like to encourage other investigators to use these cell cultures in their studies of human aging. It is hoped that information obtained from these studies will then be used for further formulations of *in vitro* indices of human aging.

Another important aspect of these studies is that they may provide a unique type of longitudinal study. It is anticipated that a small number of individuals will consent to repeated skin biopsies over 5- to 10-year intervals. Skin fibroblast cultures will be established from these biopsies and the resultant cells frozen in our cell bank. At a later time point, cells from the same individual obtained at increasing chronological age can be thawed, returned to tissue culture, and examined in parallel under identical conditions.

In conclusion, we have explored a potential alternate approach to examining human biological aging. Measurements of a number of parameters in skin fibroblast cultures derived from volunteer members of the Baltimore Longitudinal Study have revealed a significant decline in replicative capabilities in those cultures derived from older donors. These results would suggest that tissue culture can be utilized to examine human cellular aging. Future studies will be directed at examining the correlations between these tissue culture determinations and *in vivo* physiological and psychological measurements as well as the formulation of a longitudinal analysis of cellular aging.

References

GOLDSTEIN, S., LITTLEFIELD, J. W., and SOELDNER, J. S. (1969). *Proc. Nat. Acad. Sci., USA*, **64**, 155–9.

KOHN, R. R. (1975). *Science, N.Y.*, **188**, 203–4.

MARTIN, G. M., SPRAGUE, C. A., and EPSTEIN, C. J. (1970). *Lab. Invest.*, **23**, 86–92.

SCHNEIDER, E. L. and MITSUI, Y. (1976). *Proc. Nat. Acad. Sci., USA*, **73**, 3584–8.

—— and CHASE, G. A. (1976). In *Interdisciplinary topics in gerontology* (ed. R. G. Cutler), Vol. 10, pp. 62–9. Karger, Basel.

SMITH, J. R., SMITH, O. M. P., and SCHNEIDER, E. L. (1978). *Proc. Nat. Acad. Sci., USA*, **75**, 1353–6.

Session 18

Immunology

Immunoregulatory systems and aging Roy L. Walford

Introduction

The importance of gerontology, the study of the aging process, for modern medicine can best be illustrated by reference to certain actuarial data. Fig. 1 shows survival curves of populations from several countries in the twentieth century, and from ancient Rome. In the more advanced industrial societies, and increasingly with more recent times, the 50 per cent survival point has shifted progressively to a later age. This shift is due to improved sanitation and nutrition, cure of specific diseases, and general 'public health' measures. However, the age of the longest-lived survivor or, as a more workable assessment, of the 10th decile of survivorship, has in fact remained about the same not only irrespective of place but even since ancient times. Now longest-lived survival data provide the best measure of the actual aging rate in a population or species (Sacher 1959). All our medical and public health efforts since antiquity have only succeeded in rotating the survival curve about its terminal, fixed point (Fig. 1). On the average, therefore, people live longer today but they still age at the same rate as in the past. And because, in modern times, the curve is approaching a

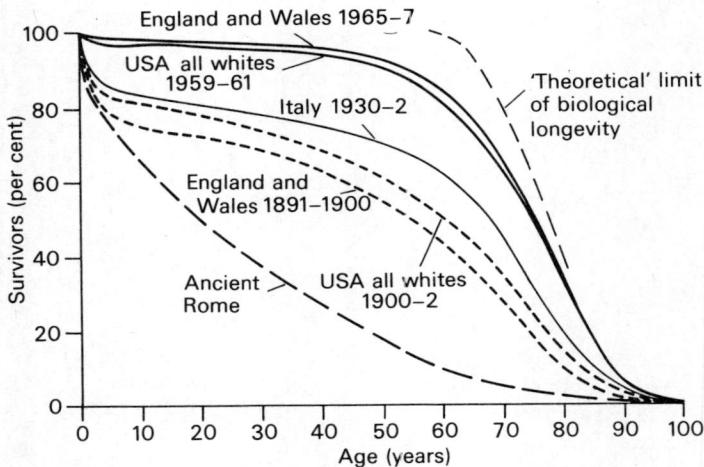

FIG. 1. Survival curves in human populations, ancient Rome → modern Europe and USA.

rectangularized form, complete eradication of vascular disease, maturity-onset diabetes, cancer, and indeed all major 'diseases of aging' will only extend average human life span by half a dozen or so years (the main killer of persons of very advanced age is not disease *per se* but accident, secondary to the augmenting feebleness of age).

Figure 2 further illustrates the concept I am developing, by showing the life expectancy of humans once the age of 60 years has been reached. Surprisingly there has been little betterment since the year 1789! The obvious conclusion is that on a population basis, although not of course on an individual basis, occidental societies are in a sense nearing the end of medical progress unless the process of aging itself can be influenced.

The 'diseases of aging' are not the cause but to a considerable degree the sequelae of the increasing vulnerability of the aging organism. As shown in Fig. 3, these maladies as a class demonstrate an age-specific peak incidence in

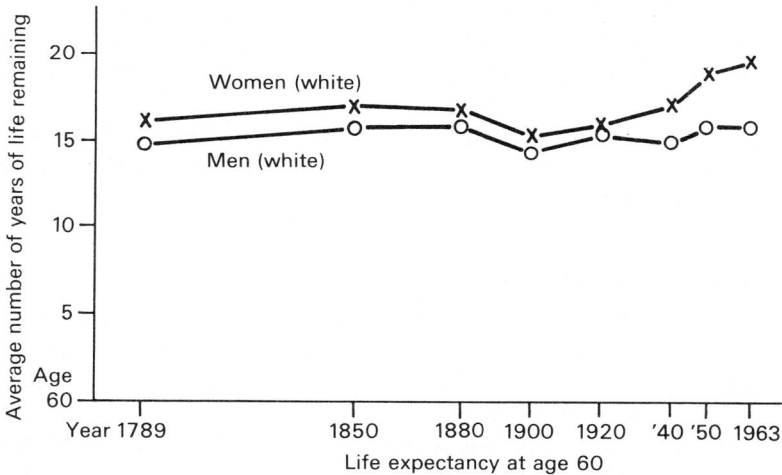

FIG. 2. Life expectancy once 60 years has been reached, 1789 to 1963.

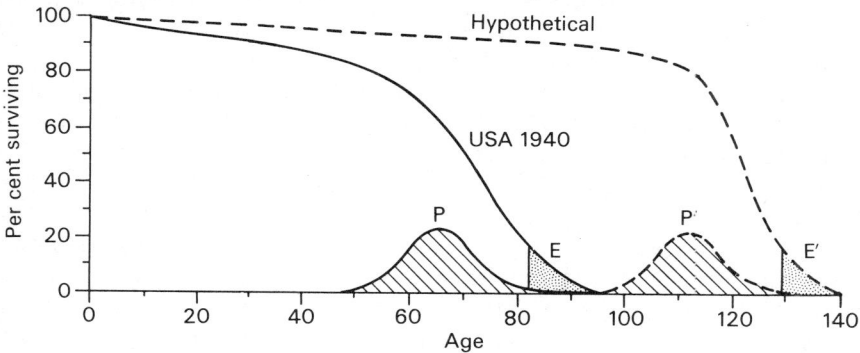

FIG. 3. Effect on age-specific incidence (P, P′) of the 'diseases of aging' of extension of the tenth decile of survivorship, and on percentages of enfeebled or senile oldsters in the population (E, E′).

relation to the downswing of the survival curve. If the terminal portion of the curve could be shifted to a later age, the peak incidence would also shift, thus P→P' in Fig. 3. If substantial postponement of disease be regarded as cure, then excessive direct preoccupation with prevention or treatment of specific age-related diseases, rather than with the biology of aging itself, must be regarded as undue emphasis, an example of putting the cart before the horse. Extend life span and you automatically cure all these diseases, but curing all the diseases will not greatly extend life span, which is the paradox of gerontology.

So long as the survival curve be kept rectangularized, retardation of the aging rate can only be achieved by stretching out the young and middle years, not the terminal years. The last small segment of survivors of curve A, Fig. 3 (the shaded area) may be considered feeble or senile. An equal (shaded) area is seen towards the end of curve B, Fig. 3. But note that the shaded area of curve B is a smaller proportion of the total area subsumed under that curve than the shaded area of curve A. The actual per cent of senile persons in the general population will thus be *decreased* by a significant deceleration of the rate of aging. The popular nightmare of an increasing army of senile oldsters does not accord with informed expectations.

Given the theoretical importance of gerontology as a discipline at this point in time, what are its prospects? Are we still groping in the dark or close to real progress? I believe the latter is the case.

Theories of aging: genetic restriction

Theories of aging resolve into either stochastic processes (random events, perhaps with autocatalytic secondary effects, 'error catastrophe'; Orgel 1963) or programmed events. Programmed events would in particular be assumed to display a classical genetic base, the code written in the genome. But at what level? At the same time we may inquire whether aging reflects broad-spectrum phenomena—for example, changes along the whole DNP molecule such as might be induced by cross-linking—or more localized processes involving relatively few genes. I have opted for the latter concept in a so-called 'limited gene theory of aging' (Walford 1972, 1974), and will pursue it further here.

Normal cells in tissue culture eventually undergo senescence-like changes, with decreasing ability to divide, and finally extinction of the clone (Hayflick 1966). Transformed or malignant cells, on the other hand, however annoying they seem to our aesthetic priorities, are a legitimate form of living matter. They do not die out on culture. They are potentially immortal. Now transformation may be induced by the introduction of only a few viral genes into a normal cell. Transformation by carcinogenic chemicals, such as benzopyrene, may likewise require only a restricted target, equivalent in this instance to about 20 genes (Huberman, Mager, and Sachs 1976). The target could even be smaller if the transformation genes were located at hot spots with higher than average mutation potentials. (Some of the histocompatibility genes in fact appear to show such an increased mutation rate; Bailey and Kohn 1965.) The point is that transformation, which eliminates aging from cells in culture, involves only a limited number of genes.

To support the thesis from another side: analysis of the genetic basis for the increasing life span of hominid species in the last several hundred thousand years led to the conclusion that mutations of no more than about 0.6 per cent of the total genome could be responsible for the increase (Cutler 1975; Sacher 1975).

It seems to me that if only a few discrete 'structural' genes were involved in aging, one might expect the occurrence of mutational aging freaks: individuals with very extended life span, or disease conditions with greatly accelerated aging rates. The former at least have clearly not been observed. As to the latter, a highly instructive analysis by Martin (1977) has made clear that while many syndromes in the human show features of accelerated aging, none display the complete spectrum. (The oftenest quoted example, the disease progeria, lacks the following features of aging, among others: senile dementia, increase in lipofuchsin 'aging' pigment, amyloidosis, cataracts, increase in frequency of tumours, diabetes mellitus, and degenerative arthritis.) If a relatively small number of genes be involved in aging, and if these are not primarily structural genes, they may well be regulatory genes.

The main histocompatibility complex (MHC)

A limited gene approach to aging seems therefore to be most consistent with the above facts and ideas if complex regulatory genes, or so-called 'supergene' systems, be invoked. The main histocompatibility complex (MHC)—for example, the H-2 system in mice or the HLA system in humans—represents such a major regulatory system. It controls, influences or regulates at least the following functions (for references see Walford 1977): the recognition phase of cellular immunity as manifested in the mixed lymphocyte reaction; cell-mediated lymphocytotoxicity; the development of specific suppressor cells important for immunoregulation; susceptibility to a number of viruses; susceptibility or resistance to a number of spontaneously occurring malignancies including lymphomas and cancers of the breast, lungs, and liver; susceptibility to the development of different auto-immune diseases; the ability to mount an immune response to certain specific antigens (via the immune-response genes); the age-specific maturation rates, peaks and rates of decline of different immune response capacities; components of the complement system; T/B cell collaboration (helper cells); the expression of the theta-antigen; levels of plasma testosterone and testosterone-binding protein. In addition, the gene products located at the D and K loci of the H-2 system may be required for recognition of 'self' (Bevan 1975; Doherty and Zinkernagel 1975). Furthermore, the H-2 system is in strong linkage disequilibrium with the highly complex T/t system, which has an important but as yet little understood influence on differentiation (Klein and Hammerberg 1977).

It has been suggested that the MHC may be fundamentally involved in the aging process (Walford 1970, 1974). Recent studies in congenic mice lend support to this surmise (Smith and Walford 1977). Congenic strains differ from another at a relatively short chromosomal region. Mice congenic for the H-2 region, which is the MHC in mice, can be prepared by selective breeding experiments upon any particular background; for example upon C57BL, C3H, or A strain backgrounds. Analysis of the aging patterns of 14 strains congenic for H-2 upon these backgrounds led us to the observation that for 50 per cent survival and also for 10th decile survivorship the variation in life span was as great as that observed between non-congenic strains. One might have expected much greater uniformity within a congenic set unless the H-2 region itself exerts a significant effect upon the rate of aging. A portion of these data are shown in Tables 1 and 2.

Although genetically identical except for the short H-2 region on the 17th chromosome, the mice within each set demonstrated considerable variation of

Table 1 Effect of H-2 alleles on tenth decile survivorship in mice congenic on a C57BL/10 background (adapted from Smith and Walford (1977))

Strain	H-2 allele	Life span (in weeks)						
		1	2	3	4	5	6	7
1. B10.AKM	m	139						
2. B10.Br/Sg	k	†	149					
3. B10.PL	u	†	—	153				
4. B10.A/Sg	a	†	†	—	154			
5. B10.D2/n	d	†	†	—	—	155		
6. C57BL/10	b	†	†	—	—	—	155	
7. B10.RIII	r	†	†	†	†	†	†	170

†Denotes statistically significant differences: for strain B10.R111, $p < 0.002$ for all comparisons; for other comparisons $p < 0.03$.

Table 2 Survival data and incidences of commonest tumours for groups of male mice congenic at the H-2 histocompatibility region upon three separate backgrounds (adapted from Smith and Walford (1977)†

Strain	H-2 allele	Mean survival (in weeks)	Mean of tenth decile (in weeks)	Tumour incidences (per cent) Lymphoma hepatoma lung tumours		
B10.AKM/Sn	m	99	139	53	5	0
C57BL/10Sn	b	134	155	29	2	3
B10.RIII(7INS)/Sn	r	141	170	23	0	10
C3H.JKSn	j	112	136	3	50	14
C3H/HeDiSn	k	98	138	5	51	10
C3H.SW/Sn	b	108	150	3	38	0
A.BY/Sn	b	85	114	10	2	10
A.CA/Sn	f	85	127	0	14	28
A/WySn	a	97	134	13	15	26

†B10.AKMSn mice have statistically significantly shorter mean and tenth decile survivorships ($p < 0.05$, generally much less) than both congenic partners, and C57BL/10Sn a significantly shorter 10th decile survivorship than B10.R111(7INS)/Sn mice. On the C3H background C3H.JKSn mean survival is significantly different from C3H/HeDiSn but not from C3H.SW/Sn. C3H.SW/Sn has a significantly longer tenth decile than its partners. On the A-strain background all strains differ significantly from one another at 10th decile and A/WySn from its two partners for mean survival.

mean and 10th decile survivorship. Evidence of a complex interplay between the particular H-2 allele and the over-all genetic backgrounds was additionally provided by the observation that H-2^b might promote either longer or shorter life span depending upon the several backgrounds (Table 2). In a study by Popp (1977) the allele H-2^n on a C56BL background correlated with greatly shortened survival, premature greying of hair, and other evidence perhaps interpretable as accelerated aging.

In our study (Smith and Walford 1977) the particular H-2 allele exerted also a striking influence upon the incidence of different tumours within the background of the congenic lines, although there was no consistent relationship between the over-all tumour incidence and life span (Table 2). Strain A/WySn, for example, showed the highest tumour incidence among the A lines, but clearly the longest survival by both mean and 10th decile criteria.

Insight into the relationship between age-related immune function and life span in some of these same strains of congenic mice can be garnered from the data of Meredith and Walford (1977) illustrated in Fig. 4, which shows the age-related response of the strains to phytohemagglutinin (PHA), purified protein derivative (PPD), and pokeweed mitogen (PWM). PHA is known to be a T-cell specific mitogen, PPD a B-cell specific mitogen, and PWM to stimulate B-cells and cortisone-resistant T-cells. For the C3H strains there was no consistent relationship between the mortality data given in Table 1 and the age-specific response to several mitogens. For the C57BL strain, however, the longest-lived line, namely B10.RIII/Sn, displayed the highest PHA response throughout most of life, and the shortest-lived line, namely B10.AKM/Sn, the lowest response. The survival patterns of the A strain mice also accorded with the age-specific PHA response, with the longer-lived A/WySn line showing a higher PHA response throughout life than its partners. The response to the thymus-independent mitogen, PPD, did not correlate with strain-specific life span, although differences on the basis of the H-2 type were noted. With regard to PWM mitogen, the very long-lived B10.RIII/Sn mouse clearly displayed higher responses than its congenic partners. No significant differences were noted for A or C3H strains for this mitogen.

The above studies indicate that given any particular genetic background, the MHC in mice exerts a significant influence upon life span as determined by mean or 10th decile survival statistics, and this influence might be mediated at least in part by preservation of the functional integrity of genes within the MHC. Since the MHC is in fact the master genetic control region for a wide variety of immune functions, particularly the thymus-dependent functions, it would be strong evidence against a major role for the immune system in the aging process if such an influence could not be demonstrated.

Because of the desirability of making an aging hypothesis as general as possible, it is worth noting that self/non-self recognition, histocompatibility reactions, and specific immunocompetence with components of memory are not limited to vertebrates but have been described in echinoderms, annelids, and coelenterates (Hildemann 1977). Furthermore, cell surface markers of the

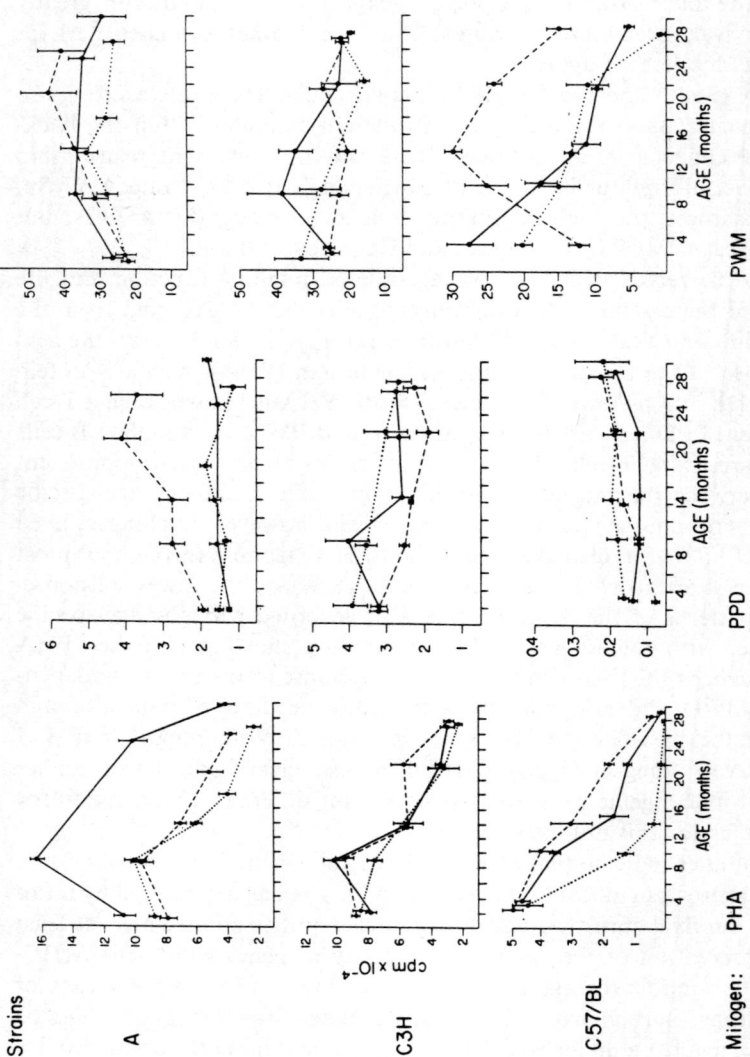

FIG. 4. Age-related mitogenic responses of spleen cells from groups of mice congenic at the H-2 histocompatibility region and upon three different genetic backgrounds. (●——●) A/WySn (H−2ᵃ), C3H.SW/Sn (H−2ᵇ), C57BL/10Sn (H−2ᵇ); (●−−−●) A.CA/Sn (H−2ᶠ), C3H.JK/Sn (H−2ʲ), C57BL10.RIII/Sn (H−2ʳ); (●·····●) A.By/Sn (H−2ᵇ), C3H/HeDiSn (H−2ᵏ), C57BL10.AKM/Sn (H−2ᵐ). (Adapted from Meredith and Walford (1977).)

MHC such as H-2 in mice or HLA in man are expressed on all nucleated cells of the body. I believe that most requirements which might be conceptualized to make us think that a particular regulatory system is involved in aging can be met by the MHC.

Immune dysfunction and aging

The response of the host lymphoid cells to non-self, altered self, or foreign alloantigens—be they tissue grafts, indigenous malignancy, or virus-altered cells—is characterized by a recognition phase during which a subpopulation of host cells undergoes blastogenesis. The recognition phase, measured in the mixed lymphocyte reaction, is mediated in mice most strongly by genes at the IA locus of the MHC. Recognition is followed by the development of 'killer' cells responsible for cell-mediated lymphocytotoxicity in which the foreign or altered cells are lysed. This cytotoxic reaction is not I-region controlled but is dependent upon genetic factors present at the K and D ends of the H-2 in the mouse or the A and B loci of HLA in man. Both stimulator and effector aspects of what one may regard as classical transplantation immunity—which to some degree is present in every metazoan animal so far studied in detail—are therefore influenced by the MHC.

With age in mice the mixed lymphocyte reaction declines to about a third of its peak youth value (Konen, Smith, and Walford 1973; Gerbase-DeLima, Liu, Cheney, Mickey, and Walford 1975), and cell-mediated lymphocytotoxicity to a considerably greater extent (Goodman and Makinodan 1975). Both these reactions may involve more than one T-cell subset, such as T_1 (precursor) cells and T_2 (amplifier) cells. Utilizing the *in vivo* graft-versus-host reaction, Asofsky, Tigelaar, and Cantor (1971) demonstrated that T_1 and T_2 cells would 'synergize' with one another in producing a response greater than that shown by the sum of responses of the cells taken singly. We were able to demonstrate that this ability to synergize also declines significantly with age (Gerbase-DeLima *et al.* 1975).

The humoral immune response involving the manufacture of immunoglobulin antibodies, to the extent that it requires T/B-cell co-operation, also declines markedly with age. The most thorough studies of this decline are those of Makinodan, Perkins, and Chen (1971) and Kishimoto, Takahama, and Mizumachi (1976).

Certain mitogens, chiefly phytohaemagglutinin (PHA) and concanavallin-A (con-A) stimulate T-dependent lymphoid cells to undergo blastogenesis and incorporate tritiated thymidine. The response to these mitogens declines markedly with advanced age in mice (Mathies, Lipps, Smith, and Walford 1973; Hori, Perkins, and Halsall 1973; Meredith and Walford 1977). It has been shown, however, that the lymphoid cells of an old mouse possess just as many combining sites for PHA as those from a young mouse (Hung, Perkins, and Yang 1975). Despite receptor site equality, the old lymphoid cell population gives a diminished response, signifying either that many cells respond to a lesser degree or that a lower percentage of cells among the old population respond.

So-called 'suppressor cells' are lymphoid cells which suppress another immune reaction or potential reaction. Important in regulatory control of the immune system and in mitigating against auto-immunity, they are coded for by a locus in the I-region of the MHC in mice (Shreffler 1977). There is evidence for the existence of both thymic and splenic suppressor cells which act in different ways (Talal 1976). Suppressor cells for the mixed lymphocyte reaction and for the response to dinitrophenyl hapten tend to increase with normal aging in long-lived strains of mice (Gerbase-DeLima *et al.* 1975; Segre and Segre 1976).

While the subject is too complex for detailed presentation here, a strong case can be made that all the major 'diseases of aging' such as cancer, senile amyloidosis, vascular disease, cerebral deterioration, and maturity-onset diabetes are to a variable but significant degree influenced or potentiated by age-related immune functional decline (Walford 1969, 1974; Matthews, Whittingham, and Mackay 1974; Blumenthal and Alex 1975).

Auto-immunity and aging

Age-related functional decline or imbalance is especially prominent in, but of course not unique to the immune system. However, as the normal immune response declines, auto-immune manifestations greatly increase, and it is this duality of phenomena going in opposite directions (Fig. 5) that is unique and interesting and not obviously present in other organ systems undergoing aging alterations. There occurs with aging a striking increase in the incidence of auto-antibodies both in humans and mice (Mackay 1972; Siegel, Braun, and Morton 1972; Yunis, Stutman, Fernandes, Teague, and Good 1972), and probably including brain-reactive antibodies (Nandy 1972). Longitudinal studies in

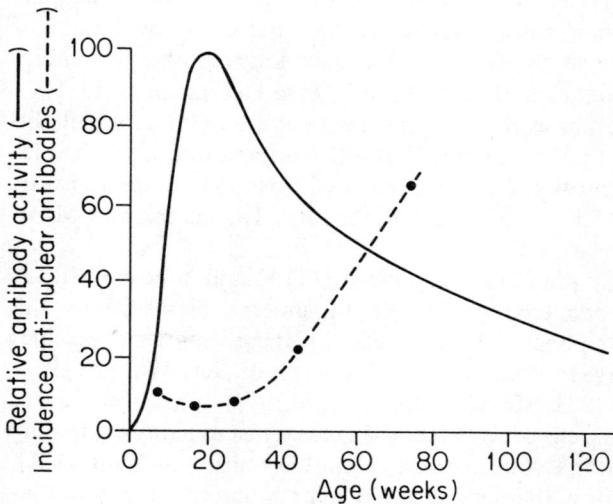

FIG. 5. Relative immune functional capacity (smooth curve) and incidence of auto-immune manifestations in relation to age in mice (dotted curve).

humans indicate that individuals with auto-antibodies in their sera show an increased mortality rate (Mathews, Whittingham, Hooper, and MacKay 1973).

Consideration of auto-immunity inclines one to the possibility that aging may be not entirely a process of programmed, passive wearing-out of systems, but of active self-destruction (Walford 1969; Denckla 1975). This distinction or duality of active and passive processes requires to be kept in mind, because most current theories of aging have postulated purely deteriorative processes, either stochastic or programmed.

One possible experimental model for aging is the chronic graft-versus-host reaction (Walford 1962). When immunocompetent cells are introduced into a tolerant host, a graft-versus-host reaction ensues in which the introduced cells react against the recipient animal. This reaction, which is also obviously a model for a form of auto-immune state, is characterized by lymphoid depletion and hypoplasia, fibrosis, eosinophilic deposits, an increased number of plasma cells in lymphoid organs, hyaline changes in renal glomeruli, renal atrophy, immune-complex formation, weight loss, arteriosclerosis, changes in skin and hair, thymic atrophy, amyloidosis, decreased responsiveness to isoantigenic stimuli, positive tests for auto-antibodies, a decrease in the ratio of soluble to insoluble collagen (Liu and Walford 1970), disturbances in T and B cell collaboration, increased numbers of suppressor cells, and activation of latent viruses (Grebe and Streilein 1976). All these phenomena are also found in normal aging. The parallelism can hardly be regarded as other than striking.

Conceptually related to the decline in normal immune functions as set against the rise in auto-immunity is an age-related imbalance in the ability to distinguish self from non-self. Naor, Bonvida, and Walford (1977) demonstrated that the response of mice to a 'modified-self' antigen, trinitrophenylated syngeneic mouse red blood cells, persists in the face of a drastic decline with age in the response to the 'non-self' antigen, trinitrophenylated sheep red blood cells. TNP-mouse red blood cells can legitimately be regarded as an auto-antigen (Cunningham 1976). Thus the ratio of the response of auto- to alloantigen increased with age. Such disturbances in regulatory function, or in the homeostatic control of tolerance as postulated some years ago (Walford 1969), may be of critical importance for aging. The auto-antibody response to the liver-specific F-antigen in mice is thought to be under control of two genes, one being linked to H-2 (Silver and Lane 1975). The ability of mice to respond to mouse thyroglobulin is determined by a gene linked to H-2 (Allison and Denman 1976).

It is appropriate now to emphasize that as a class the auto-immune diseases in humans demonstrate a high statistical correlation with a number of gene products of the HLA system (Dausset, Degos, and Hors 1974; Vladutiu and Rose 1974; Svejgaard, Platz, Ryder, Nielsen, and Thomsen 1975). The commonest HLA specificity whose frequency is significantly increased in various auto-immune diseases is HLA-B8, which suggests that this or more probably a closely linked gene could be regarded as an auto-immune-susceptibility gene. Interestingly enough, it has recently been noted by Yunis and Greenberg (1977) that the frequency of HLA-B8 is decreased in older cohorts of human females, suggesting the possibility of an increased mortality rate in females carrying this marker.

Diabetes mellitus presents many features of accelerated aging (Goldstein, Niewiarowski, and Singal 1975) including a shift in the incidence of severe arteriosclerosis to a younger age, an increased frequency of auto-antibodies to gastric, thyroid, and nuclear antigens (Whittingham, Mathews, MacKay, Stocks, Ungar, and Martin 1971), amyloidosis, and a sharply decreased replicative potential of fibroblasts in tissue culture (Vracko and Benditt 1975). Juvenile diabetes at least is clearly influenced by the genetic make-up of the MHC, although the precise formulation is not yet apparent. A number of studies report an increased frequency of HLA-B8, as well as certain MLR determinants in juvenile diabetes (Thomsen, Platz, Anderson, Christy, Lyngsoe, Nerup, Rasmussen, Ryder, Nielsen, and Svejgaard 1975). An increased frequency of recombination or of homozygosity at the HLA region has also been claimed (Rubenstein, Suciu-Foca, Nicholson, Fotino, Malinaro, Harisiadis, Hardy, Reemtsma, and Allen 1976), and an increased rate of death occurs in those older diabetics who demonstrate auto-antibodies (Whittingham *et al.* 1971). L. Greenburg and E. Yunis (personal communication) observed that in maturity onset familial diabetes, inheritance may segregate with one of the HLA haplotypes. A suggestive case can therefore be made for the role of immunogenetic factors in diabetes, which is one of the most characteristic 'diseases of aging'.

The information about HLA in man may be interpreted to lend support to conclusions derived from the congenic mouse data cited above, namely, that the MHC influences aging rates. The situation in humans is simply less clear due to the genetic heterogeneity of the species.

Life span shortening and prolongation

Whereas a number of experimental models such as post-thymectomy wasting, chronic parabiotic rejection, low-dosage total body irradiation, and various diseases (see Martin 1977) manifest features of accelerated aging, the fit is never exact. While irradiation shifts peak incidence of malignancy to a younger age, the types of malignancies seen are not percentagewise the same, nor is the ratio of insoluble/soluble collagen (a good biochemical criterion for aging) correspondingly altered. Interestingly enough for our present thesis, the model showing the closest fit is the auto-immunity of NZB/W mice (Yunis *et al.* 1972). The problem with using these various experimental or natural models as probes is that one is never sure he is dealing with true aging, instead of a partial semblance thereof. Investigators are still arguing whether irradiation-induced life span shortening is true aging or not.

The prolongation of the life span (measured by longest-lived or tenth decile survival statistics) of a long-lived strain is a more clear-cut experiment. The terminal portion of the life curve of a long-lived strain can be moved to the right *only* by influencing the basic aging rate (Fig. 3), and not by better hygiene, better animal husbandry, or avoidance or cure of specific disease.

Two methodologies are known which clearly and dramatically decelerate the aging process according to longest-lived survivor as well as other assessments, and two additional approaches may at least in part serve to rejuvenate or reconstitute the immune system of old animals, although their effect on life span has not yet been adequately determined.

(1) *Controlled caloric undernutrition, the classical McCay rat experiment* (McCay, Crowell, and Maynard 1935). When animals from the time of weaning or early youth are maintained on a nutritionally adequate but sharply calorically restricted diet (i.e., *under*nutrition but not *mal*nutrition), life span may be prolonged from 20 to as much as 100 per cent. Later work, largely of a biochemical nature and also confined to the rat, confirmed that controlled dietary restriction decelerates the rate of aging (Ross 1969). We have shown that in long-lived strains of mice a similar dietary regime delays maturation of the immune response capacity, slows the normal age-related fall-off in that capacity, and prolongs life span (Walford, Liu, Gerbase-DeLima, Mathies, and Smith 1974; Gerbase-DeLima *et al.* 1975). At a young age the cells of dietarily restricted mice show a diminished immune response to mitogens; however, by one year of age and continuing through a later period they respond better than cells from control mice (Fig. 6). A similar relationship obtains with the response to injected sheep red blood cells. Skin allograft survival is greatly prolonged in dietarily restricted mice and does not reach normal values until over 1 year of age. These studies add up to a 'reversal effect', as illustrated schematically in Fig. 7.

(2) *Mild long-term lowering of core body temperature.* Early observations by naturalists, e.g., that fence lizards live longer in the northern than southern

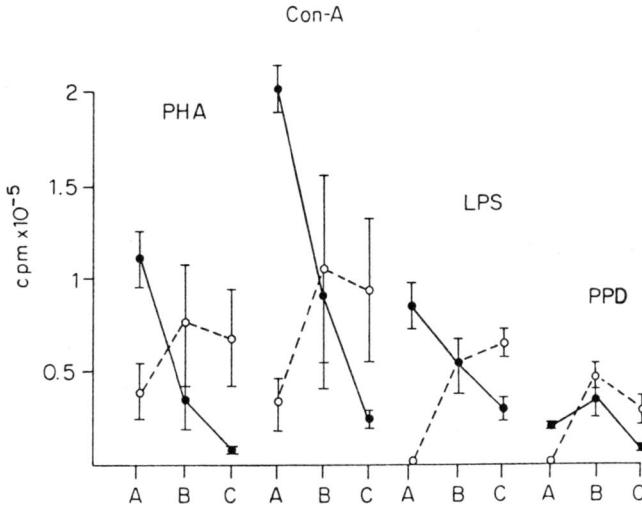

FIG. 6. Tritiated thymidine uptake of PHA, Con-A, LPS, and PPD stimulated spleen cells from restricted (O——O) and non-restricted (●——●) mice of three different ages (A = 31–4 weeks; B = 56–61 weeks; C = 75–85 weeks). (Adapted from Gerbase-De Lima *et al.* (1975).)

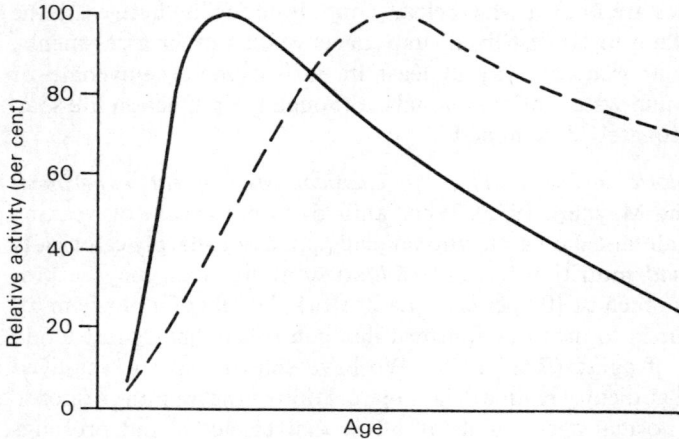

FIG. 7. The reversal effect. Solid line represents immune response of control mice, dotted line of dietarily restricted mice. If restriction delays maturation of immune response capacity and maintains a 'younger' immune system into a later age, then young restricted mice would show a decreased and older restricted mice an increased reactivity compared to controls.

United States, prompted us to undertake laboratory investigations of the effect of body temperature on life span in poikilothermic vertebrates. We were aware from work by Hildemann and associates (Hildemann and Cooper 1963) that the immune system is extremely sensitive to variations in body temperature. Using several species of annual fish of the genus *Cynolebias*, we noted that populations retained at 15 °C lived substantially longer than those at 20 °C and showed deceleration of the aging rate as estimated by collagen solubility (Liu and Walford 1966; Walford, Liu, Troup, and Hsi 1969). The life span prolongation by reduced temperature could not be attributed merely to general metabolic slowdown (Lieu and Walford 1972). Finally, the prolongation effect of reduced temperature was exerted maximally during the last half or two-thirds of life (Lieu and Walford 1975).

The temperature phenomenon is paradoxical in terms of the relation between immunology and aging. Lowering body temperature greatly suppresses both humoral and cellular immunity. This would seem likely to accentuate the immunodeficiency of aging; nevertheless, life span is greatly prolonged. The fact that reduced body temperature especially prolongs the last half of life may indicate that suppression of age-related auto-immunity overrides any disadvantages accruing from adding, by such a regime, to the general immunodeficiency of aging. Lending mild support to this view is the observation that long-term, late-life administration of immunosuppressive drugs may, despite toxic side-effects, favourably influence the 50 per cent survival point of mouse populations (Walford 1969).

It seems reasonable to emphasize that the life span-prolonging effects of caloric undernutrition and of lowering body temperature are maximally effective at the opposite periods of life span: nutritional manipulation during the first half and temperature lowering during the last half. One of these regimes delays the immunodeficiency of normal aging, the other probably ameliorates the autoimmunity that develops with age. The situation may reflect the operation of dual, age-related, immune dysfunctional processes.

(3) A few chemical agents such as 2-mercaptoethanol (Makinodan, Deitchmau, Stoltzner, Kay, and Hirokawa 1975), polynucleotides (Han and Johnson 1976), and thymic hormone (Goldstein, Hooper, Schulof, Cohen, Thurman, and McDaniel 1974) may restimulate in part the lapsed immune potential of old animals (Walford, Meredith, and Cheney 1977). The possible effects of these agents on life span and disease patterns have not yet been assessed.

(4) The immune system of an old animal may be in whole or in part reconstituted by injection or grafting of young immunocompetent cells, with or without total body irradiation to make space for the injected cells to home into. Preliminary experiments with injection of young T_2 cells (which show the greatest immune functional decline with age) into 200-R-irradiated animals yielded mild lifespan prolongation (Walford *et al.* 1977). Sublethal total body irradiation of old mice followed by bone marrow transplantation and neonatal thymus grafting may be expected to yield quite a remarkable reconstitution of immune potential (Hirokawa and Makinodan 1976) but the effect on life span is not known.

Suffice it to say that the known life span extension and age-deceleration induced by categories (1) and (2) above are consistent with action via an immunoregulatory mechanism but, being complex experiments, could be otherwise interpreted. Significant extension by categories (3) and (4) would yield a much narrower range of interpretive possibilities. Extension of the tenth decile of survivorship of a long-lived strain by a method susceptible to only one interpretation constitutes in my view the critical test of any aging hypothesis. The current state-of-the-art in immunology is sufficiently advanced that tests of this nature can and are being undertaken.

Addendum

Studies by Hart and Setlow (1974) provided the intriguing information that the maximum life spans of different species show a positive correlation with the DNA repair capacities of cells from that species. Using different strains of congenic mice, we have recently presented evidence that the main histocompatibility complex influences the DNA repair capacity as measured either as excision repair capacity after ultraviolet irradiation or a bleomycin sensitivity (Walford and Bergmann 1979). It seems therefore that a complex relationship may exist between the main histocompatibility complex, DNA repair capacity and maximum life span potential.

Acknowledgement

These investigations were supported by NIH Grant AG00424.

References

ALLISON, A. C. and DENMAN, A. M. (1976). Self-tolerance and autoimmunity. *Brit. Med. Bull.*, **32**, 124–9.

ASOFSKY, R., TIGELAAR, R., and CANTOR, H. (1971). Cell interaction in the graft-versus-host response. In *Progress in immunology* (ed. D. B. Amos), pp. 369–81. Academic Press, New York.

BAILEY, D. W. and KOHN, H. I. (1965). Poop on spontaneous mutation rate of histo-compatibility site. Inherited histocompatibility changes in progeny of irradiation and unirradiated inbred mice. *Genetics Res.*, **6**, 330–40.

BEVAN, M. J. (1975). Interaction antigens detected by cytoxic T cells with the major histocompatibility complex as modifier. *Nature*, **256**, *(Lond.)*, 419–21.

BLUMENTHAL, H. T. and ALEX, M. (1975). Special issue on athero-arteriosclerosis. *Gerontologia*, **21**, 131–75.

CUNNINGHAM, A. J. (1976). Self-tolerance maintained by active suppressor mechanisms. *Transpl. Rev.*, **31**, 23–43.

CUTLER, R. G. (1975). Evolution of human longevity and the genetic complexity governing aging rate. *Proc. Nat. Acad. Sci.*, *USA*, **72**, 4664–8.

DAUSSET, J., DEGOS, L., and HORS, J. (1974). The association of the HL-A antigens with diseases. *Immunol. Immunopathol.*, **3**, 127–49.

DENCKLA, W. D. (1975). A time to die. *Life Sci.*, **16**, 31–44.

DOHERTY, P. C. and ZINKERNAGEL, R. M. (1975). A biological role for the major histocompatibility antigens. *Lancet*, ii, 1406–9.

GERBASE-DELIMA, M., MEREDITH, P., and WALFORD, R. L. (1974). Age-related changes including synergy and suppression in the mixed lymphocyte reaction in long-lived mice, *Fed. Proc.*, **34**, 159–61.

——, LIU, R. K., CHENEY, K. E., MICKEY, R., and WALFORD, R. L. (1975). Immune function and survival in a long-lived mouse strain subjected to undernutrition. *Gerontologia*, **21**, 184–202.

GOLDSTEIN, A. L., HOOPER, J. A., SCHULOF, R. S., COHEN, G. H., THURMAN, G. B., and McDANIEL, M. C. (1974). Thymosin and the immunopathology of aging. *Fed. Proc.*, **33**, 2053–6.

GOLDSTEIN, S., NIEWIAROWSKI, S., and SINGAL, D. P. (1975). Pathological implications of cell aging *in vitro*. *Fed. Proc.*, **34**, 56–63.

GOODMAN, S. A. and MAKINODAN, T. (1975). Effect of age on cell-mediated immunity in long-lived mice. *Clin. Exp. Immunol.*, **19**, 533–47.

GREBE, S. C. and STREILEIN, J. W. (1976). Graft-versus-host reactions: a review. *Adv. Immunol.*, **22**, 120–221.

HAN, I. H. and JOHNSON, A. G. (1976). Regulation of the immune system by synthetic polynucleotides. VII. Amplification of the immune response in young and aging mice. *J. Immunol.*, **117**, 423–7.

HART, R. W. and SETLOW, R. B. (1974). Correlation between deoxyribonucleic acid excision repair and lifespan in a number of mammalian species. *Proc. Nat. Acad. Sci.*, *USA*, **71**, 2163–73.

HAYFLICK, L. (1966). Cell culture and the aging phenomenon. In *Topics in the biology of aging* (ed. P. L. Krohn), pp. 83–100. Interscience, New York.

HILDEMANN, W. H. (1978). Phylogenetic and immunogenetic aspects of aging. In *Genetic effects on aging* (ed. D. Bergsma and D. E. Harrison), pp. 97–108. The National Foundation, March of Dimes.

—— and COOPER, E. L. (1963). Immunogenesis of homograft in fishes and amphibians. *Fed. Proc.*, **22**, 1145–51.

HIROWKAWA, K. and MAKINODAN, T. (1975). Thymic involution: effect of T cell differentiation. *J. Immunol.*, **114**, 1659–64.

HORI, Y., PERKINS, E. H., and HALSALL, M. K. (1973). Decline in phytohemagglutinin responsiveness of spleen cells from aging mice. *Proc. Soc. exp. Biol. Med.*, **144**, 48–53.

HUBERMAN, E., MAGER, R., and SACHS, L. (1976). Mutagenesis and transformation of normal cells by chemical carcinogens. *Nature, (Lond.)*, **264**, 360–1.

HUNG, C., PERKINS, E. H., and YANG, W. (1975). Age-related refractoriness of PHA-induced lymphocyte transformation. II. ^{125}I-PHA binding to spleen cells from young and old mice. *Mech. Aging Develop.*, **4**, 103–12.

KISHIMOTO, S., TAKAHAMA, T., and MIZUMACHI, H. (1976). *In vitro* immune response to the 2, 4, 6-trinitrophenyl determinant in aged C57BL/6J mice: changes in the humoral immune response to, avidity for the TNP determinant and responsiveness to LPS effect with aging. *J. Immunol.*, **116**, 294–300.

KLEIN, J. and HAMMERBERG, C. (1977). The control of differentiation by the T complex. *Immunol. Rev.*, **33**, 70–104.

KONEN, T. G., SMITH, G. S., and WALFORD, R. L. (1973). Decline in mixed lymphocyte reactivity of spleen cells from aged mice of a long-lived strain. *J. Immunol.*, **110**, 1216–21.

LIU, R. K. and WALFORD, R. L. (1966). Increased growth and lifespan with lowered ambient temperature in the annual fish, *Cynolebias adloffi. Nature, (Lond.)*, **212**, 1277–8.

—— and —— (1970). The influence of runt (wasting) disease on skin collagen ratios in laboratory mice. *The Gerontologist*, **10**, 21.

—— and —— (1972). The effect of lowered body temperature on lifespan and immune and non-immune processes. *Gerontologia*, **18**, 363–88.

—— and —— (1975). Mid-life temperature-transfer effects on lifespan of annual fish. *J. Gerontol.*, **30**, 129–31.

MACKAY, I. R. (1972). Ageing and immunological function in man. *Gerontologia*, **18**, 239–304.

MAKINODAN, T., PERKINS, E. H., and CHEN, M. G. (1971). Immunological activity of the aged. *Adv. Gerontol. Res.*, **3**, 171–98.

——, DEITCHMAU, J. W., STOLTZNER, G. H., KAY, M.-M., and HIROKAWA, K. (1975). Restoration of the declining normal immune functions of aging mice, *10th Internat. Congr. Gerontol., Jerusalem*, Vol. 2, p. 23.

MATHEWS, J. D., WHITTINGHAM, S., HOOPER, B. M., and MACKAY, I. R. (1973). Association of autoantibodies with smoking, cardiovascular morbidity, and death in the Busselton population. *Lancet*, i, 754–8.

——, ——, and MACKAY, I. R. (1974). Autoimmune mechanisms in human vascular disease. *Lancet*, ii, 1423–6.

MATHIES, M., LIPPS, L., SMITH, G. S., and WALFORD, R. L. (1973). Age-related decline in response to phytohemagglutinin and pokeweed mitogen by spleen cells from hamsters and a long-lived mouse strain. *J. Gerontol.*, **28**, 425–30.

MARTIN, G. M. Genetic syndromes in man with potential relevance to the pathobiology of aging. In *Genetic effects on aging* (ed. D. Bergsma and D. E. Harrison) pp. 5–40. The National Foundation, March of Dimes (In press.)

McCAY, C. M., CROWELL, M. F., and MAYNARD, L. A. (1935). The effect of retarded growth upon the length of lifespan and upon the ultimate body size. *J. Nutr.*, **10**, 63–79.

MEREDITH, P. and WALFORD, R. L. (1977). Effect of age on response to T and B cell mitogens in mice congenic at the H-2 region. *Immunogenetics*, **5**, 109–29.

NANDY, K. (1972). Brain reactive antibodies in mouse serum as a function of age. *J. Gerontol.*, **27**, 173–7.

NAOR, D., BONVIDA, B., and WALFORD, R. L. (1976). Autoimmunity and aging, the age-related response of mice of a long-lived strain to trinitrophenylated syngeneic mouse red blood cells. *J. Immunol.*, **117**, 2204–8.

ORGEL, L. E. (1963). The maintenance of the accuracy of protein synthesis and its relevance to aging. *Proc. Nat. Acad. Sci., USA*, **49**, 517.

POPP, D. M. Use of congenic mice to study the genetic basis of degenerative disease. In *Genetic effects on aging* (eds. D. Bergsma and D. E. Harrison) pp. 261–80. The National Foundation, March of Dimes (In press.)

ROSS, M. H. (1969). Aging, nutrition, and hepatic enzyme activity patterns in the rat. *J. Nutrition, Suppl. 1*, **97**, Part 2, 565–601.

RUBENSTEIN, P., SUCIU-FOCA, N., NICHOLSON, J. F., FOTINO, M., MOLINARO, A., HARISIADIS, L., HARDY, M. A., REEMTSMA, K., and ALLEN, F.H., Jr (1976). The HLA system in the families of patients with juvenile diabetes mellitus. *J. exp. Med.*, **143**, 1277–82.

SACHER, G. A. (1959). Relation of lifespan to brain weight and body weight in mammals. In *The lifespan of animals, Ciba Foundation Colloquium on Aging,* Vol. 5, p. 115. Little, Brown and Co., Boston.

—— (1975). Maturation and longevity in relation to cranial capacity in hominid evolution. In *Antecedents of man and after. Primates: functional morphology and evolution* (ed. R. Tuttle), Vol. 1, pp. 417–41. Mouton, The Hague.

SEGRE, D. and SEGRE, M. (1976). Humoral immunity in aged mice. II. Increased suppressor T cell activity in immunologically deficient old mice. *J. Immunol.*, **116**, 735–46.

SHREFFLER, D. C. (1977). The H-2 model: genetic control of immune functions. In *HLA and disease* (ed. J. Dausset and A. Svejgaard), pp. 33–45. Munkgaard, Copenhagen.

SIEGEL, B. V., BRAUN, M., and MORTON, J. I. (1972). Detection of antinuclear antibodies in NZB and other mouse strains. *Immunology*, **22**, 457–63.

SILVER, D. M. and LANE, D. P. (1975). Dominant nonresponsiveness in the induction of autoimmunity to liver-specified F-antigen. *J. exp. Med.*, **142**, 1455–62.

SMITH, G. S. and WALFORD, R. L. (1978). Influence of the H-2 and H-1 histocompatibility systems upon lifespan and spontaneous cancer incidences in congenic mice. In *Genetic effects on aging* (eds D. Bergsma and D. E. Harrison), pp. 281–312. The National Foundation, March of Dimes. (In press.)

SVEJGAARD, A., PLATZ, P., RYDER, L. P., NIELSEN, L. S., and THOMSEN, M. (1975). HL-A and disease associations—a survey. *Transpl. Rev.*, **22**, 3–43.

TALAL, N. (1976). Disordered immunologic regulation and auto-immunity. *Transpl. Rev.*, **31**, 240.

THOMSEN, M., PLATZ, P., ANDERSON, O. C., CHRISTY, M., LYNGSOE, J., NERUP, J., RASMUSSEN, K., RYDER, L. P., NIELSEN, L. S., and SVEJGAARD, A. (1975). MCL typing in juvenile diabetes mellitus and idiopathic Addison's disease. *Transpl. Rev.*, **22**, 125–47.

VLADUTIU, A. O. and ROSE, N. R. (1974). HL-A antigens: association with disease. *Immunogenetics*, **1**, 305–28.

VRACKO, R. and BENDITT, E. P. (1975). Restricted replicative lifespan of diabetic fibroblasts *in vitro*: its relation to microangiopathy. *Fed. Proc.*, **34**, 68–70.

WALFORD, R. L. (1962). Auto-immunity and aging. *J. Gerontol.*, **17**, 281–5.

—— (1969). *The immunologic theory of aging.* Munksgaard, Copenhagen.

—— (1970). Antibody diversity, histocompatibility systems, disease states, and aging. *Lancet*, **ii**, 1126–229.

—— (1972). Introduction to special issue, 'Immunology and aging', *Gerontologia*, **18**, 243–6.

—— (1974). The immunologic theory of aging, current status. *Fed. Proc.*, **33**, 2020–7.

—— (1977). Human B-cell alloantigens, their medical and biological significance. In *Proc. Internat. Congr. of the HLA System—new aspects, Sept. 1976, Bergamo, Italy*, pp. 105–27. Elsevier, North-Holland.

—— and BERGMANN, K. (1979). Influences of genes associated with the main histocompatibility complex on deoxyribonucleic acid excision repair capacity and bleomycin sensitivity in mouse lymphocytes. *Tissue Antigens*, **14**, 336–42.

——, LIU, R. K., GERBASE-DELIMA, M., MATHIES, M., and SMITH, G. S. (1974). Longterm dietary restriction and immune function in mice: response to sheep red blood cells and to mitogenic agents. *Mech. Aging Develop.*, **2**, 447–54.

——, ——, TROUP, G. M., and HSI, J. (1969). Alterations in soluble/insoluble collagen ratios in the annual fish, *Cynolebias bellottii*, in relation to age and environmental temperature, *Exp. Gerontol.*, **4**, 103–9.

——, MEREDITH, P., and CHENEY, K. E. (1977). Immunoengineering: prospects for correction of age-related immunodeficiency states. In *Immunology and aging* (ed. T. Makinodan and E. Yunis), pp. 183–201. Plenum Press, New York.

WHITTINGHAM, S., MATHEWS, J. D., MACKAY, I. R., STOCKS, A. E., UNGAR, B., and MARTIN, F. I. R. (1971). Diabetes mellitus, autoimmunity and aging. *Lancet*, **i**, 763–6.

——, STUTMAN, O., FERNANDES, G., TEAGUE, P. C., and GOOD, R. A. (1972). The thymus, autoimmunity and the involution of the lymphoid system. In *Tolerance, autoimmunity and aging* (ed. R. A. Good and M. Siegel), pp. 62–119. Charles C. Thomas, Springfield, Illinois.

The status of cells in the immune system during aging
Amiela Globerson and David Friedman

Introduction

Various immunological functions have been shown to decline during aging, both in mice and in humans. In parallel, it has been noted that the incidence of auto-immune manifestations increases with age (Walford 1969). These striking phenomena have led to the hypothesis that such changes in the immune system may in fact underlie various pathological manifestations of aging (Walford 1969). Analysis of the mechanisms of immunity and auto-immunity is thus of dual importance in that it may lead to understanding of the pathogenesis and establishment of an appropriate methodology for the repair of immune disorders.

Modern immunology, as it stands today, reveals that immune responses are performed and controlled by several distinct cell-types: the T and B cells and their subpopulations, and the macrophages. Each of these cell types fulfils a specific function and can be distinguished by membrane properties (Greaves, Owen, and Raff 1973). Accordingly, whether an immune response will manifest in production of antibodies or in delayed type hypersensitivity, for instance, depends on the type of cells participating in the response and on their mode of interaction. Furthermore, whether a response will or will not occur may depend on the existence and function of suppressor cells which can interfere with the response (Gershon 1974). Obviously, understanding the cellular basis of the disorders in the immune system which occur with age requires a critical analysis of the status of each of the participating cell types. Indeed, research performed in a number of laboratories in the past few years has followed this line of thought. In this chapter, we shall present the results of our studies on the cells involved in immune responses and shall discuss the state of knowledge as reflected from our results and the reports of others.

Materials and methods

1. *Mice*. (C3H/eb × C57BL/6J)F_1 male mice were obtained from the Animal Breeding Center of the Weizmann Institute of Science, Rehovot. The mice were kept at a constant temperature (25 °C) and fed Purina and water *ad libitum*.

2. *Studies of antibody response. Antigens and immunization.* SRBC: *in vivo*, 0.2 ml of 10 per cent SRBC was injected i.p. *In vitro*, 10 μl of 1 per cent SRBC was applied to each culture. α-Dnp-polylysine: mean molecular weight 7500; 10 μg of antigen solution of 10 μg/ml was added to each culture. Polyvinylpyrrolidone (PVP, K-90): molecular weight 360 000 (Fluka, Switzerland); 0.26 μg of the antigen solution in PBS was injected i.p.

3. *Organ culture technique*. We used the method of Bernstein and Globerson (1974) which is a modification of the filter well technique of Globerson and Auerbach (1966). The response to Dnp-polylysine was tested in medium samples collected at 2-day intervals. The response to SRBC was tested by determining the number of PFC after teasing the spleen cultures into cell suspensions.

4. *Antibody assays*. Antibody response to SRBC was determined in the spleens of the immunized mice or in spleen cultures by the assay of haemolytic plaque-forming cells (PFC) in agar, by Arrenbrecht's (1973) modification of Jerne's technique (Jerne and Nordin 1963). Indirect plaques representing IgG antibodies were developed by rabbit anti-mouse IgG antiserum. The response to PVP was tested by a similar method; the target cells in this case were SRBC coated with PVP K-15 (Andersson and Blomgren 1971). The response to Dnp-polylysine was determined by inactivation of DNP-T4 modified bacteriophage (Segal, Globerson, Feldman, Haimovich, and Sela 1970).

5. *Cell transfer*.

a. *Irradiation*. Mice received 800 R total body irradiation from a ^{60}Co source.

b. *Cell preparation and transfer*. Spleen or thymus tissues were teased and passed through fine mesh. The bone marrow cells were obtained from the tibiae and femura. Cells were injected into the lateral vein of the tail within 2 h after irradiation. Subsequently, the mice were immunized by the appropriate antigen, i.p.

6. *Assay of the GVH response.* We used the filter well technique for organ cultures developed by Auerbach and Globerson (1966) to determine the capacity of spleen cells to induce a graft-versus-host reaction *in vitro*.

7. *THF.* Thymus humoral factor (THF) prepared from calf thymus (Trainin and Small 1970) was kindly obtained from Professor N. Trainin of our department.

Results and discussion

The bulk of evidence indicating that immune reactivity declines with age is based on studies performed on intact animals (Walford 1969). Accordingly, a low response may be attributed to changes occurring in one or more of the cell-types comprising the reacting apparatus or to interference of environmental mediators. To distinguish between such possibilities it is necessary to remove the test cells from the aged animals and to examine them when isolated. An experimental system partially meeting these requirements, the '*in vivo* culture model', was extensively employed by Makinodan and Peterson (1964), who transplanted test spleen cells from aged mice into young irradiated recipients. Production of antibodies was found to be limited under such conditions too. Further assessment of the cellular defect, performed in an *in vitro* cell culture system (Heidrick and Makinodan 1973), indicated that the macrophage compartment of the spleens of aged mice functioned normally whereas the lymphoid cell population expressed reduced activity. It should be emphasized, however, that these observations do not rule out the possibility that other functions of macrophages may deteriorate with age. For instance, macrophages of aged mice (18–24 months old) manifest higher rates of phagocytosis of SRBC, as compared to those of young ones (Globerson and Razin, in preparation). The next question thus raised was as to whether the defect in the lymphocytes is in the T or the B cell compartment. We approached this question by examining the reactivity of spleen cells of aged mice with respect to distinct T and B cell functions.

In the first series of experiments we studied the potential of spleen cells of aged mice to induce a GVH response (Friedman, Keiser, and Globerson 1974). We employed for that purpose the *in vitro* model of this reaction (Auerbach and Globerson 1966), to ensure that the results reflect the potential of the test cells, without any involvement of mechanisms which may be associated *in vivo* in an intact organism. The ability of spleen cells to elicit this reaction *in vitro* (Auerbach and Globerson 1966) was found to decline with age; the cells of 24–36-month-old mice failed to react (Table 1). The inability of cells of aged mice to produce this reaction may be related to the fact that the thymus involutes with

Table 1 *In vitro* GVH response induced by spleen cells of aged mice

Age (months)	Total no. of cultures	Per cent positive cultures
2–3	33	76
12–15	20	60
23–26	16	19
32–33	16	19

age, rendering T cells, which are normally developing in the thymus, deficient. Such deficiency could be the result of one of two alternative mechanisms:

(a) The stem cell pool is exhausted and thus the mature T cell pool is depleted.
(b) There exists a sufficient number of stem cells yet maturation is arrested due to thymus malfunction.

Now, Hirokawa and Makinodan (1975) demonstrated that the thymus of aged mice is inefficient in inducing T-cell maturation. If the first possibility were correct, then activation of T-cell function would be triggered by exposure of the cells of aged mice to the effect of the thymus. Yet, if the target cells for thymus influence were unavailable, in accordance with the second hypothesis, such activation would be impossible. To elucidate this point we performed experiments in which test spleen cells were incubated with a thymic extract (THF) (Trainin and Small 1970) under conditions previously found appropriate for the induction of reactivity of spleen cells from neonatally thymectomized (Trainin, Small, and Globerson 1969) or adult sublethally irradiated (Globerson, Umiel, and Friedman 1975) animals. As shown in Table 2, treatment with THF led to a significant increase in splenomegaly indices (Friedman, Keiser, and Globerson 1974). It was thus concluded that the spleen of the aged mouse contains cells with the potential to react, but that these are incapable, *a priori*, of expressing this potential and THF treatment renders them reactive. It is of interest to note in this respect that attempts to rejuvenate the immune system of aged mice by grafts of young thymuses have failed in the past (Metcalf, Moulds, and Pike 1966; Micklem, Ogden, and Payne 1973). One might argue that the thymic grafts did not function in the aged animals because they encountered inhibitory environmental or homronal effects. Dependency of the thymus on hormonal control of the pituitary has indeed been indicated (Pierpaoli and Sorkin 1969; Fabris 1977). But recent studies by Makinodan suggest that thymus grafts can, in fact, restore immunological activity to aged mice (Hirokawa, Albright, and Makinodan 1976). In Makinodan's studies however, lethally irradiated aged recipients were grafted, in parallel, with normal young bone marrow cells. Under such conditions, the reactive system obtained is of donor origin and is not based purely on activated cells originating in the aged recipient. Critical studies are necessary to investigate this point.

Next we conducted experiments to determine whether reduction in antibody response with age is based on a deficiency in other manifestations of the T-cell

Table 2 *In vitro* effect of THF on induction of a GVH response by spleen cells of aged mice

Age (months)	Treatment	No. of cultures assayed	Per cent positive cultures
23–26	THF	24	63
	None	23	17
2–3	THF	24	75
	None	24	79

compartment as well. We attempted to assess the status of the T-cell types involved as helper cells in antibody production, during aging. In such an assessment, the production of IgG-type antibodies has been found to be more T-cell-dependent than that of IgM-type antibodies (Taylor and Wortis 1968; Schrader 1975). Indications that the decline in IgG antibody response during aging is more pronounced than that of IgM have been reported (Makinodan and Peterson 1966; Rann 1967). Yet, the cellular basis of this phenomenon was not thoroughly examined.

We studied the production of antibodies of these two immunoglobulin classes during aging. Our study involved analysis of the response to a variety of antigens, *in vivo* and *in vitro*. At first, mice of various age groups were injected with SRBC and production of antibodies was measured by assaying for the number of direct and indirect PFC in their spleens. On days 5 and 10 after immunization, a remarkable reduction in the responses, as compared to that of young mice, was recorded (Figs. 1 and 2). The reduction was noted on the two different days of assay, thus ruling out the possibility that the low number of PFC on day 5 reflected a delay in the peak level of response.

To examine whether low reactivity in this case is due to mechanisms interfering with production of antibodies in the aged animal or whether it reflects a deficiency intrinsic to the spleen, further studies were performed *in vitro*. Spleens of mice aged 3 and 36 months were explanted to organ cultures and stimulated *in vitro* with SRBC (Globerson and Auerbach 1966). Then, 5 days later, the cultures

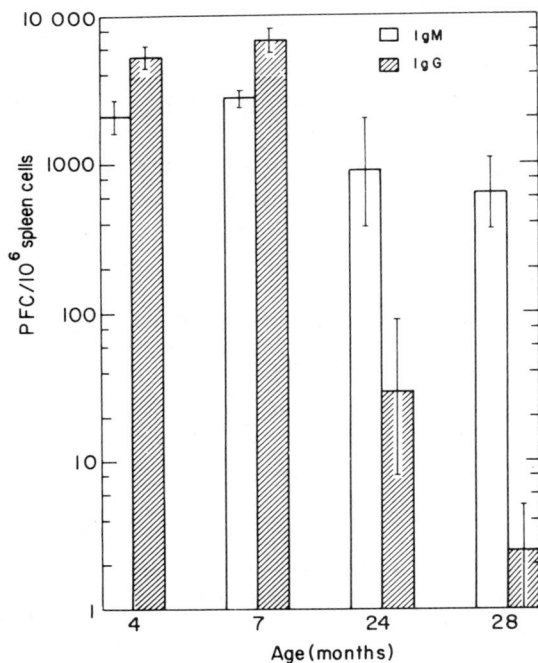

FIG. 1. IgM and IgG antibody response to SRBC *in vivo*, in mice of different ages. Each column represents the geometric mean of the results obtained in 6–7 mice of the same age group, ± standard error.

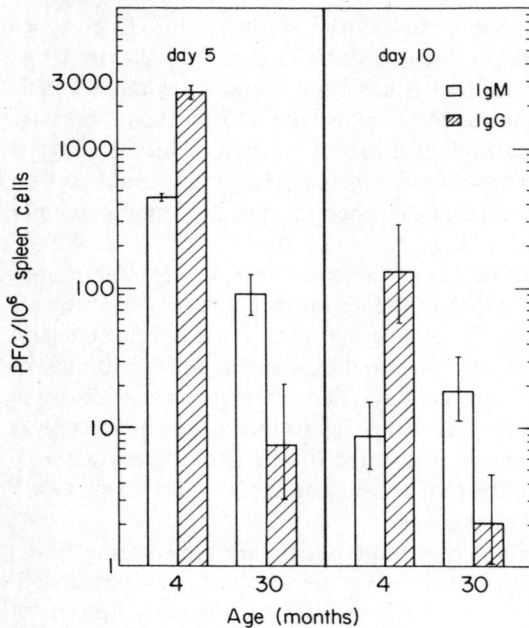

Fig. 2. IgM and IgG antibody response to SRBC *in vivo*, in 4- and 30-month-old mice. Each column represents the geometric mean of the results obtained in 5 mice of the same age group ± standard error.

were assayed for the number of PFCs. As shown in Table 3, the response of cultures originating in the aged mice was remarkably low.

Similar results were obtained when cell culture techniques were employed (Heidrick and Makinodan 1973). However, one should take into account the fact that under certain conditions, when no response was expressed in cell cultures, it did manifest in organ cultures (Globerson 1976). Accordingly, onset of antibody response to SRBC in cell cultures was noted at the age of 2 weeks (Fidler, Chiscon, and Golub 1972) whereas in the organ culture technique spleens of 3–5-day-old mice reacted (Alter 1969). The integrity of the spleen tissue may be important for reactivity. The observation that even organ cultures of spleens of aged mice failed to react is thus significant.

Table 3 *In vitro* antibody response to SRBC by spleens of young and old mice

Age (months)	PFC/10^6 spleen cells	
	+SRBC	−SRBC
3	290 (230–366)	13 (8–23)
36	9 (5–16)	1.7 (1.2–2.3)

PFCs were counted in cell suspensions prepared from 20 cultures from the same spleen, which were immunized (+SRBC) or untreated (−SRBC). The values represent geometric means of the results obtained in 4 individual spleens of the same age group. Numbers in parentheses are the upper and lower limits of the standard error of the mean.

In a further experiment, spleen organ cultures from mice of various age groups were stimulated with a chemically-defined synthetic antigen, Dnp-polyly-sine, and the response was followed for the entire period of antibody production. As shown in Fig. 3 which represents the peak levels of response measured on day 6 of culture a gradual decrease in intensity of response occurs with age. Spleen cultures of 30-month-old mice exhibited no response, as compared to those of mice aged 28 and 23 months and young mice (7 and 4.5 months). The kinetics of the response of spleen cultures of aged mice is given in Fig. 4, showing that such cultures did not produce any significant reaction during the entire period of culture. It was thus concluded that the low reactivity is based on intrinsic defi-ciency in the spleen itself. The next studies were thus focused on analysis of the cellular basis of this defect.

Since production of antibodies is based on co-operation between T and B cells, a low response could be attributed to either of these cell populations. The possibility that the T-cell compartment is deficient in aged animals has been pointed out in various studies in the past (Konen, Smith, and Walford 1973; Hori, Perkins, and Halsall 1973) as well as in experiments which we performed, as described above. It was therefore inviting to determine whether the lowered antibody response is based on deficiency in the T-helper-cell population. Our reasoning was that if these low responses resulted from inadequate T-cell help in the aged spleen, then reactivity might be expected to be regained when the system was supplemented with active T cells from young donors. A cell transfer system was deemed to be a most suitable experimental set-up to examine this possibility. We transferred spleen cells of aged mice into young irradiated recipients, together with thymocytes from young mice. As shown in Fig. 5, this procedure led to a

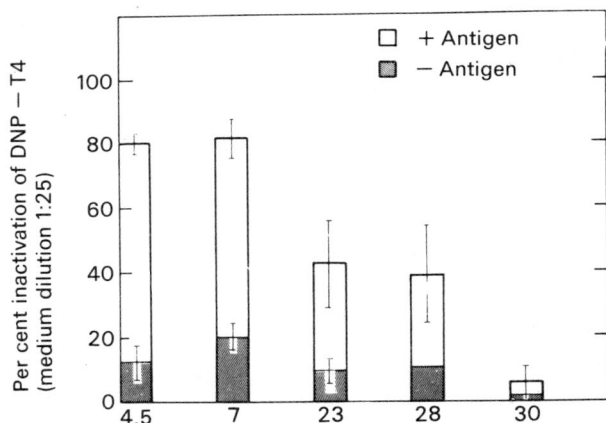

FIG. 3. Antibody response to Dnp-polylysine *in vitro*, in mice of different ages. Four spleens from each age group were tested. 10 cultures from each spleen were stimulated with antigen and 10 cultures served as untreated controls. The response to Dnp was tested 6 days after immuniza-tion in 1 : 25 dilution of medium collected from 10 stimulated or untreated cultures from the same spleen. Each column represents the arithmetic mean of the response obtained in 4 samples pooled from 4 individual spleens of the same age group ± standard error.

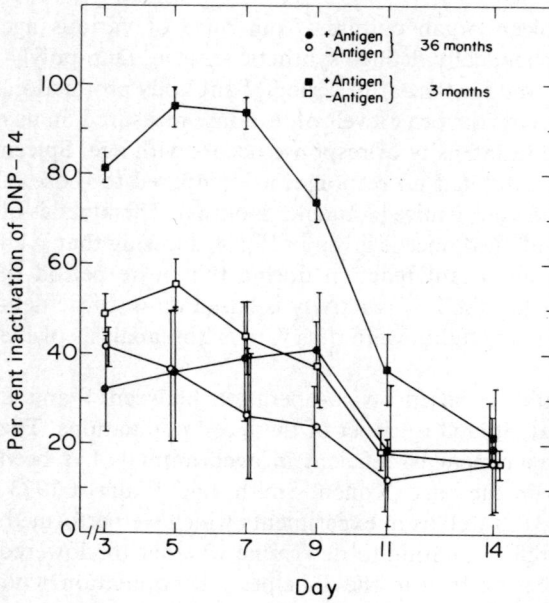

FIG. 4. Kinetics of the antibody response to Dnp-polylysine *in vitro* and 3- and 36-month old mice. Details as in Fig. 5.

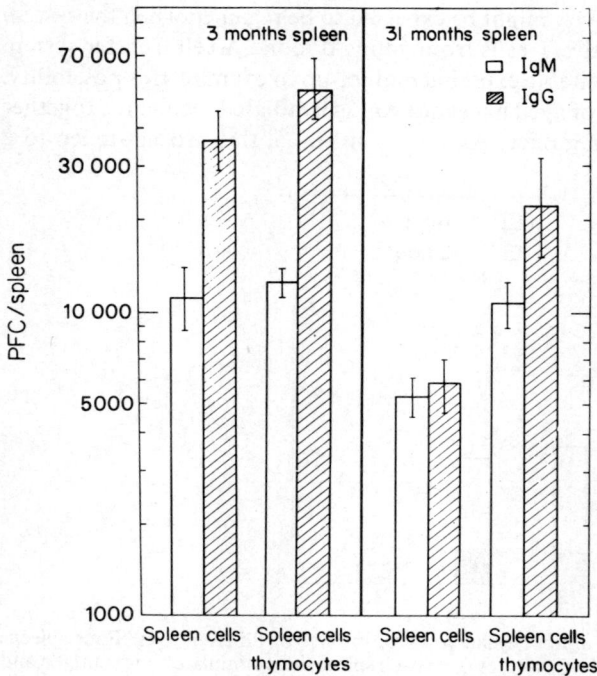

FIG. 5. Reconstitution of IgM and IgG antibody response to SRBC in irradiated mice with 10⁷ spleen cells from young or old mice with or without 10⁸ thymocytes from young mice. Each column represents the geometric mean of response obtained in 6–8 mice of the same group, ± standard error.

higher antibody response than that obtained in the absence of thymocytes. However, it was noted that even under these conditions the response did not reach the levels observed in the control group which received young spleen cells. A variety of parameters were examined to investigate whether these results stemmed from technical procedures (e.g., inefficient T-cell dose, etc.), but the same observation was recorded in all of these experiments. It was thus inferred that in addition to the T-cell deficiency, the B-cell compartment is also affected during aging. These results can be explained on the basis of two alternative hypotheses:

(a) The relatively low response of B cells from aged mice under these conditions is related to their possible failure to co-operate with the T helper cells.
(b) The low response reflects a defect in the B-cell function in production of antibodies.

To distinguish between these two possibilities we employed the antigen polyvinylpyrrolidone which is known to evoke a response independently of T helper cells (Möller and Michael 1971). Thus, mice of various age groups were immunized with PVP and their response was followed, as shown in Fig. 6. The old mice manifested a poor response as compared to the young mice, suggesting that the impaired B-cell activity during aging is not based on a defect in co-operation with T helper cells.

The possibility that a low B-cell response is actually due to an excess of suppressor cell function in this case was thoroughly investigated. Increase in suppressor cells in aging has been documented in a variety of studies (Gerbase-De Lima *et al.* 1975; Segre and Segre 1976, 1977; Gershon and Metzler 1977). Furthermore, the response to PVP has been found to be regulated by T-suppressor cells (Rotter and Trainin 1974). Therefore, the response to PVP was

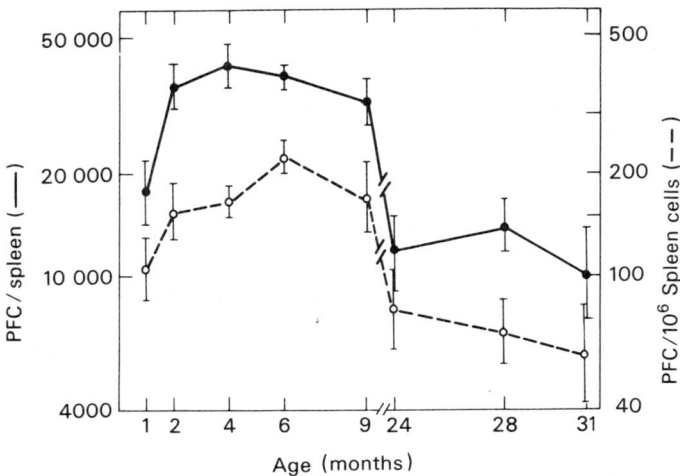

FIG. 6. Antibody response to PVP *in vivo*, in mice of different ages. Each point represents the geometric mean of the response obtained in 7–8 mice of the same age group, ± standard error.

measured in 24-month-old mice which had been thymectomized at the age of 2 months, as well as in thymectomized, irradiated mice treated with T-cell-depleted spleen cells of aged mice. However, the response to PVP was low even under these conditions (Friedman and Globerson 1978, and unpublished data). It was thus deduced that the B-cell comportment itself is probably deficient in the aging mice.

Deficiency in the B-cell compartment could be pictured by assuming that the stem cell pool in the bone marrow is exhausted with age and that as a result of this, the B-cell population residing in the spleen is limited. Alternatively, the stem cell pool in the bone marrow of old animals may be of the same size as that of young mice; yet differentiation of the bone marrow stem cells may be arrested in the aged animal. We therefore decided to assess the status of the B precursor cells in the bone marrow of aged as compared to young mice. Hence, test bone marrow cells were transferred into young irradiated recipients receiving thymus cells from young donors and the antigen SRBC simultaneously. Production of antibodies was then measured as in the previous experiments. As shown in Fig. 7, the same level of response was obtained in groups receiving bone marrow cells from old as from young donors. It was thus concluded that bone marrow of aged mice does contain cells capable of differentiating into antibody-producing cells when transferred into young recipients. The results of studies performed in other laboratories have pointed to the same conclusion. Thus, Micklem *et al.* (1973) and Farrar, Loughman, and Nordin (1974) observed that, *a priori*, bone marrow of aged mice can give rise to antibody-producing cells at a level similar to that of bone marrow from young animals. What, then, is the nature of impairment in the B-cell compartment during aging? It may be argued that although the number of cells in the bone marrow having the potential to give rise to PFC in the spleen remains the same during aging and is similar in old and young mice, the bone marrow cells do differ in certain properties. For instance, as Farrar *et al.* (1974) noted, they are more sensitive to ALS treatment. How this is reflected in the intact aged animal is, as yet, unclear. The capacity of bone marrow cells to migrate and/or home to the spleen within the aged organism may be limited. Alternatively, they may home to the spleen, yet fail to differentiate there. Indication that in the aged mouse the spleen micro-environment does not support differentiation of B cells has been noted by Hanna, Nettesheim, and Peters (1971). On the other hand, more recent studies by Hirokawa and co-workers (1976) showed that bone marrow cells from young donors develop in lethally irradiated aged recipients and resume normal function. The ideal approach to solving the question of whether the spleens of aged mice contain precursor cells of B antibody-producing cells, the differentiation of which was arrested at some stage, is subjecting such spleen cells to agents affecting B-cell maturation. Unfortunately, our knowledge in this respect is still inadequate and performance of such experiments will have to be delayed. More extensive investigation is still needed to reveal the mechanisms underlying B-cell differentiation and the agents inducing it under normal conditions. Likely candidates for differentiation-inducing agents worth mentioning here are the B-cell maturation-inducing

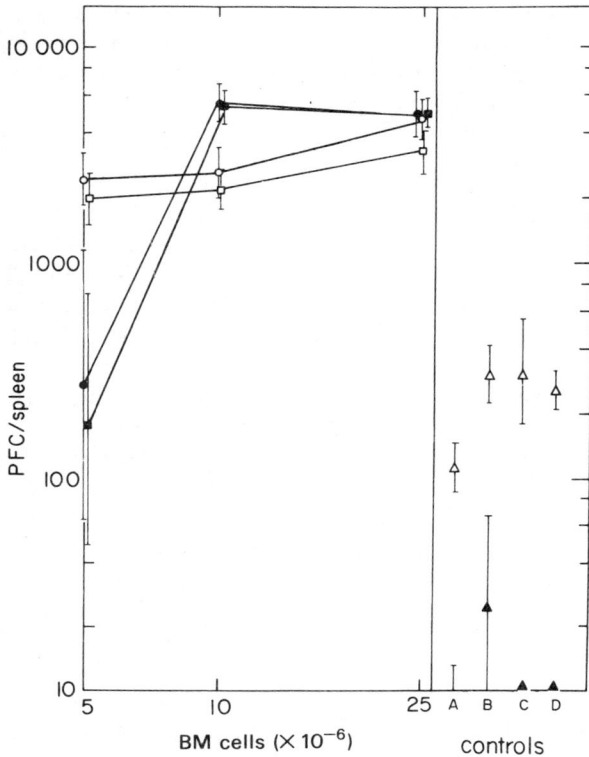

FIG. 7. Reconstitution of antibody response to SRBC in irradiated mice by different doses of bone marrow cells from young or old mice together with 10^8 thymocytes from young mice. Each point represents the geometric mean of response obtained in 6–8 mice of the same group ± standard error. Open symbols: IgM; closed symbols: IgG. Squares: 30 months; circles: 6 months; triangles, controls, as follows: (A) 25×10^6 bone marrow cells from 6-month-old mice; (B) 25×10^6 bone marrow cells from 30-month-old mice; (C) 10^8 thymocytes from 2-month-old mice; (D) no cells.

hormone of bursa origin in chicken (Jankovic and Leskowitz 1965) and the T-cell factors which affect B, and suppressor cell maturation prior to antigen stimulation (Schimpl and Wecker 1972). It is maintained that a better knowledge of the normal embryonic development of the various immune reactive and immunosuppressor cells will enlighten us regarding the status of these cells in aging. Extensive ontogenetic studies are under way in our laboratory, focusing on the normal B-cell development in the mouse embryo (Globerson 1976; Globerson *et al.* 1977; Rabinowich *et al.* 1979).

Other mechanisms prevailing in the aged organism which may have a pronounced effect on immune reactivity should not be disregarded. For instance, it has been indicated in our laboratory that increased levels of cholesterol in the serum may have an influence on the lymphocyte cell membrane and on the reactivity of lymphocytes to mitogens *in vitro* (Rivnay, Shinitzky, and Globerson

1976; Rivnay, Globerson, and Shinitzky 1978, Rivnay *et al.* 1980). Accordingly, critical studies on the possibility that the low activity manifested by immune reactive cells in the aged organism is due to high cholesterol levels in the serum are currently being performed in our laboratory.

Summary

Analysis of the cellular basis of decreased immune reactivity to foreign antigens during senescence indicates that it is related to deficiency in both T and B lymphocyte compartments. These deficiencies can be explained on the basis of impairment of maturation rather than exhaustion of stem cell pools. T cell activity can be conferred *in vitro* by exposing spleen cells of aged mice to thymic hormone (THF). Concerning the B cells, experimental evidence indicates that bone marrow cells of aged mice can differentiate into antibody-producing cells if they have the opportunity of homing to spleens of young recipients but the precise contribution of this micro-environment is as yet unclear.

We have not touched on the cellular mechanisms of increase in auto-immune reactions in senescence, nor in the status of suppressor cells. These points undoubtedly deserve appropriate attention, but they are beyond the scope of this presentation.

List of abbreviations

T cells, thymus processed cells; B cells, cells of bone marrow origin, not processed by the thymus; SRBC, sheep red blood cells; Dnp-polylysine, dinitrophenyl poly-L-lysine; PVP, polyvinylpyrrolidone; PFC, hemolytic plaque-forming cell; GVH, graft versus host; THF, thymus humoral factor; ALS, antilymphocytic serum.

Acknowledgements

This work was supported by the Minerva Foundation. We thank Mrs M. Lev-Ran, Mrs L. Abel, and Mrs S. Leib for their technical assistance. Mrs M. Baer provided editorial assistance.

References

ALTER, B. (1969). MSc. Thesis, University of Wisconsin.
ANDERSSON, B. and BLOMGREN, H. (1971). *Cell Immunol.*, **2**, 411.
ARRENBRECHT, S. (1973). *Eur. J. Immunol.*, **3**, 506.
AUERBACH, R. and GLOBERSON, A. (1966). *Exp. Cell Res.*, **42**, 31.
BERNSTEIN, A. and GLOBERSON, A. (1974). *Cell Immunol.*, **10**, 173.
FABRIS, N. (1977). In *Comprehensive Immunology, Vol. I: Immunology and Aging* (ed T. Makonodan and E. Yunis), pp. 73–89, Plenum Med. Book Co., New York.
FARRAR, J. J., LOUGHMAN, B. E., and NORDIN, A. A. (1974). *J. Immunol.*, **112**, 1244.

FIDLER, J. M., CHISCON, M. O., and GOLUB, E. S. (1972). *J. Immunol.*, **109**, 136.

FRIEDMAN, D. and GLOBERSON, A. (1978). *Mech. Aging Dev.*, **7**, 299.

——, KEISER, V., and GLOBERSON, A. (1974). *Nature*, **251**, 545.

GERBASE–DELIMA, M., MEREDITH, P., and WALFORD, R. L. (1975), *Fed. Proc.*, **34**, 159–61.

GERSHON, R. K. (1974). In *Contemporary topics in immunology* (ed. M. D. Cooper and N. L. Warner), pp. 1–40, Plenum Press, New York.

—— and METZLER C. M. (1977). In *Comprehensive Immunology, Vol. I: Immunology and Aging* (ed. T. Makinodan and E. Yunis), pp. 103–10. Plenum Med. Book Co., New York

GLOBERSON, A. (1976). *Curr. Top. Microbiol. Immunol.*, **75**, 1–43.

——, and AUERBACH, R. (1966). *J. exp. Med.*, **124**, 1001.

GLOBERSON, A., RABINOWICH, H., and UMIEL, T. (1977). In *Developmental Immunobiology* (ed. J. B. Solomon and H. D. Horton), pp. 331–7. Elsevier/North Holland Biomed. Press, Amsterdam.

——, UMIEL, T., and FRIEDMAN, D. (1975). *Ann. NY Acad. Sci.*, **249**, 248.

GREAVES, M. F., OWEN, J. J. T., and RAFF, M. C. (Eds.) (1973). *T and B lymphocytes: origins, properties and roles in immune responses*. Excerpta Medica, Amsterdam; American Elsevier Publ. Co., Inc., New York.

HANNA, M. G. Jr., NETTESHEIM, P., and PETERS, L. C. (1971). *Nature New Biol.*, **232**, 204.

HEIDRICK, M. L. and MAKINODAN, T. (1973). *J. Immunol.*, **111**, 1502.

HIROKAWA, K. and MAKINODAN, T. (1975). *J. Immunol.*, **114**, 1659.

——, ALBRIGHT, J. W. and MAKINODAN, T. (1976). *Clin. Immunol. Immunopathol.*, **5**, 371.

HORI, Y., PERKINS, E. H. and HALSALL, M. K. (1973). *Proc. Soc. exp. Biol. Med.*, **144**, 48.

JANKOVIC, B. D. and LESKOWITZ, S. (1965). *Proc. Soc. exp. Biol.* (NY), **118**, 1164.

JERNE, N. K. and NORDIN, A. A. (1963). *Science, N.Y.*, **140**, 405.

KONEN, T. G., SMITH, G. S., and WALFORD, R. L. (1973). *J. Immunol.*, **110**, 1216.

MAKINODAN, T. and PETERSON, W. J. (1964). *J. Immunol.*, **93**, 886.

—— and —— (1966). *Dev. Biol.*, **14**, 112.

METCALF, D., MOULDS, R., and PIKE, B. (1966). *Clin. exp. Immunol.*, **2**, 109.

MICKLEM, H. S., OGDEN, D. A., and PAYNE, A. C. (1973). In *Ciba Foundation symposium on haemopoietic stem cells*, pp. 285–301.

MÖLLER, G. and MICHAEL, G. (1971). *Cell Immunol.*, **2**, 309.

PIERPAOLI, W. and SORKIN, E. (1969). In *Lymphatic tissue and germinal centers in immune response* (ed. L. Fiore-Donati and M. G. Hanna, Jr.), pp. 397–401. Plenum Press, New York.

RABINOWICH, H., UMIEL, T., REISNER, Y., SHARON, N., and GLOBERSON, A. (1979). *Cell. Immunol.*, **47**, 347.

RANN, J. S. (1967). *J. Gerontol.*, **22**, 92.

RIVNAY, B., BERGMAN, S., SHINITZKY, M., and GLOBERSON, A. (1980). *Mech. Aging Dev.*, **12**, 119.

——, GLOBERSON, A., and SHINITZKY, M. (1978). *Eur. J. Immunol.*, **8**, 185.

——, SHINITZKY, M., and GLOBERSON, A. (1976). *Israel J. Med. Sci.*, **12**, 1253.

ROTTER, V. and TRAININ, N. (1974). *Cell. Immunol.*, **13**, 76.

SCHIMPL, A. and WECKER, E. (1972). *Nature New Biol.*, **237**, 15.

SCHRADER, J. W. (1975). *J. Immunol.*, **114**, 1665.

SEGAL, S., GLOBERSON, A., FELDMAN, M., HAIMOVICH, J., and SELA, M. (1970). *J. exp. Med.*, **131**, 93.

SEGRE, D. and SEGRE, M. (1976). *J. Immunol.*, **116**, 735.

—— and —— (1977). *Mech. Aging Dev.*, **6**, 115.

TAYLOR, R. B. and WORTIS, H. H. (1968). *Nature, (Lond.)*, **220**, 927.

TRAININ, N. and SMALL, M. (1970). *J. exp. Med.*, **132**, 885.

——, ——, and GLOBERSON, A. (1969). *J. exp. Med.*, **130**, 765.

WALFORD, R. L. (1969). *The immunologic theory of aging*. Munksgaard, Copenhagen.

Studies on the humoral immune response on aging men and mice

W. Hijmans, J. J. Haaijman and J. Radl

The association of aging with changes in the immune system has been well documented. Makinodan, Albright, Good, Peter, and Heidrick (1976) have emphasized its decline in function, while Walford (1969) has focused on the regular occurrence of the presence of auto-antibodies with increase in age. These results are only apparently contradictory, since it is recognized that the normal immune system should be regarded as a balanced system with positive and negative signals and feedback mechanisms. A defect may disturb the balance, and depending on its location lead to different abnormalities, e.g. a deficiency and/or the production of auto-antibodies.

A third characteristic immunological phenomenon of the aged individual is the restricted heterogeneity of the immunoglobulins and idiopathic paraproteinaemia. The relationship of idiopathic paraproteinaemia to age was the outcome of a screening programme of serum samples with electrophoresis as part of a population study in Sweden (Axelsson, Bachmann, and Hällén 1966).

The aetiology and the significance of these phenomena are still largely unknown, nor is it possible to predict the development of the immune deviations in the individual case. The final situation depends on a number of variables such as species, strain, antigen, and sex. Our experience on these aspects will be reviewed here. These findings will be discussed, as observed on three different levels: serum, cells, and organs.

Serum

Immunoglobulins

(a) *Men*. In a population study on serum immunoglobulin levels Kalff (1970) found an increase of the levels with age throughout adult life of IgG and IgA with no significant differences between the sexes; IgM levels showed no changes but were significantly higher for females than for males. His graphs clearly show the increase of variation with age. The same pattern was found when this study was extended to a group of persons older than 95 years (Radl, Sepers, Skvaril, Morell, and Hijmans 1975). The elevated level of IgG was caused by an increase in the IgG_1 and IgG_3 subclasses. This detail may be of more than just passing interest, because these two subclasses are more effective in binding complement than IgG_2 and IgG_4.

(b) *Mice.* The CBA strain, bred under conventional conditions, was chosen because it is a long-lived strain with no known tendency to age-related pathology of the immune system itself. For the quantification of the immunoglobulin levels a fluorescent micromethod was developed, in which antibodies, bound to sepharose beads were reacted with the serum samples. Details on the methods and the results have been published (Haaijman, van den Berg, and Brinkhof 1977a). There were no major changes in the levels of the respective Igs, with the exception of the IgG_1 and IgG_{2b} levels, which showed an increase with age. No systematic differences between males and females were observed. A striking phenomenon was the increased variation with age, but this did not apply to IgM—in contrast to the findings in men.

Idiopathic paraproteinaemia

(a) *Men.* In a group of 73 volunteers older than 95 years, a para-proteinaemia was found in 19 per cent of the individuals (Radl *et al.* 1975), in addition to an indication of restricted heterogeneity of the serum immuno-globulins in a further 15 per cent. The distribution of these abnormalities over the three major classes did not show special features. The figure of 19 per cent is the same as the figure reported by Englisovà, Englis, Kyral, Kourilek, and Dvorak (1968).

(b) *Mice.* A promising development to further our insight into the significance of idiopathic paraproteinaemia in men was provided by Radl and Hollander (1974), when they described analogous findings in mice of the C57BL strain. The incidence of idiopathic paraproteinaemia rises to over 50 per cent at about two years of age, whereas it is much lower in other strains studied. Several lines of investigation have been initiated, with an emphasis on recon-stitution experiments. These suggest that a deficiency in the T-cell system may play an important role in the development of paraproteins (Muiswinkel, Radl, and van der Wal 1976). This hypothesis (Radl 1976) receives support from observations in patients and animals with thymic deficiency in whom para-proteins have been detected regularly (Radl 1979a, 1980).

On the other hand, transplantation experiments in mice with idiopathic paraproteinaemia demonstrated that this condition in its final stage represents an intrinsic cellular defect in one B-cell alone and might be considered to be a benign neoplasm of the B-immune system (Radl *et al.* 1979).

Antibodies

In mice the humoral immune response to both thymus dependent and thymus independent antigens was analysed. In mice of the Balb/c strain there was no decrease in the number of plaque forming cells in the spleen against the thymus independent lipopolysaccharide (LPS) and in the aged animals the anti-LPS level in the serum was higher than in the young mice of this strain.

In the NZB strain of mice, which is characterized by the development of generalized auto-immune disease and early death, the reaction to lipopoly-saccharide was already impaired when these animals were two months old (Blankwater, Levert, and Hijmans 1975).

The reaction to thymus-dependent antigens was studied with human serum albumin in CBA mice (Haaijman and Hijmans 1978). The antibody level in the pre-immune sera increased during the first half year of their life. It showed a slight decrease thereafter. A clear age-related decline was observed of the primary reaction and the two-year-old mice generally failed to show any reactivity. Again an increased variability was recorded, which in this case started around the first year. The response after the booster dose of human serum albumin was less susceptible to alterations with age than the primary response, which is in agreement with the data of Morton and Siegel (1969) obtained for the NZB strain and those of Finger, Beneke, Emmerling, Bertz, and Plager (1972) for the NMRI strain. For 2-year-old animals the increase in variability of the booster response was evident. Unfortunately only two 3-year-old animals survived the experiment. In both a very slight reactivity was found.

Auto-antibodies

The sera which were available on the study of the group of healthy individuals over 95 years of age were investigated in Dr Doniach's laboratory (unpublished observations). The results are summarized in Table 1. It is clear that the increase with age of the incidence of auto-antibodies, as reported in a large number of studies, cannot be extrapolated to our group of highly aged persons. The number of positive sera is not excessively high and the titre is low. For several of the auto-antibody systems the results are equal to those seen in healthy young adults. Also in this instance, therefore, the deviating pattern occurs on the basis of selectivity.

The cause of the levelling off of the auto-antibody titres is not clear. As suggested by MacKay, Wells, and Fudenberg (1975) it could be due to the fact that individuals with high levels have in general a shorter life expectancy. In our study we may have covered only the survivors, who show less inclination for the formation of high levels of auto-antibodies. From a clinical point of view

Table 1 Auto-antibodies in 70 persons ⩾ 95 years†

Test	Positive per cent	Titre
Antigammaglobulin	35	low
ANA	25	low
Thyroid	23	low
Stomach	6	
Kidney	1	
Muscle (smooth)		as in controls
Muscle (striated)		as in controls
Purkinje		as in controls
Liver		no mitochondrial

†Data from A. Florin-Christensen, D. Doniach, and W. Hijmans (unpublished).

the conclusion may be drawn that also in the very aged the presence of auto-antibodies in high titres calls for further investigation and should not be regarded as merely a sign of aging.

Cells

A basic rule in immunology states that one plasma cell synthesizes immunoglobulins of single specificity only. This implies that the gene products are immunoglobulin molecules, with affinity for only one antigen, that they belong to one class, one type, etc. Exceptions, however, do occur.

In men a few per cent of the plasma cells contain immunoglobulins of different classes and types even under normal conditions (Hijmans, Schuit, and Radl 1973). Recently we reported on bone marrow samples from sixteen individuals with double paraproteinaemia, which were studied with immunofluorescence to investigate the cellular origin of these paraproteins (Van Camp, Schuit, Hijmans, and Radl 1978). In the majority of these cases separate cell populations were responsible for this phenomenon, confirming data in the literature. In some our findings indicated a second possibility in which both paraproteins were synthesized by the cells of one clone. Evidence for a third possibility was also obtained, namely a proliferation of 'switch' precursor cells leading to the formation of two clones.

In mice two strains were studied. The results in the CBA strain are published in detail (Haaijman and Hijmans 1978). They are summarized in Table 2. The large number of double cells in the 6-week-old animals is an unexpected finding; the decrease with age was a surprise. The C57BL strain of mice was also studied, because of its tendency to form paraproteins. The preliminary results in this strain indicate an increase in double cells with the age.

Table 2 Number of C-Ig cells ($\times 10^{-3}$) containing two Ig classes or subclasses in male CBA mice

	6 weeks	2 years
No. of slides	160	160
Slides with double cells	67	20
Total no. of double cells	386	59
X	2.4	0.4

Organs

Evidence has been adduced that in adult man the bone marrow is the major site of the formation of immunoglobulins (Hijmans 1975; Benner and Oudenaarden 1976), who have extended these studies to mice, showed that, after a second administration of antigen, antibody formation in the bone marrow greatly exceeds that by the spleen.

Haaijman, Schuit, and Hijmans (1977b) reported that in CBA mice the spleen is the major site of the synthesis of immunoglobulins up to about six months of age as judged from the number of Ig-containing cells. In older animals, the relative contribution of the bone marrow to the total number of C-Ig cells increases with age, possibly due to a gradual shift in the individual animal from primary-type responses to a pattern of secondary-type responses. As can be seen from Table 3 the contribution by the mesenteric lymph nodes and the Peyer plaques is negligible in older animals. No indication of a decreased over-all immunological activity in senescence was obtained. If the shift was, however, studied in more detail (Haaijman and Hijmans 1978), it was observed that it did not apply to the IgG_3 subclass.

Table 3 Contribution in per cent of different lymphoid organs to the total number of C-Ig cells in young and old male CBA mice

Age	Bone marrow	Spleen	Mesenteric lymph nodes	Peyer's patches
6 weeks	22	54	8	16
2 years	68	31	0	1

Summary

We have presented here in summary form a number of studies, performed in our laboratory. Their basis is the generally accepted relationship between decreased humoral immunity and aging. This includes a decline in the immune reaction and an increase in auto-immunity. Another regular immune phenomenon in men with a positive correlation with aging is paraproteinaemia. An analogous condition has now been observed in mice, especially of the C57BL strain.

So far it is not possible to predict which pathway an individual will follow. It is clear that age, sex, and strain are determinative factors in this highly selective process. It is also clear that the enormous flexibility of living organisms and the complexity of the immune system will have to be taken into account in every theory of immunological aging.

References

AXELSSON, U., BACHMAN, R., and HÄLLEN, J. (1966). Frequency of pathological proteins (M-components) in 6, 995 sera from an adult population. *Acta med. Scand.*, **179** (2), 235–45.

BENNER, R. and OUDENAARDEN, A. (1976). Antibody formation in mouse bone marrow. V. The response to the thymus-independent antigen Escherichia coli lipopolysaccharide. *Immunol.* **30**, 49–58.

BLANKWATER, M. J., LEVERT, L. A., and HIJMANS, W. (1975). Age-related decline in the antibody response to E. coli lipopolysaccharide in New Zealand mice. *Immunol.*, **28**, 847–54.

ENGLISOVA, M., ENGLIS, M., KYRAL, V., KOURILEK, K., and DVORAK, K. (1968). Changes of immunoglobulin synthesis in old people. *Exp. Gerontol.*, **3**, 125.

FINGER, H., BENEKE, G., EMMERLING, P., BERTZ, R., and PLAGER, L. (1972). Secondary antibody forming potential of aged mice, with special reference to the adjuvant on priming. *Gerontologia*, **18**, 77–95.

—— and HIJMANS, W. (1978). The influence of age on the immunological activity and capacity of the CBA mouse. *Mech. Aging Devolop.*, **7**, 375–98.

——, VAN DEN BERG, P. and BRINKHOF, J. (1977a). Immunoglobulin class and subclass levels in the serum of CBA mice throughout life. *Immunol.*, **32**, 923–7.

——, SCHUIT, H. R. E., and HIJMANS, W. (1977b). Immunoglobulin containing cells in different lymphoid organs of the CBA mouse during its life span. *Immunol.*, **32**, 427–37.

HAAIJMAN and HIJMANS, W. (1975). The immunological basis of connective tissue disorders. In *Proceedings of the fifth Lepetit Colloquium held in Madrid, Spain, 11–13 November 1974;* (ed. L. G. Silvestri), pp. 203–7. North-Holland, Amsterdam.

——, SCHUIT, H. R. E. and HULSING-HESSELINK, E. (1971). An immunofluorescence study on intracellular immunoglobulins in human bone marrow cells. *Ann. NY Acad. Sci.*, **177**, 290–305.

——, ——, and RADL, J. (1973). Deviation in the balance of intracellular heavy- and light-chain determinants in human plasma cells. In *Protides of the biological fluids—20th colloquium* (ed. H. Peeters), pp. 181–4. Pergamon Press, Oxford and New York.

KALFF, M. W. (1970). Quantitative determination of serum immunoglobulin levels by single radial immunodiffusion. *Clin. Biochem.*, **3**, 91–104.

MACKAY, I. R., WELLS, J. V., and FUDENBERG, H. H. (1975). Correlation of Gm allotype, antibody response, and mortality. *Clin. Immunol. Immunopathol.*, **3**, 408–11.

MAKINODAN, T., ALBRIGHT, J. W., GOOD, P. I., PETER, P. I., and HEIDRICK, M. L. (1976). Reduced humoral immune activity in long-lived old mice: an approach to elucidating its mechanisms. *Immunol.*, **31**, 903–11.

MORTON, J. I. and SIEGEL, B. V. (1969). Secondary antibody response of overtly autoimmune NZB mice. *Immunol.*, **16**, 481–4.

MUISWINKEL, W. B., RADL, J., and VAN DER WAL, D. J. (1976). The regulatory influence of the thymus-dependent immune system on the heterogeneity of immunoglobulins in irradiated and reconstituted mice. *Adv. exp. Med. Biol.*, **66**, 617.

RADL, J. (1979a). The influence of the T immune system on the appearance of homogeneous immunoglobulins in man and experimental animals. In *Proceedings of the Advanced Study Institute on Humoral Immunity in Neurological Diseases* (ed. A. Lowenthal), p. 517. Plenum Press, New York.

—— (1979b). Idiopathic paraproteinaemia—a consequence of an age-related deficiency in the Timmune system. Three stage development—a hypothesis. *Clin. Immunol. Immunopathol.*, **14**, 251.

—— (1980). Immunoglobulin levels and abnormalities in aging humans and mice. In *Immunology of aging* (ed. W. H. Adler and A. A. Nordin). Uniscience Series on Methods in Aging Research, Vol. 5. CRC Press, Florida.

—— and HOLLANDER, C. F. (1974). Homogeneous immunoglobulins in sera of mice during aging. *J. Immunol.*, **112**, 2271–3.

——, DE GLOPPER, E., SCHNIT, H. R. E., and ZURCDER, C. (1979). Idiopathic paraproteinemia II. Transplantation of the paraprotein-producing clone from old to young C 57 BL/KaLw Rij mice. *J. Immunτl.*, **122**, 609.

——, SEPERS, J. M., SKVARIL, F., MORELL, A., and HIJMANS, W. (1975). Immunoglobulin pattern in humans over 95 years of age. *Clin. exp. Immunol.*, **22**, 84–90.

VAN CAMP, B. G. K., SCHUIT, H. R. E., HIJMANS, W., and RADL, J. (1978). The cellular basis of double paraproteinaemia in man. *Clin. Immunol. Immunopathol.*, **9**, 111–19.

WALFORD, R. L. (1969). *The immunologic theory of aging.* Munksgaard, Copenhagen.

Index

Note: Figures in *italics* refer to pages on which illustrations or tables appear.